S0-BSN-547

Nanotechnology Environmental Health and Safety:
Risks, Regulation and Management

Published titles

9780815515432	Nam-Trung Nguyen	*Micromixers* (2008)
9780815515449	Jean Berthier	*Microdrops and Digital Microfluidics* (2008)
9780815515777	Behraad Bahreyni	*Fabrication and Design of Resonant Microdevices* (2008)
9780815515739	Francois Leonard	*The Physics of Carbon Nanotube Devices* (2009)
9780815515784	Mamadou Diallo, Jeremiah Duncan, Nora Savage, Anita Street & Richard Sustich	*Nanotechnology Applications for Clean Water* (2009)
9780815515876	Rolf Wüthrich	*Micromachining Using Electrochemical Discharge Phenomenon* (2009)
9780815515791	Matthias Worgull	*Hot Embossing* (2009)

Forthcoming titles

9780815515838	Waqar Ahmed & M.J. Jackson	*Emerging Nanotechnologies for Manufacturing* (2009)
9780080964546	Richard Leach	*Fundamental Principles of Engineering Nanometrology* (2009)
9780815520238	Jeremy Ramsden	*Applied Nanotechnology* (2009)
9780815515944	Veikko Lindroos, Markku Tilli, Ari Lehto & Teruaki Motooka	*Handbook of Silicon Based MEMS Materials and Technologies* (2009)
9780815515869	Matthew Hull & Diana Bowman	*Nanotechnology Environmental Health and Safety: Risks, Regulation and Management*

Nanotechnology Environmental Health and Safety:

Risks, Regulation and Management

Edited by

Matthew Hull

Diana Bowman

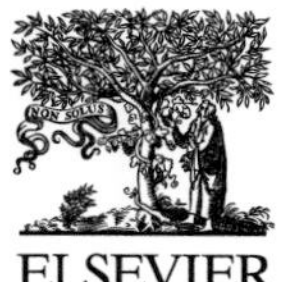

AMSTERDAM • BOSTON • HEIDELBERG • LONDON • NEW YORK • OXFORD
PARIS • SAN DIEGO • SAN FRANCISCO • SINGAPORE • SYDNEY • TOKYO
William Andrew is an imprint of Elsevier

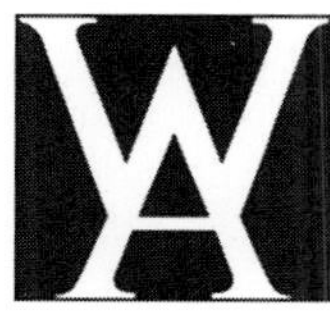

William Andrew is an imprint of Elsevier
The Boulevard, Langford Lane, Kidlington, Oxford OX5 1GB, UK
Radarweg 29, PO Box 211, 1000 AE Amsterdam, The Netherlands

First edition 2010

British Library Cataloguing in Publication Data
A catalogue record for this book is available from the British Library

Library of Congress Cataloging-in-Publication Data
A catalog record for this book is availabe from the Library of Congress

ISBN: 978-0-8155-1586-9

For information on all William Andrew publications
visit our web site at books.elsevier.com

Printed and bound in the USA

10 11 12 13 14   10 9 8 7 6 5 4 3 2 1

Contents

Micro- and Nanotechnologies

Series Editor: Jeremy Ramsden

Professor of Nanotechnology, Microsystems and Nanotechnology Centre, Department of Materials, Cranfield University, United Kingdom

The aim of this book series is to disseminate the latest developments in small-scale technologies, with a particular emphasis on accessible and practical contents. These books will appeal to engineers from industry, academia, and government sectors.

Foreword

Andrew D. Maynard

Back in 2001, I had the privilege of visiting Richard Smalley's laboratory at Rice University. I was working with a team measuring the airborne release of single walled carbon nanotubes as they were produced and handled. The work led to some of the first published data on possible inhalation exposures to nanotubes, but my abiding memories of that visit are of Rick's overwhelming enthusiasm for this innovative new material, and a rather relaxed attitude among his research team to prevent exposure. Wipe your finger along any surface in the lab it seemed, and it would come away black.

Carbon nanotubes epitomize the tension between realizing the promise of emerging engineered nanomaterials and avoiding possible new risks. Carbon nanotubes are quite unlike anything else we have had in our materials construction set—strong, lightweight, highly conductive of heat and electricity, and able to be combined with other materials in innovative new ways. They have uses as wide ranging as better batteries to stronger materials and transparent conductors to anti-radiation sickness drugs. Yet there are hints that they could be uniquely harmful to humans and the environment if they get to the wrong place, in the wrong form. Successful and much-needed carbon nanotube-based applications will depend on identifying and managing these possible risks.

Carbon nanotubes are just one of countless new engineered nanomaterials being developed though. And while the tension between benefits and risks may not be as pronounced in many cases, using these new materials successfully will still depend on understanding how to handle them safely.

In *Nanotechnology Environmental Health and Safety: Risks, Perspectives and Management,* Matthew Hull and Diana Bowman have succeeded in bringing together a strong cast of authors with a variety of perspectives to shed light on uncertainties currently being faced by an expanding nanomaterial community. By outlining the issues confronting researchers and manufacturers, as well as some of the nascent risk management options available, they have produced a practical resource for anyone grappling with the challenge of using engineered nanomaterials as safely as possible.

Following that first visit to Richard Smalley's lab, there was a marked change in attitudes. Enthusiasm for the potential uses of carbon nanotubes remained unabated. But work practices were tightened up beyond all recognition. Using knowledge on possible risks together with advice on good hygiene practices, the team successfully slashed the chances of potentially harmful exposures occurring.

My sense is that this book is set to have the same impact, but on a broader audience. It won't tell you everything you need to know on how to use engineered nanomaterials safely—that would be an impossible task, given all that we still don't know. But it will help researchers, producers, and users of these materials take steps toward significantly reducing the chances of harm occurring.

Andrew D. Maynard
July 12, 2009

Series Editor's Preface

Whereas, formerly, societies stumbled upon their consensuses seemingly through a series of accidents with much backtracking, in our present globalized society we feel that they should be reached through a much more rational process, informed by reliable and comprehensive knowledge. This book has been assembled very much in that spirit of promoting such rational decision-making. The object of discussion is the impact, focusing on health and safety aspects, of nanotechnology on the human environment. Uniquely, it combines technological aspects (i.e., the toxicology of nano objects) with issues of regulation (i.e., legal aspects, covering both the USA and the European Union) and management of the risks. As is customary in the series, there is a strong emphasis on practical matters rooted in reality—for example, the book includes several case studies in the section on risk management.

The authors point out that in some situations current knowledge is too scanty to be able to make a fully rational decision. Indeed, with a technology as new as nanotechnology, this situation is rather common. Individual inventors and companies will nevertheless press ahead, without waiting for the rationally designed regulatory framework to be in place. This somewhat chaotic reality must be encompassed in any practically useful risk assessment, making it a much more complex matter than in well-established industries.

It is sobering, even alarming, to realize that although Strabo the Greek and Pliny the Elder documented the health dangers arising through contact with asbestos about 2000 years ago, this knowledge was not sufficient to prevent the ghastly diseases resulting from exposure to amphibole asbestos that became such a prominent part of occupational medicine in the latter part of the twentieth century. In fact, formal risk assessment is a relatively new area, the first one being carried out by the US Environmental Protection Agency in 1975. This inability, or unwillingness, to learn from knowledge accumulated in the past intrudes, seemingly irrationally, into the orderly vision of the knowledge-based economy. Before the invention of printing, knowledge was indeed a rare commodity that could only be shared with difficulty. Nowadays, in principle at least one can conveniently access a vast quantity of scientific and technical literature from a desktop computer, thanks to the World Wide Web. Yet, paradoxically, citation patterns in the primary research literature increasingly provide evidence that researchers read less, and are generally less aware of past and even contemporary knowledge. This problem will also need to be addressed, if it is not to become a real barrier to the responsible development and use of advanced technology in the twenty-first century.

As the authors point out, the overarching question is how to maximize the benefits of nanotechnology while minimizing the risks. The contributions in this book provide a wealth of information and analysis that will be of immense value to companies, government departments, and other organizations involved in insurance, developing regulatory and legal frameworks, and in guarding their workforces against undue hazards. It will also serve as an important milestone in the further development of the theoretical basis of the subject.

Jeremy Ramsden
September 2009

Preface

Matthew S. Hull, Diana M. Bowman and Steffi Friedrichs

Risk is a reality. And while innovative management frameworks, policies, protective strategies, and regulation can do much to reduce the risks associated with certain products or activities, seldom can they eliminate those risks entirely. Technological advancements in a modern age, ranging from the introduction of the automobile through to, for example, biotechnology and the comforts that accompany them, are no different. Such advancements come pre-packaged with their own unique set of risks and trade-offs.

Indeed, *progress has never been a bargain; you have to pay for it*.[1] Exactly how much we are willing to "pay" for progress—new technologies and the products derived from them—is usually established through risk tolerance thresholds that materialize through society's perceptions (factual or otherwise) of the technology. While this will vary over time and between jurisdictions, it will nevertheless involve a complex interplay between social attitudes and culture, economics, politics, history and science. What is acceptable to some in terms of risk may not therefore be acceptable to all.

Some thresholds, usually those that have developed over time and with input from practical experience or hard data, can be quite clear and well established. Such thresholds readily lend themselves to translation into legislative instruments, regulations (state or non-state based), or standards. Other thresholds, however, particularly those still in their formative stages, can be remarkably amorphous and dynamic. In these latter situations, there is simply too little information available to fully assess the actual risks or even the benefits to society, and the decision of whether or not to proceed is likely to become increasingly clouded and complex.

It is the inseparable nature of risk and reward that underlies the current debate surrounding the emergence of nanotechnologies. And it is the manner in which stakeholders in different jurisdictions have risen to address this issue that motivates the present work. The aim of this book is to provide

[1] Quote from 'Inherit the Wind', 1960, Stanley Kramer Productions.

readers with a snapshot of perspectives on the potential environmental health and safety (EHS) risk, posed by some facets of the technology and risk management strategies from individuals who have helped shape the evolving nanotechnology EHS landscape.

According to an oft-cited definition, nanotechnology is the study of phenomena governed by novel properties arising from the diminutive size of an object, which includes at least one dimension of 1–100 nm (National Nanotechnology Initiative, 2001). For reference, the common flu virus is 40 nm in diameter, while the width of a human hair is typically more than a thousand times larger. From nano-scale size and control arise extraordinary new properties not found at other size scales; for example, carbon nanotubes (a cylindrical shape with a diameter of up to 100 nm, and a lengths of up to several microns) possess tensile strength many times that of steel, but with only a fraction of the weight; nanoscale titanium particles offer novel photo-catalytic properties; and nanoscale quantum dots possess tunable fluorescent properties attributable to quantum confinement effects.

Over the last two decades, and during a period that many would suggest represents only its infancy, the field of nanotechnology has spurred some of the most exciting advancements in science, engineering, and manufacturing since the industrial revolution. According to some commentators we are in the midst of a 'Nano Revolution' (see, for example, Merkle, 2000; Drexler, Peterson and Pergamit, 2003; Sparrow, 2008). This so-called [r]evolution has 'erupted' or 'evolved'—depending on one's view—from the development of new instruments and the subsequent convergence of enhanced capabilities to visualize and manipulate materials at the molecular scale with large-scale investment by the public and private sectors on nanotechnology initiatives.

Given the current rate of progress, it is difficult to predict precisely what nanotechnology-enabled innovations will emerge in the years ahead. However, as evidenced by talk of space elevators (Appell, 2002; Pugno, 2006) and Crichton's (2002) shape-shifting nanoassemblers, the absence of a clear development trajectory certainly has not stifled imaginations. For curious readers seeking a more pragmatic perspective on forthcoming nanotechnologies, Roco (2004) has described four distinct generations of nanotechnology-enabled structures and devices whose emergence coincides to some degree with the acquisition of the scientific and engineering capabilities necessary to actually produce them. Of course, technology is disruptive by nature and sometimes imaginations rule the day!

Amidst the excitement over undeniable progress in nanoscale science and engineering, one fact remains: *in the past, society has been taught some cruel and lasting lessons by the promise of new technologies*. Such lessons have been comparatively frequent and hard-learned for new classes of chemicals or materials and examples abound in recent history: while extremely effective at controlling insect-borne disease, DDT and similar pesticides had unintended negative effects on reproduction of avian predators; although regarded as exceptional coolants and aerosol propellants, chlorofluorocarbons (CFCs) have been linked to depletion of the earth's protective ozone layer; and finally, while once hailed as a miracle mineral of natural origin, with applications in myriad products ranging from building materials to automotive products, asbestos—as discussed by Mullins in his chapter – has become synonymous with a legacy of chronic respiratory disease and class-action litigation.

What is perhaps most interesting about these cases is that they are all relatively recent and their effects are still rippling through society. Unlike previous generations, it would appear that modern society has been conditioned to question not only the acute risks of emerging technologies, but also those potential risks that may lie just beyond the grasp of current scientific understanding. We have become highly sensitized to the societal risks of new technologies, and while this new-found sensitivity is accompanied rightly or wrongly by a degree of cynicism, it also fosters a level of *techno-trepidation* that can be put to good use to usher in advancements in science and engineering in a safe and responsible manner.

It would be unbalanced, however, to consider in this discussion only those examples or aspects of technologies that had unintended negative consequences on society. Just as the past century has highlighted the potential dangers of new technologies, they have also demonstrated technology's extraordinary utility in overcoming many of humankind's greatest challenges. DDT, for example, has been credited with saving millions of lives in developing countries ravaged by malaria. Such facts cannot be ignored. But what if those lives could be saved without potentially catastrophic consequences to ecosystems? What if advanced materials could be created without compromising the health of millions of workers who manufacture them? These are the questions that must be considered when weighing the potential benefits and risks of any new technology.

As remarkable as recent advancements in nanotechnology have been, the world's proactive engagement of emerging nanotechnology EHS risks—both known and unknown—has been remarkable in its own right. Internationally, governments have included in national nanotechnology research initiatives language specifically mandating funding of risk-related research. While the adequacy, effectiveness, and legitimacy of many of these activities have been questioned (see, for example, Powell and Colin, 2008; Friends of the Earth Australia, 2009), they nevertheless represent a dramatic shift from the development-focused paradigm of the past. Along with government-led programs, a number of corporations, non-profit organizations and academic research institutions have developed their own nanotechnology-specific risk management initiatives. While not completely altruistic in nature, some of these initiatives demonstrate industry's recognition of the fact that when it comes to the risks of new technologies and products, a sound business case can be made for behaving proactively rather than reactively. Trade organizations, international standards committees, and professional services providers have also weighed in on the nanotechnology EHS debate, expressing both concerns about risk and potential measures to mitigate them.

Nanotechnologies are no longer confined to the laboratory, and industrial-scale nanomanufacturing is a commercial reality around the globe. In Africa, the South African Nanotechnology Initiative (SANi) (2009) includes efforts to synthesize nanoscale particles for applications in solar cells, catalysis, fuel cells, and composite materials. In Asia, companies are now manufacturing multi-ton quantities of carbonaceous fullerenes and nanoscale silver particles. Firms in Australia manufacture nanotechnology-enabled products ranging from metal oxide nanoparticle sunscreens to highly branched, nanoscale materials known as dendrimers. In North America and the European Union, a diverse and robust nanomanufacturing industry has emerged, with the capability of producing anything from semiconducting quantum dots to multi-ton quantities of metallic oxide nanoparticles and carbon nanotubes. And in South America, an extensive network of government and industry supported nanotechnology research centers has emerged, along with strong nanotechnology-focused collaborations with international partners in India, Africa, and the European Union.

To conclude, the question before us is this: *How do we extract and ensure the benefits of nanotechnology, while minimizing potential and often ill-defined risks?* The chapters that follow consider this question through the experiences of representatives from academia, trade unions, Fortune 500 corporations, entrepreneurs, insurers, nanotechnology facility managers, and experts in product liability and environmental law. The result, we trust, is a balanced discussion of the emerging nanotechnology EHS landscape, coupled with practical strategies developed to manage these risks in nanotechnology facilities of varying size and complexity.

REFERENCES

Appell, D., 2002. Nanotechnology: Wired for Success. Nature 419 (6907), 553–555.

Crichton, M., 2002. Prey. HarperCollins, New York.

Drexler, K., Peterson, C., Pergamit, G., 2003. Unbounding the Future: the Nanotechnology Revolution. Quill Books, New York.

Friends of the Earth Australia, accessed May 28, 2009. Questioning government's role as chief nanotechnology proponent—a biased adjudicator? Available at: <www.nano.foe.org.au/node/307>

Merkle, R.C., 2000. Are we prepared for the nanotechnology revolution? Proceedings of the IEEE 88 (1), 107–108.

National Nanotechnology Initiative, 2001. Nanotech Facts: What is Nanotechnology? NNI, Washington, DC. Available at: <www.nano.gov/html/fats/whatIsNano.html>, accessed May 28, 2009.

Powell, M., Colin, M., 2008. Meaningful citizen engagement in science and technology: what would it really take? Science Communication 30 (1), 126–136.

Pugno, N.M., 2006. On the strength of the carbon nanotube-based space elevator cable: from nanomechanics to megamechanics. Journal of Physics: Condensed Matter 18, S1971–S1990.

Roco, M.C., 2004. Nanoscale science and engineering: unifying and transforming tools. AlChE Journal 50 (5), 890–897.

South African Nanotechnology Initiative, 2009. Welcome to the South African Nanotechnology Initiative. SANi, Johannesburg. Available at: <http://sani.org.za/index.php>, accessed May 27, 2009.

Sparrow, R., 2008. Talkin' 'Bout a (Nanotechnological) Revolution. IEEE Technology and Society Magazine 27 (2), 37–43.

List of Contributors

Robert Blaunstein

Dr Blaunstein is the past President of Nanotech Risk Management, providing technical, underwriting, and risk management advisory services. Clients include the insurance and reinsurance industry, financial entities, and technology developers to identify and implement risk management solutions to the EHS, product liability, and general liability risks associated with nanotechnologies. Dr Blaunstein is currently the Director of Environmental Underwriting at Markel Insurance Company, West Coast Regional Office. Previous positions have included Vice President for Risk Assessment at AIG Consultants, American International Group, and Managing Director for Seneca Insurance Company's Environmental Casualty Profit Center. Dr Blaunstein was an Assistant Professor of Physics at the University of Tennessee and a Consulting Scientist to the Oak Ridge National Laboratory where he lectured and conducted research in the area of atomic and molecular physics. He is a frequent lecturer at nanotechnology conferences and has published extensively in the area of nanotechnology risk management.

Diana M. Bowman

Diana M. Bowman is a Senior Research Fellow in the Center for Regulatory Studies, Faculty of Law, Monash University. Diana is also a Visiting Scholar in the Faculty of Law, K.U. Leuven, and the Center for Technology, Ethics, and Law in Society, King's College, London. Diana's research has focused primarily on legal and regulatory and public health policy issues relating to new technologies, with a particular focus on nanotechnologies. She is a co-editor (along with Graeme Hodge and Andrew Maynard) on the forthcoming book *International Handbook on Regulating*

Nanotechnologies. Diana has published widely in the area of regulating new technologies, with over 50 articles and book chapters in this field.

Steffi Friedrichs

Dr Steffi Friedrichs is the Director of the Nanotechnology Industries Association (NIA), globally the only industries-focused trade association in nanotechnology, providing a sector-independent, responsible voice for the industrial nanotechnologies supply chains. In this capacity, she has given evidence to numerous expert committees and regulatory organizations; she initiated in-depth programs in support of the ongoing advancement of nanotechnologies and participated in many stakeholder debates and citizen's engagement panels. Steffi joined the NIA from The Technology Partnership, where, as a Senior Nanotechnology Consultant, she was responsible for the development of nanotechnology innovations and contributed to the tendering and due diligence processes for the MNT Network (Department of Trade and Industry, UK Government).

Steffi started her scientific career with an undergraduate degree in "Diplom-Chemie" at the Technical University of Braunschweig (Germany), before taking a DPhil at the University of Oxford (UK), specializing in single-walled carbon nanotubes (both synthesis and toxicology). She subsequently held a Fellowship at Oxford University and a Lectureship in Nanotechnology at Cambridge University.

Matthew S. Hull

Matthew S. Hull is the President of NanoSafe, Inc., a nanotechnology environmental health and safety services company headquartered in Blacksburg, Virginia (US). He is also a doctoral student and National Science Foundation IGERT Fellow in the Virginia Tech Department of Civil and Environmental Engineering. Prior to returning to Virginia Tech, Matthew directed and participated in research programs exploring applications and implications of nanotechnology for agencies ranging from the US Department of Defense to the UK Department of Environment, Food, and Rural Affairs (DEFRA). In 2005, while working with a commercial nanomanufacturer, Hull developed the NANOSAFE™ risk management framework for commercial nanotechnology companies. That framework would go on to spin-off programs focused on web-enabled nanotechnology EHS management systems, nanotechnology waste recovery and recycling processes, and life-cycle ecotoxicological studies of nanomanufacturing.

Igor Linkov

Dr Igor Linkov is an Adjunct Professor of Engineering and Public Policy at Carnegie Mellon University and a Research Scientist with the US Army Engineer Research and Development Center. Dr Linkov has managed multiple ecological and human health risk assessments and risk management projects. Many of his projects have included application of the state-of-the-science modeling and software tools to highly complex sites and projects (e.g., restoration and remediation planning, insuring emerging risks, risk-based prioritization of engineering projects). He has published widely on environmental policy, environmental modeling, and risk analysis, including 10 books and over 100 peer-reviewed papers and book chapters. Dr Linkov has served on many review and advisory panels for DHS, EPA, NSF, EU and other US and international agencies. He is DOD representative at the Interagency Working Group on Nanotechnology Environmental and Health Implications (NEHI). The Governor of Massachusetts has appointed Dr Linkov to serve as a Scientific Advisor to the Toxic Use Reduction Institute. He is the recipient of the 2005 SRA Chauncey Starr Award for exceptional contribution to risk analysis.

John C. Monica, Jr.

John C. Monica, Jr has considerable litigation experience in defending national and international products liability claims for Fortune 500 companies. He is a nationally recognized authority on nanotechnology product liability issues. As a member of American National Standards Institute and American Society for Testing and Materials, John participates in the development of voluntary international nomenclature and EHS standard for the nanotechnology industry. Additionally, he has successfully represented numerous clients in a variety of general commercial litigation matters in state and federal courts. John is the Associate Editor for legislative/regulatory affairs, *Nanotechnology Law & Business*, and has authored numerous articles on nanotechnology. John has a JD with honours from George Washington University School of Law and a BA from Northwestern University.

Steve Mullins

Steve started in the union movement 10 years ago as an Industrial Officer at the Actors and Journalist Union. For the past 7 years he has worked at the

Australian Council of Trade Unions in the ACTU's commercial arm and then filling the Acting International Officer role before taking up the ACTU's OH&S Policy Officer position in 2004. Steve represents the interests of working people on Safe Work Australia and on other government and non-government bodies. Steve is also an Al Gore-trained Climate Project presenter.

Michele L. Ostraat

Dr Michele L. Ostraat, Senior Director for the Center for Aerosol Technology at RTI International, has expertise in aerosol technology, nanoparticle applications, submicron particle processing, micro- and nanofiber filtration, portable nanoparticle detection, occupational safety and health of nanoparticles, and inhalation toxicology. Before joining RTI, Dr Ostraat worked at DuPont's Experimental Station with primary responsibilities in the aerosol synthesis and characterization of submicron and nanoparticles for a variety of electronic and materials applications. She earned her PhD (2001) and MS (1998) degrees in Chemical Engineering from the California Institute of Technology. Dr Ostraat has authored numerous research publications in the areas of aerosol nanoparticle synthesis, characterization, and electrical properties, holds six patents, and has given over 45 conference presentations and invited talks.

Annette B. Santamaria

Dr Annette B. Santamaria is a Senior Manager in the Health Sciences Practice of ENVIRON International Corporation and is located in Houston, Texas. She is a board-certified toxicologist and has extensive experience evaluating human health risks associated with exposure to a variety of consumer products, pharmaceuticals, medical devices, food additives, personal care products, nanomaterials, and industrial chemicals. She developed the Nanotoxicology Specialty Section of the Society of Toxicology. Dr Santamaria has an MPH from the Johns Hopkins School of Public Health and Hygiene and a PhD in toxicology from the University of Texas School of Public Health.

Christie M. Sayes

Dr Christie M. Sayes is an Assistant Professor at Texas A&M University with appointments in Veterinary Physiology and Pharmacology, Biomedical

Engineering, and the Institute for Biosciences & Technology. Her training includes a post-doctoral fellowship in pulmonary toxicology at DuPont, a PhD in chemistry and nanoscience from Rice University, and a BS in chemistry from LSU. She is actively studying the health effects of various nanomaterials in in vitro and in vivo systems and has made significant correlations between physicochemical properties and toxicological profiles. Dr Sayes has authored over 40 publications, reviews, and book chapters and has ongoing collaborations with academia, industry, and government.

Geert van Calster

Professor Geert van Calster (LLM, PhD) is the Director of the Institute for Environmental and Energy Law and Director of the Master program on Energy and Environmental law at the K.U. Leuven. Geert is a Chair/Research Associate of the Research Fund, K.U. Leuven (2003–2013), a visiting lecturer at Oxford University (September 2006 onward), and counsel (practicing) at DLA Piper (Brussels). His expertise covers EC environmental law and EC economic law, EC and international energy law, international trade law, and international environmental law, subjects on which he publishes and speaks extensively. His most current research interests include the regulation of new technologies (nanotechnologies in particular) and climate change law. His editorial works include the Editorial Board of *Carbon & Climate Law Review*; *Nanotechnology Law & Business*; and Associate editor, *Law, Probability and Risk*.

John Weaver

John R. Weaver serves as the Facility Manager for the Birck Nanotechnology Center at Purdue University, responsible for the cleanroom and laboratory operations, facility infrastructure, training, and safety. John was involved from the conceptual stages of the BNC through design, construction, equipment installation, and startup. Building on 35 years in the semiconductor industry with roles ranging from process development to contamination control engineering, John is well established in nanotechnology-facility design and operation. He is a Fellow of the Institute of Environmental Sciences and Technology and holds a variety of leadership positions in the field. His work is extensively published and John is a well-known instructor of nanotechnology and cleanroom short courses.

SECTION 1

Risks

CHAPTER 1

Toxicological Studies with Nanoscale Materials

Annette B. Santamaria

Christie M. Sayes

CONTENTS

1.1 INTRODUCTION

The use of nanomaterials is expected to have great potential to improve consumer and industrial products, address critical energy needs, enhance security systems, and improve the medical field. This opportunity is based on the unique physical properties (e.g., magnetic, optical, mechanical, and electrical) and quantum mechanics (e.g., electron configuration and confinement) that vary continuously or abruptly with changes in the size of some materials produced at the nanoscale (1–100 nm). However, as with any new technology, the identification of potential health risks is a prerequisite for a proper assessment of the usefulness and safety of the new chemicals, materials, and products that may be developed. Both hazard and exposure potential will vary widely for different nanomaterials and for different products that incorporate nanomaterials and the human and environmental health risks will be determined by the hazards posed and the potential exposures to the nanomaterials. As new nanotechnology-based materials are developed, it is important to have a framework that may be followed to evaluate their potential toxicity, exposure levels, and for obtaining information that will be useful for conducting future safety and risk assessments.

The unusual or new properties of nanomaterials are predominantly associated with their nanometer-scale size, structure-dependent electronic configurations, and an extremely large surface area-to-volume ratio relative to larger sized chemicals and materials. The main characteristic of nanomaterials is their size, which falls in the transitional zone between individual atoms or molecules and the corresponding bulk materials (Nel et al., 2006). Particle size and surface area are important material characteristics from

Nanotechnology Environmental Health and Safety

a toxicological and health perspective because as the size of a particle decreases, its surface area increases, which allows a greater proportion of its atoms or molecules to be displayed on its surface rather than within the interior of the material. These atoms or molecules on the surface of the nanomaterial may be chemically and biologically reactive, potentially contributing to the development of adverse health effects. Other physical and chemical properties such as shape, surface coating, aggregation potential, and solubility may also affect the physicochemical characteristics and transport properties of the nanomaterial, with the possibility of negating or amplifying any associated size-related effects.

Although impressive from a physicochemical viewpoint, the novel properties of nanomaterials raise concerns about potential adverse effects on biological systems. Some studies suggest that some nanomaterials can affect biological behaviors at the cellular (e.g., membrane) and subcellular (e.g., protein, DNA) levels. There is also a concern that some nanoparticles may readily travel throughout the body, deposit in target organs, penetrate cell membranes, lodge in mitochondria, and may trigger a variety of damaging responses such as inflammation or reactive oxygen species generation. However, in many cases, nanomaterials will be components of larger scale products such as nano-composites, surface coatings, or may be embedded in a product matrix, so the potential for direct exposure will be negligible. As the field of nanotechnology continues to evolve and produce nanomaterials, the human and environmental health implications associated with exposure to nanomaterials will need to be considered and evaluated through the conduct of carefully designed toxicological and exposure studies. Several studies are currently being conducted to evaluate many of the theoretical capabilities and any associated effects of nanomaterials for penetrating biological membranes (e.g., lung, skin, gut), eliciting cellular toxicity, and being systemically distributed and localized in tissues or organs.

This chapter will briefly describe the evolving field of nanotoxicology and why nanomaterials may be of toxicological concern, what physicochemical characteristics of nanomaterials may impact their toxicological potential and dosimetry issues that may need to be considered when designing toxicological studies. This will be followed by a brief discussion of the safety assessment process that is currently used to evaluate the safety of chemical substances developed for use in consumer products, such as foods, food packaging, personal care products, pesticides, drugs, and medical diagnostics and how this process may or may not need to be modified for nanomaterials. Because of the importance of characterizing the physicochemical properties of nanomaterials for toxicological evaluation, the process and techniques available to accomplish this will be explained in detail. A general overview of the types of toxicological studies that may be required to perform a hazard evaluation of nanomaterials and suggested frameworks for evaluating nanomaterials is described. Finally, some limitations and challenges faced by scientists, academicians, regulators, and industry personnel when evaluating the human and environmental health risks of nanomaterials are articulated.

1.2 NANOTOXICOLOGY

The evaluation of the safety of nanomaterials will likely require a multidisciplinary approach between toxicologists and experts in materials science, chemistry, physics, biotechnology, engineering, and/or other appropriate disciplines. Identifying precisely what qualifies as a nanoscale material is difficult and currently a subject of substantial discussion in the scientific, regulatory, and standards-setting communities. However, it is generally accepted that nanomaterials may include structures, materials, devices, and systems with fundamentally new properties and functions, which result from their size in the range of about 1–100 nanometers (nm). Concerns about the health implications of nanomaterials have been expressed because particles and materials in the nanosize range may pose toxicological hazards due to their enhanced reactivity (for example, chemical, electrical, and magnetic) and potential for systemic availability. The physicochemical properties of nanomaterials can modify cellular uptake, protein binding, translocation from portal-of-entry to the target site, and the potential for causing tissue injury (Oberdörster et al., 2005a). The theoretical ability for nanomaterials to interact with biological systems in adverse ways is creating intense interest in the scientific, toxicology, and regulatory communities, and several studies addressing health and safety issues associated with the development and use of nanomaterials have been published in the scientific literature (Warheit et al., 2004, 2007a; Lam et al., 2004, Shvedova et al., 2003, 2008, 2009; Monteiro-Riviere et al., 2005, 2008; Sayes et al., 2004, 2007; Gopee et al., 2007; Park et al., 2007; Baker et al., 2008; Hagens et al., 2007; Ji et al., 2007; Helland et al., 2007; Ryman-Rasmussen et al., 2007; Park et al., 2008; Poland et al., 2008; Takagi et al., 2008; Zhang and Monteiro-Riviere, 2008; Guo et al., 2009; Nygaard et al., 2009).

By studying the toxicological potential of nanomaterials (an emerging field known as "nanotoxicology"), data may be obtained that will be useful for conducting future safety and risk assessments for these novel substances. Because of their size, nanomaterials may theoretically be able to deposit in the respiratory tract, penetrate intact skin, be absorbed through the gastro-intestinal tract, or pass directly into or through cells and ultimately translocate to various tissues and organs. The available data support the ability of the lung, gastrointestinal tract, and skin to act as a significant barrier to the systemic exposure of many chemical substances and nanomaterials and the acute systemic toxicity of many nanomaterials appears to be low (Stern and McNeil, 2008). Based on our current understanding of ultrafine particles (typically defined as ambient particles smaller than 100 nm), traditional approaches and study protocols currently used for routine toxicological evaluation of chemicals or larger particles are likely to be sufficiently robust to provide meaningful toxicological characterization of nanomaterials. Research on ambient ultrafine particles has laid the foundation for the emerging field of nanotoxicology, with the goal of studying the biokinetics and the potential of engineered nanomaterials (nanoparticles, nanotubes, nanoshells, quantum dots, etc.), to cause adverse effects (Oberdörster et al., 2005a). Some concepts of nanoparticle kinetics, such as absorption, distribution, metabolism, cell interactions, and excretion, will most likely be similar for these two groups of ambient and engineered typically insoluble nanoscale particles.

It is important to develop a balance between the development of nanomaterials and the conduct of research necessary to identify potential health hazards and develop critical data for conducting future safety assessments of nanomaterials and the products that incorporate them. At this point, it appears that the research, development, and production of nanomaterials are greatly outpaced by the speed in which toxicological and exposure information is being acquired and published in the scientific literature. Initially, an understanding of the mammalian and ecological toxicity profiles of nanomaterials will be necessary to prioritize those nanomaterials that are safe for use and to establish appropriate safety procedures for handling those nanomaterials that may pose potential health hazards, if there is sufficient exposure. For newly developed nanomaterials, it may be necessary to conduct a broad range of in vitro and in vivo studies to evaluate potential toxicological effects following oral, dermal, inhalation, and/or injection as routes of exposures.

The unique chemical and physical properties of nanomaterials may present special challenges to the toxicologist or ecotoxicologist when designing studies to accurately and reproducibly identify adverse biological interactions or effects. Nevertheless, it is anticipated that the types of biological interactions and toxicological effects of nanomaterials will be similar to those observed for any potentially hazardous chemical agent following injection, inhalation, dermal, or oral exposure. That is, it is not likely that nanomaterials will produce new or unusual health effects. Therefore, the types of endpoints that are typically evaluated in existing toxicological study protocols (acute and chronic effects, genotoxicity, carcinogenicity,

1) The need to characterize nanomaterials during several stages of toxicological testing (e.g., before, during, and after test substance administration, in cells or tissues);
2) How to properly express and/or administer the dose of nanomaterials (e.g., by mass, surface area, shape, particle number);
3) How to confirm that the nanomaterial is within the nano size scale or in the desired form during administration;
4) Potential analytical difficulties in detecting and quantifying nanomaterials in cells and tissues;
5) Difficulty in selecting the most appropriate endpoints to evaluate;
6) Whether it is reasonable and accurate to extrapolate observed in vitro results to the in vivo situation.

FIGURE 1.1 *Variables that may impact the toxicological evaluation of nanomaterials.*

immunological, reproductive, and developmental effects) may not need to be modified when evaluating the hazard potential of nanoscale materials (Figure 1.1).

Much can be learned and utilized from available research on similar substances for conducting hazard evaluations of nanomaterials. The identification of hazards depends on the diverse physicochemical characteristics of nanomaterials and the hazards of novel materials and structures will be less predictable than smaller scale versions of previously studied larger sized substances that may have well-characterized toxicity profiles (for example, nanoscale versus microscale particles of metal oxides such as titanium dioxide or zinc oxide) (Tsuji et al., 2006). The inhalation and dermal routes of exposure have been the primary focus for health effects research of nanomaterials; however, research on the use of nanomaterials in medical devices (see, for example, Williams, 2007; Christenson et al., 2007), diagnostics (Yang, 2007), and therapeutics (see, for example, Wang et al., 2007; Bai et al., 2006; Lockman et al., 2004) is also contributing to the understanding of the toxicokinetics and toxicodynamics of nanomaterials. The field of ultrafine particle research has a long history of studying the administration of test substances and evaluating the mechanisms of lung injury caused by ultrafine particles. The research available on the relationship between size and surface area on the deposition, translocation, and toxicity of small particles found in the ambient environment may also be useful for modeling the behavior and toxicological potential of nanoparticles. However, there are significant differences between ambient ultrafine particles and nanomaterials. These differences include the heterogeneous chemical composition and polydisperse particle size distribution of ambient ultrafine particles versus the homogeneous composition and monodisperse particle size distribution of nanomaterials. Further, the method of production for nanomaterials is significantly different than the generation of heterogeneous ambient ultrafine particles. In addition, it may be possible to alter the production process or the physicochemical properties (e.g., different functional groups) of nanomaterials to ameliorate or reduce their toxicity. Because of the apparent differences between ambient ultrafine particles and specific engineered nanoparticles, it will be necessary to conduct toxicological studies to evaluate potential hazards following inhalation exposure for most, if not all, engineered nanomaterials.

There is also a large body of research available on the factors that contribute to the ability of a substance to be able to penetrate skin. Research has been conducted in the pharmaceutical industry for many years to develop drugs that can be administered dermally and penetrate skin (Hadgraft and Lane, 2005; Kogan and Garti, 2006). The epidermal layer of skin represents a formidable protective barrier and it is very difficult for chemicals and particles to penetrate the skin (Kanikkannan et al., 2000; Nohynek et al., 2008). Most of our knowledge about the dermal penetration of chemicals in vesicle-type and other micro- or nano-sized formulations has been gained by the research on transdermal drug delivery (TDD) techniques (Nohynek et al., 2007). Several studies that have attempted to identify TDD systems have reported that the passive drug delivery by occlusive patches, vesicle-type formulations, gels, or creams may only yield significant skin penetration and therapeutic effects of drug substances that have a combination of parameters, including a high pharmacological potency, a suitable log octanol/water partition coefficient value (1–3), a melting point below 200°C, and a molecular mass of $<$500 daltons (Nohynek et al., 2007). Drug substances marketed today in passive TDD systems all fit into these limits, and they have molecular weights between 160 and 360 daltons and a molecular size between 0.75 and 1.6 nm. Therefore, the dermal penetration potential of nanomaterials may be dependent on variables other than particle size, such as molecular size and partition coefficients. Currently, there is little evidence that nanomaterials penetrate through the skin barrier into the living tissue (i.e., dermal compartment) and the potential for nanomaterials to penetrate skin has been a topic of continued investigation (Zhang and Monteiro-Riviere, 2008; Mavon et al., 2007; Gamer et al., 2006).

Moreover, considering the impacts of dermal exposures and corresponding hazard concerns of nanomaterials, it must be taken into consideration that the dermal uptake of nanoparticles will be an order of magnitude smaller than the uptake via the inhalation or oral routes of exposure (Warheit et al., 2007b). However, damaged skin or sites with skin flexing may be areas of increased risk for the penetration of nanoparticles (Levin and

Maibach, 2005; Rouse et al., 2007; Zhang and Monteiro-Riviere, 2008). So far there is not sufficient evidence to conclude that dermal absorption occurs for nanomaterials, and more importantly, whether or not nanomaterials can cause adverse local or systemic effects even if they do penetrate skin (Nanoderm, 2007; Nohynek et al., 2008; Borm et al., 2006; Tran et al., 2005; Gopee et al., 2007; Ryman-Rassmussen et al., 2007; Murray et al., 2009). In many cases, it will likely be necessary to evaluate the dermal penetration potential and dermal toxicity of nanomaterials on a case-by-case basis.

Studies have also been conducted to evaluate the potential for nanomaterials to be absorbed systemically following ingestion, primarily for the development of orally administered drugs (Malik et al., 2007; Galindo-Rodriguez et al., 2005; des Rieux et al., 2007). The development of orally bioavailable dugs delivered in nanomaterials or as nanoparticles has been difficult because of the ability of the gastrointestinal and intestinal mucosa to serve as a significant barrier to systemic availability. For example, obstacles to nanomaterial bioavailability after oral administration include particle or molecular size, intestinal membrane permeability, intestinal and hepatic metabolism, and particle solubility. In addition, nanomaterials in the gastrointestinal tract may be scavenged by cells overlying the intestinal mucosa and in this way circumvent active uptake by intestinal epithelium. Oral exposure to nanomaterials may result from the ingestion of foods, water, drugs, or exposure to food-contact products that may contain nanomaterials. In addition, nanomaterials may be ingested incidentally when they are transferred from hand to mouth (for example in occupational settings) and ingestion of inhaled particles may occur when they are cleared from the respiratory tract via the mucosociliary escalator. Nanoparticles and microparticles (0.1–3 μm) are ingested at high levels every day and it is estimated that 10^{12}–10^{14} microparticles are ingested per person per day in the Western world (Borm et al., 2006). Although nanoparticles in food are infrequently taken up into gut lymphatics and distributed to other organs, most nanoparticles are rapidly eliminated via feces (Nel et al., 2006). A gastrointestinal route of translocation of ingested ultrafine particles to the blood, is supported by studies in rats and humans that have shown that TiO_2 particles (150–500 nm) taken in via food can translocate to the blood and are taken up by the liver and spleen (Bockmann et al., 2005). However, there is insufficient evidence to determine whether nanoparticles adversely affect the gut or the organs they may be distributed to if they are able to pass through the gastrointestinal or intestinal mucosa (Tran et al., 2005).

Some studies indicate that nanoparticles can enter the brain, possibly via nerves in the nose or via the blood through the blood–brain barrier, however, the potential impact of nanoparticles on the human brain and neural tissue is not clear at this time (Oberdörster et al., 2005a; Borm et al., 2006). Inhaled nanoparticles may be able to gain access to the brain by two different mechanisms: (1) transsynaptic transport after inhalation through the olfactory epithelium, and (2) uptake through the blood–brain barrier (Borm et al., 2006). The first pathway has been studied primarily with model particles such as carbon, gold, and manganese oxide in experimental inhalation animal models and the second pathway has been evaluated through extensive research and particle surface manipulation in drug delivery, as an approach to try to get drugs to the brain (Agarwal et al., 2009; Juillerat-Jeanneret, 2008; Borm et al., 2006; Aschner et al., 2007; Kreuter, 2004; Silva, 2007). The pharmaceutical studies suggest that the physiological blood–brain barrier may limit the distribution of some proteins and viral particles (which may be smaller than nanoparticles) after transvascular delivery to the brain, suggesting that the healthy blood–brain barrier contains defense mechanisms protecting it from blood-borne nanoparticle exposure (Borm et al., 2006). There have been a few studies that reported the potential for nanoparticles to enter the brain and adversely affect neuronal tissue, either by traversing the blood–brain barrier or by traveling along neurons (e.g., olfactory or trigeminal nerves) (Wang et al., 2008a, 2008b). For example, in a study with largemouth bass, Oberdörster (2004) reported that carbon fullerenes dissolved in tetrahydrofuran caused increased lipid peroxidation in the fish brain tissue, but not in the gills or liver. However, the relevance of this study to human and/or environmental health risks has been questioned because of several methodological issues (e.g., vehicle, dose) and further research is needed to understand the potential for nanomaterials to reach the brain and what associated adverse effects may result.

Long-term exposures to inhaled particulate matter (PM) has been reported to be associated with an increased risk of a variety of cardiovascular diseases, including myocardial ischemia and infarctions, heart failure, arrhythmias, strokes, and increased cardiovascular mortality (Brook, 2008; Stone et al., 2007; Sint et al., 2008). Cardiovascular effects of PM have been described in epidemiological and toxicological studies, although the cardiovascular effects as described in human epidemiological studies have not yet been definitively linked to the nanoparticle component (Borm et al., 2006). Toxicological studies with combustion nanoparticles have reported that high exposures to nanoparticles may cause observable cardiovascular effects or thrombosis (Borm et al., 2006). The effects are invariably seen in experimental animals given high doses, often by instillation directly into the lungs or the blood. Evidence from in vitro and in vivo toxicological studies and controlled human exposure studies have demonstrated several mechanisms by which ultrafine particle exposure may trigger acute events as well as

prompt the chronic development of cardiovascular diseases. For a number of nanoparticles, oxidative stress-related inflammatory reactions have been observed (Borm et al., 2006). PM inhaled into the pulmonary tree may cause remote cardiovascular health effects via three general pathways: instigation of systemic inflammation and/or oxidative stress, alterations in autonomic balance, and potentially by direct actions on the vasculature of particle constituents capable of reaching the systemic circulation. However, additional research is necessary to understand the potential for inhalation exposure to engineered nanomaterials to result in the elicitation of cardiovascular effects.

Unlike gases, liquids, and many solid materials, the desirable properties of engineered nanomaterials closely depend on size, shape, and structure (both physically and chemically) at the nanoscale. Although quantitative toxicity studies on engineered nanomaterials are still relatively sparse, published data on fullerenes, single- or multi-walled carbon nanotubes, nanoscale metal oxides such as TiO_2 and quantum dots support the need to carefully consider how nanomaterials will be characterized when evaluating potential biological activity (Warheit et al., 2007c; Teeguarden et al., 2007; Sayes et al., 2007; Powers et al., 2006, 2007). At this time, appropriate approaches for characterizing nanomaterials and for detecting them during and after administration in toxicological studies are being developed for use in study protocols. Because of the potentially diverse and complex physical and chemical characteristics of nanomaterials, the level of characterization that will be required when evaluating them in vitro and in vivo will be more sophisticated and technically challenging than what has traditionally been done to evaluate microscale particles and other chemicals (Powers et al., 2006). When possible, it is desirable that the physical and chemical characteristics that are potentially associated with the mechanism of toxicity are measured or can be determined in toxicity screening tests. In addition, it is desirable to collect sufficient information to allow retrospective interpretation of toxicity data in the light of new or future findings (for example, total surface area, mass, and shape). Complete characterization of nanoparticles includes measurements such as size and size distribution, shape and other morphological features (for example, crystallinity, porosity, and surface texture), chemistry of the material, solubility, surface area, state of dispersion, surface chemistry, and other physicochemical properties. Exhaustive characterization of test materials may be time consuming, expensive, and complex, and to some extent, the amount of characterization required will depend on the objectives of the study. Clearly, characterizing every physicochemical parameter of a test material will be impractical for most toxicological studies. Given the wide range of analytical techniques available in many disciplines associated with nanotechnology, multi-disciplinary collaborations with research and analysis groups offering state-of-the-art nanomaterial characterization capabilities are strongly recommended when conducting toxicological studies with nanomaterials.

In vitro studies, which have become an essential component of risk assessment-directed research paradigms for chemicals, pharmaceuticals, consumer products, and fine and ultrafine particulates, are an essential element of all tiered approaches for toxicity assessment of nanomaterials that have been proposed (Teeguarden et al., 2007). In general, in vitro techniques are seen as an important adjunct to in vivo studies for evaluating mechanism of toxicity, providing rapid and cost-effective screening, and to reduce the use of live animal models in research. These studies allow specific biological pathways or toxicological endpoints to be tested under controlled conditions, as well as the isolation of mechanistic pathways that is not feasible in vivo. They can serve as rapid screening assays for a broad range of toxicological endpoints and are more rapid and less expensive than in vivo studies. However, there are several problems or limitations with in vitro approaches for evaluating the toxicity of substances such as nanomaterials, including a lack of validation against in vivo adverse effects, dosimetry mismatch, over-simplicity as compared to actual in vivo conditions, and the difficulty in extrapolating observations and exposure levels to in vivo conditions. In addition, in vitro methods do not provide the balanced environment of the whole body, where feedback mechanisms in different organs and tissues involving different cell types maintain the homeostasis of the organism and the ability of in vitro methods to metabolize and clear the chemical and its derivatives is usually limited and does not replicate the situation in the whole body (Purchase, 2000). However, in many cases, nanomaterials may be difficult to obtain in large quantities; therefore, it may be necessary to conduct in vitro studies to identify preliminary toxicological endpoints of concern and to estimate in vivo starting doses for toxicity testing. At least three to four dose levels with controls should be used in all in vitro systems to obtain information on dose–response however, the use of high doses in in vitro studies without any consideration or discussion of realistic in vivo exposures may lead to erroneous conclusions about the hazard potential of a nanomaterial.

In vitro assays may be best used to:

1. screen some parameters that drive the toxicity potential of the nanomaterial;
2. rank potential toxicities of many nanomaterials to assist in the selection of candidates for further development;

3. screen specific endpoints that may be evaluated in future in vivo studies (e.g., cytotoxicity, genotoxicity, generation of reactive oxygen species, cytokine release, reproductive effects);
4. provide information that may be useful for selecting appropriate doses for in vivo studies; and
5. reduce the number of animals necessary to characterize the toxicity of nanomaterials.

There are several important attributes to consider when designing in vitro studies for evaluating nanomaterials, including the selection of appropriate types of cells that may be exposed to the material (e.g., lung or skin epithelia, macrophages or other elements of the reticuloendothelial system) and measuring common modes of action such as oxidative stress and inflammation that may be extrapolated to in vivo effects (Nel et al., 2006).

Requirements for in vitro and in vivo screening studies will differ according to the potential route of exposure for the nanomaterial (for example, ingestion, dermal, and inhalation) and an understanding of potential human exposures will be necessary for developing appropriate screening strategies. Another variable that needs to be carefully considered when designing toxicological studies for nanomaterials is the choice of an appropriate dosimetry for the quantitative evaluation of the administered test material in the in vitro or in vivo system. Dosimetry is the measurement of the amount of material in the environment (e.g., administered dose or exposure) or in the body. Although toxicological response may be associated with a wide range of physicochemical characteristics, measuring dose against a physical metric of mass, surface area, or particle number for a well-characterized material will enable quantitative interpretation of data (Oberdörster et al., 2005a). The appropriate selection of the dose metric will depend on the hypothesized parameter most closely associated with anticipated response (e.g., surface area) or the metric which may be most accurately measured. When possible, it is recommended that sufficient information about the test material be collected to be able to evaluate dose in three metrics (mass, surface area, particle number).

Despite the considerable attention that in vitro systems have received and their growing application to nanomaterial toxicity assessment (Braydich-Stolle et al., 2005; Hussain et al., 2005), little attention has been devoted to a critical examination of their suitability, particularly when it comes to particle solution dynamics and dosimetry (Teeguarden et al., 2007). In contrast to soluble chemicals, particles can settle, diffuse, and aggregate differentially according to their size, density, and surface physicochemistry, which can significantly affect the cellular dose (Teeguarden et al., 2007). The definition of dose for nanoparticles in an in vitro system is therefore more dynamic, more complicated, and less comparable across particle types than it is for soluble chemicals. Therefore, it is critical to develop a more complete understanding of these processes, how particle and media characteristics affect them, and their potential impact on cellular dose in vitro before dose–response assessment for certain nanomaterials may be conducted adequately. Development and deployment of a validated computational model for in vitro dosimetry would provide a tool for calculating cellular dose for in vitro studies to be used prospectively in research planning or retrospectively for interpretation of studies (Teeguarden et al., 2007). Such a model would allow researchers to estimate more relevant measures of cellular dose from primary particle characteristics (particle size, density, concentration, and if available, surface charge) reveal more accurate dose–response relationships and improve the basis for comparative toxicity assessment of nanomaterials.

Importantly, toxicological study designs should include doses that most closely reflect the anticipated exposure levels for the nanomaterial. Both in vitro and in vivo toxicological studies can provide useful data on the toxicity and mode of action of nanomaterials only if justifiable concentrations and doses are considered when designing such studies (Oberdörster et al., 2005a). A careful evaluation of exposure–dose–response relationships is critical to the toxicological assessment of nanomaterials and it is important to consider dosimetric issues:mass, number or surface of the particles and the relevance of dose levels evaluated. Very high dose levels are frequently utilized in toxicological studies to ensure that a biological effect is observed. As a result, in many instances mathematical models are then utilized to extrapolate the effects observed at high doses to low-dose levels, which more realistically represent anticipated exposures in human populations or in the environment. The evaluation of appropriate doses in the experimental design will also permit for proper identification of the dose–response curve for the nanomaterial, because when toxicological data are generated only at high concentrations/doses, it is difficult to determine whether the dose–response curve in question is best described by a linear (no threshold), supralinear threshold or hormetic mathematical model which can significantly affect how risks are evaluated for chemical substances (Oberdörster et al., 2005a).

When new engineered nanomaterials are developed, in many instances there may not be any, or limited in vitro and/or in vivo toxicological information available to evaluate potential human health risks and environmental impacts. Therefore, depending on the intended use of the nanomaterial, a battery of in vitro and in vivo studies may need to be conducted to evaluate a broad range of health endpoints, associated mechanisms of action (such as acute, chronic, reproductive, developmental, neurological, immunological, or carcinogenic effects) and the potential for any observed effects at the anticipated exposure levels. Several groups have developed suggested screening strategies and/or frameworks that include a battery of in vitro and in vivo studies for evaluating the health effects of nanomaterials and collecting data necessary for conducting a hazard evaluation—these will be discussed in more detail later in this chapter (Oberdörster et al., 2005b; Environmental Defense and DuPont, 2007; Warheit et al., 2007b).

1.3 RISK ASSESSMENT PROCESS FOR NANOMATERIALS

The number of different chemicals that are manufactured in commerce is estimated to be between 80,000 and 100,000 (for example, medicines, food additives, cosmetics, pesticides, and industrial chemicals) and this estimate does not include the multitude of naturally occurring chemicals (such as animal toxins and plant toxins) (Purchase, 2000). For the benefits of substances such as nanomaterials to be realized, they must be handled, used and disposed of safely. As nanomaterials are developed, incorporated into consumer products and disposed of, it will be necessary to evaluate whether there are any human health or environmental risks associated with their use. The potential for adverse health risks resulting from exposure to substances such as nanomaterials may be estimated by conducting a qualitative and quantitative risk assessment. Risk assessment is the systematic scientific characterization of potential adverse health effects resulting from human or environmental exposures to hazardous agents or situations (National Research Council, 1983, 1994). As with larger sized chemical substances, risk assessment will be the basis of assessing and regulating nanomaterials to protect human health and the environment. Risk assessments are conducted to provide the best possible scientific characterization of health risks to humans or the environment based on a rigorous analysis of available information and knowledge. A risk assessment consists of four components:

1. hazard identification—qualitative evaluation of the adverse effects of a substance;
2. exposure assessment—evaluation of the types (routes and media) and magnitude or levels of exposure;

3. dose–response evaluation—relationship between dose and incidence (or severity) of an adverse effect; and
4. risk characterization—quantitative estimation of the probable incidence of adverse health effects under various conditions of exposure, including a description of the uncertainties involved.

Thus, the distinction between the hazard (an inherent toxic property of a chemical that may or may not be manifested, depending on exposure potential) and risk (the consequences of being exposed to a hazardous chemical at a particular exposure level) is critical (Purchase, 2000). Each component of a risk assessment—hazard identification, dose–response evaluation, and exposure assessment—is essential for evaluating the potential risks associated with the use of a substance such as a nanomaterial. The components of a risk assessment are universal in their application for assessing the hazards and risks of chemicals or products for a variety of industries or environmental exposures, regardless of the types of chemicals of interest (such as solvents, fibers, particulates and nanomaterials).

To assess the risks associated with chemical substances such as nanomaterials, it is necessary to first identify and characterize possible hazards and estimate the likelihood and magnitude of exposure. The potential health risks of nanomaterials will be determined by their hazard potential, including dose–response relationships and exposure levels. This will require an understanding of the physicochemical properties of the nanomaterial and the conduct of appropriate and well-designed in vitro and in vivo studies to characterize the toxicological effects and associated dose–response for the nanomaterial (Figure 1.2).

The amount of toxicological research that will be required for nanomaterials will vary depending on the anticipated use of the nanomaterial and the availability of existing data. For example, the use of nanomaterials in medical devices, drugs, pesticides, foods, or food packaging will require an extensive battery of in vitro and in vivo studies to evaluate and characterize their toxicity. Many of these products involve the ingestion or direct contact with the nanomaterial, so a variety of toxicological and preclinical studies will be required to obtain regulatory pre-market approval by governmental agencies such as the United States (US) Food and Drug Administration (FDA), the US Environmental Protection Agency (EPA), European Food Safety Authority (EFSA), European Medicines Evaluation Authority (EMEA), or other agencies in various countries. The use of nanomaterials in certain consumer products that do not require pre-market approval and are typically not regulated as rigorously as food and drug products will likely not undergo such an extensive toxicological evaluation. In many cases, nanomaterials in

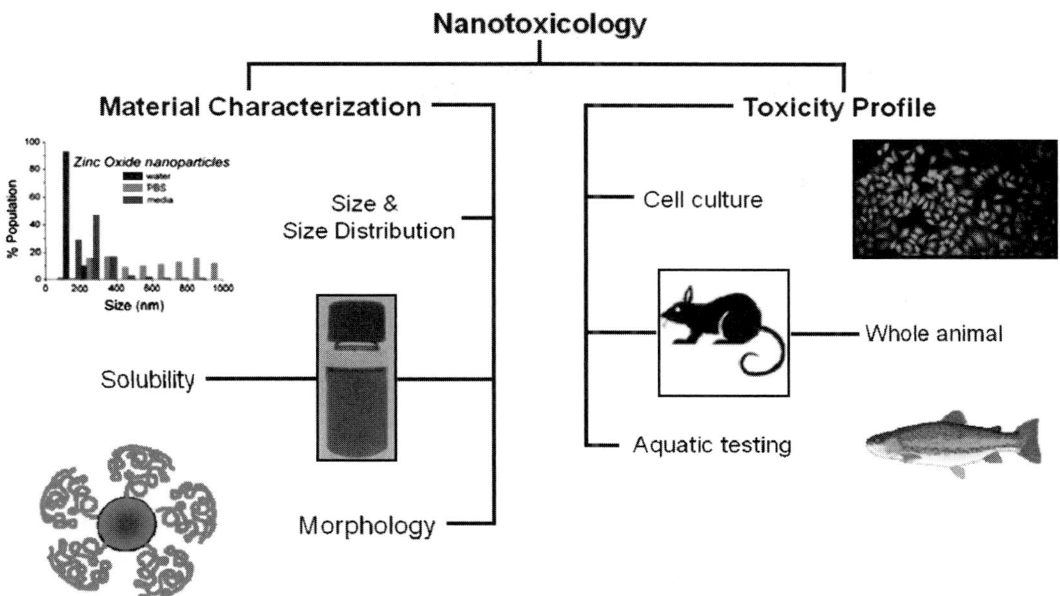

FIGURE 1.2 *Hazard Evaluation of Nanomaterials. The evaluation of the hazard potential for nanomaterials may be divided into two equally important parts: nanomaterial physicochemical characterization and toxicity profiling. The physicochemical characterization of the material should include information on size and size distribution, solubility and aggregation state, and morphological assessments (including shape, crystalline structure, surface chemistry, and allotropic state). The toxicological profile may be developed through conducting a variety of* in vitro *and* in vivo *mammalian and ecotoxicological studies.*

consumer products are embedded in a matrix, with a low potential for direct contact and exposure to free nanomaterials. However, it will be important to consider potential sources of exposure to free nanomaterials from such products (during, for example, nanomaterial production or product formulation, sanding paint, sawing, or cutting products such as pipes, plastics, or fabrics containing nanomaterials) or upon disposal of the products. There are guidance documents and regulations for a wide variety of in vitro and in vivo studies that may be followed when conducting a hazard evaluation of a nanomaterial for use in consumer products (see, for example, Organization for Economic Cooperation and Development, FDA, EPA, European Union (EU) guidelines) and the selection of appropriate and necessary studies will depend on the intended use of the nanomaterial. It may be prudent to develop decision matrixes for selecting appropriate in vitro and in vivo studies to evaluate various toxicological endpoints, using relevant routes of exposure. Ultimately, the goal of the predictive approach is to develop a series of toxicity assays that can limit the demand for in vivo studies, both from a cost as well as an animal use perspective (Nel et al., 2006). A discussion of proposed frameworks and screening studies for evaluating the toxicological potential of nanomaterials is provided later in this chapter.

As an initial evaluation for a new nanomaterial, a structure–activity evaluation (quantitative structure activity relationship (QSAR)) may identify whether any structural alerts for a toxicologically significant endpoint are evident. Given sufficient knowledge on structurally or functionally related compounds, QSAR can be used for screening virtually any reasonably well-defined biological, toxicological, or pharmacological endpoint of interest, including kinetic characteristics (i.e., absorption, distribution, metabolism, excretion (ADME)) (Doull et al., 2007). Such evaluations may be conducted with commercially available computer software. However, in the case of newly developed engineered nanomaterials, there may not be any toxicological or pharmacological information available on structurally or functionally related substances. In the case of some nanomaterials (for example, fullerenes and quantum dots), studies have reported that functional groups can have a significant impact on toxicological potential, so as data are accumulated on the impacts of chemical structure, it will be important to develop databases of such information for use in QSAR analyses for nanomaterials (Hardman, 2006; Sayes et al., 2006; Isakovic et al., 2006). In addition, the development of toxic equivalency factors (TEFs) could be useful for comparing the potential toxicological effects of different chemical structures, functional groups, or production methods for a particular class of nanomaterials (including quantum dots, fullerenes, and carbon nanotubes). The TEF methodology was developed by the EPA to estimate the hazard of a mixture of structurally related chemicals with a common mechanism of action. TEFs have been developed to compare the toxicity of members within chemical classes such as dioxins or polycyclic aromatic hydrocarbons, which include several compounds (Van den berg et al., 2006; Haws et al., 2004; Petry et al., 1996). The development of TEFs for individual members of a class of nanomaterials may be useful for conducting future risk assessments for certain types of nanomaterials (e.g., carbon nanotubes or fullerenes with different functional groups).

Of fundamental importance in conducting a risk assessment for a substance such as a nanomaterial is an understanding of the dose–response for adverse effects associated with exposure. A dose–response assessment is an evaluation of the relationship between dose and incidence (or severity) of an adverse effect. In many cases, a dose–response assessment must be conducted to extrapolate the doses associated with adverse effects observed in toxicological studies (typically in an animal model that has been treated with the nanomaterial) to exposure levels that would be considered safe for humans. If available, data in humans may also be used to determine safe exposure levels of a nanomaterial that are not associated with any adverse effects. In addition, pertinent information on the toxicokinetics (ADME) for the nanomaterial should be collected and may be incorporated into the dose–response assessment to refine the estimates of acceptable exposure levels.

In a dose–response assessment, the adverse effect which is seen at the lowest dose in a relevant experimental animal model or in a human population (e.g., occupational study) for a non-carcinogenic chemical, e.g., the Lowest Observed Adverse Effect Level (LOAEL) or No Observed Adverse Effect Level (NOAEL), is identified. Importantly, the relevance of the biological response to humans must be considered, as in some instances, the effects observed in the animal model may not occur in humans due to physiological or mechanistic differences between humans and animals. Alternatively, benchmark modeling may be conducted to establish a Benchmark Dose (BMD) from the available exposure–response data using mathematical models. The BMD may be defined as the dose of a substance that is associated with a specified increased incidence of risk, generally in the range of 1 percent to 10 percent of a health effect; or the dose associated with a specified measure or change of a biological effect. If sufficient data are available, the BMD approach provides a more quantitative alternative than the NOAEL/LOAEL process for evaluating noncancer health effects. Once a BMD, NOAEL, or LOAEL is established for a nanomaterial, safety or uncertainty factors may be applied to extrapolate the results from animals to humans (interspecies extrapolation, unless the BMD, NOAEL, or LOAEL is based on human data), to account for inter-individual variability or susceptibility within the human population, and if necessary, to extrapolate from acute to chronic exposure conditions. The BMD, NOAEL, or LOAEL may be divided by safety factors to obtain the safe exposure level or reference dose. The use of safety factors results in the establishment of an acceptable exposure level that is typically >100 times lower than the dose at which no effects are observed with the chemical of interest (such as a nanomaterial), so it is usually a very health protective and conservative value. The safety factor approach has been used for many years as the basis for conducting risk assessments by regulatory agencies to establish safe exposure levels for a variety of chemical substances, and this approach may also be used to identify safe exposure levels for nanomaterials. However, there are many inherent uncertainties associated with the application of safety factors, so as pharmacokinetic/pharmacodynamic data become available for a chemical substance, biologically based risk assessments may be conducted, reducing or eliminating the need for the application of safety factors.

Conducting a dose–response evaluation for carcinogens is more complicated because for some carcinogens, it is assumed that there is no threshold for adverse effects, so an NOAEL cannot be established. The low-dose extrapolation for carcinogens may be accomplished through the use of mathematical models such as the multistage, probit, logit, and linear extrapolation models. For carcinogens, it is important to consider whether they are considered to be genotoxic or nongentoxic and whether a threshold exists for the associated carcinogenic response. To estimate risks from carcinogens, the calculations of low-dose effects and dose–response require a more complex consideration of all the data, including information on mechanisms of carcinogenicity. The results of the calculations are values known as cancer potency factors and for carcinogens, excess lifetime risk is calculated by multiplying the anticipated dose or exposure estimate by the potency factor. The result is a value that represents an upper bound on the probability that lifetime exposure to a chemical substance, under the specified conditions of exposure, will lead to excess cancer risk. This value is usually expressed as a population risk, such as 1×10^{-6}, which means that not more than one in one million exposed individuals is expected to develop cancer as a result of exposure to the substance of interest. Risk estimates obtained in this way are not scientific estimates of actual cancer risk; they are upper bounds on actual cancer risk that are useful to regulators for setting priorities and for setting exposure limits.

In addition to obtaining information to perform a hazard and dose–response evaluation, an exposure assessment will need to be conducted to estimate and characterize any potential risks associated with nanomaterials. If the hazard identification process reveals that a nanomaterial is innocuous and does not pose a potential for eliciting any adverse human health or environmental effects, it may not be necessary to conduct additional toxicological studies or an extensive exposure assessment. In cases where the hazard evaluation determines a potential for adverse effects for the nanomaterial, in vitro and/or in vivo studies may be conducted to evaluate the potential for systemic exposure from inhalation, oral, or dermal penetration. Such information may help to refine the exposure assessment by providing estimates of internal doses. Much of the published human toxicological and epidemiology data relate to airborne exposure to nanoparticles or ultrafine particles. However, there are additional routes by which humans can be exposed to nanomaterials that may need to be considered, including: (1) ingestion (foods, food additives, and contaminants, cosmetics or other personal care products, various pharmaceuticals and medical devices); (2) dermal contact (surface finishing products, contaminants, and cosmetics); and (3) injection or implantation (pharmaceutical products) (Scientific

Committee on Emerging and Newly Identified Health Risks (SCENIHR), 2006). The exposure assessment will need to include information about the nanomaterial-containing product such as product type, frequency of use, duration of product contact, concentration of nanomaterial in the final product, use by sensitive subpopulations (i.e., babies, the elderly, pregnant women), and conditions of foreseeable misuse of the product and disposal of the products.

At this point, there is not enough knowledge regarding the toxicity of most engineered nanomaterials or information about the characteristics of nanomaterial-containing products and/or levels in the workplace to estimate safe exposure levels. Consumer products containing free nanomaterials with direct human exposure or direct emission to the environment are considered to have a high potential exposure, while products in which nanomaterials are integrated into larger scale materials with indirect human exposure or indirect emissions to the environment are considered to have a low potential exposure and associated hazard. Product categories with a high level of free nanomaterial exposure (in the workplace or to consumers) may require a higher priority for further examination of potential health risks. However, next to the likelihood and magnitude of anticipated exposure, the priority for further examination of potential risks is also determined by the toxicity of the nanomaterial. Currently, the available understanding of the probable exposure levels and toxicity profiles is insufficient to determine risks (e.g., as unacceptably high or negligible) for most engineered nanomaterials. Because this information is necessary to estimate the risks associated with each specific nanomaterial-containing consumer product or product category, it may be too early to evaluate the human health and the environmental risks for most engineered nanomaterials.

Determining anticipated route and magnitude of exposure is an important component in the overall assessment of safety and must be done on a nanomaterial-by-nanomaterial basis, with secondary exposures taken into consideration when necessary. The estimated exposure levels for a nanomaterial may then be compared with the calculated safe dose derived from the hazard identification evaluation. The procedures and factors considered in the exposure assessment process are not expected to be any different for nanomaterials than for larger particles or chemicals. The degree of hazard associated with exposure to any chemical or substance, regardless of its physicochemical characteristics, depends on several factors, including its toxicity, dose–response curve, concentration, route of exposure, duration and/or frequency of exposure. However, depending on the route of anticipated exposure (dermal, inhalation, oral) and types of associated toxicities (local or systemic), a chemical may not pose any risk of adverse effects if there is no potential for systemic exposure. A chemical will not produce adverse effects unless sufficient quantities get into the body at a concentration and for a sufficient period of time to produce a response. Importantly, measuring the concentration of a chemical in the body is not a demonstration of an adverse effect, though it may be a valid indicator of chemical exposure. In the case of dermal exposure, a chemical will not be systemically available if it does not penetrate skin, because to reach the circulation and be systemically available, chemical substances must cross several cell layers of the skin, where the rate-determining layer is considered to be the stratum corneum. However, it is possible that a chemical such as a nanomaterial can elicit a localized topical adverse effect and/or sensitization responses such as irritation, allergic contact dermatitis, contact urticaria, or phototoxicity, even if it does not penetrate the skin. It will be important to evaluate some of these endpoints in toxicological studies. As a result of the broad range of potential applications of the products of nanotechnology, a similarly broad range of environmental and human health impacts can arise from different exposure routes of nanomaterials. Currently, knowledge on the routes and magnitude of exposure to nanomaterial, as well as of the potential environmental impacts of nanomaterials, is very limited, therefore, a clear need exists to establish a full understanding of the environmental benefits and disadvantages of nanomaterials as compared with those of conventional chemicals (and products) over their complete life cycles.

The final stage of a risk assessment is called "risk characterization" in which information from the three phases is integrated to determine the probability of an adverse effect in a human population or the environment resulting from exposure to the chemical of interest. The results of the risk characterization are then communicated to the risk manager with an overall assessment of the quality of the information in the risk assessment analysis so that appropriate decisions may be made to manage any associated risks.

As scientific information is developed for nanomaterials, it will be possible to conduct safety and risk assessments to evaluate any associated human health risks and environmental impacts. It appears that the risk assessment paradigm that has been used to evaluate risks associated with traditional chemical exposures will be appropriate for evaluating nanomaterials. Groups such as SCENIHR in the EU have developed position papers on how the risk assessment process may need to be modified when evaluating the risks associated with engineered nanomaterials (SCENIHR, 2007). There do appear to be some additional data needs that should be considered early in the process when designing studies, so that there is appropriate and useful information available when conducting future risk assessments. It is anticipated that ongoing and future studies will address

1) The characterization of the mechanisms and kinetics of the release of nanoparticles from a wide range of production processes, formulations, and uses of the products of nanotechnology;
2) The actual range of exposure levels, both to humans and to the environment, and those experienced during the development, production, and use of nanomaterial-containing products;
3) The extent to which it is possible to extrapolate from the toxicology of fibers, particles and other physical forms of the same substance to the toxicology of nanoparticles;
4) Toxicokinetic data following various routes of exposure, so that information about absorption, distribution, metabolism, and excretion can be identified, and doses for hazard assessment determined. This includes dose–response data for the target organs, and knowledge of the subcellular location of nanomaterials and their mechanistic effects at the cellular level;
5) Information on the health of workers involved in the manufacture and processing of nanoparticles;
6) The fate, distribution, and persistence (including bioaccumulation) of nanoparticles in the environment; and
7) The effects of nanoparticles on various environmental species in each of the environmental compartments representative of different trophic levels and exposure routes (SCENIHR 2006).

FIGURE 1.3 *The major gaps in knowledge that need to be addressed for conducting future risk assessments of nanomaterials.*

these issues, but it is imperative that studies be designed in a manner that they will provide meaningful and useful information for conducting future risk assessments of nanomaterials (Figure 1.3).

1.4 CHARACTERIZING NANOMATERIALS FOR TOXICOLOGICAL EVALUATION

One important step in developing safety information on nanomaterials includes conducting reliable and reproducible toxicity assessment (Bucher et al., 2004) and among these issues is the characterization of materials to be tested (Powers et al., 2007). Both adequate and relevant particle characterization profiles will be essential for conducting risk assessments and safety evaluations of nanoparticles and novel engineered nanomaterials. This work is becoming increasingly important in a variety of fields, including toxicology and engineering, as well as regulatory and policy development. Physicochemical characterization of nanomaterials is pertinent for risk assessors when comparing and contrasting reports and studies addressing the potential environmental health and safety (EHS) effects of nanomaterials (Oberdörster et al., 2005a, b; Sayes et al., 2007; Tran et al., 2000). Some physical and chemical properties that are important for assessing effects of nanomaterials include particle size and distribution, morphology, chemical composition, solubility, and surface chemistry and reactivity (Powers et al., 2007).

Particle characterization can be studied on materials in solution or suspension and as the dry nanopowders, and a characterization profile of the nanomaterial recovered after exposures to in vitro or in vivo test systems should also be conducted. Nanoparticle characteristics change when exposed to normal laboratory conditions and it may further change form (structure, surface chemistry, and aggregation state) once in vivo or in vitro. Characterization of nanomaterials can be divided into three categories based on the physical state of the nanomaterial (i.e., dry, wet, or in a test system) that can be referred to as primary, secondary, and tertiary, as shown in Figure 1.4. Primary characterization is performed on particles or materials as dry powders. Secondary characterization is performed on particles or materials in the wet phase as a solution or suspension, such as in solvents, ultrapure water, environmental water (ground, fresh, marine), buffered solution (i.e., Phosphate Buffered Saline (PBS)) or cell culture media. Tertiary characterization is performed on particles or materials either in vivo or ex vivo, including characterization in cells and tissues (e.g., blood, lung fluid, liver, and kidney) as well as interactions with proteins, lipids, or specific cell types during or after treatment.

Nanomaterials are usually produced using a "bottom up" approach (particle growth, in either the liquid or aerosol phase, from a molecular precursor) to develop specific structural and functional features, resulting in highly ordered, monodisperse samples with a large surface area. Traditionally, these materials are characterized using an array of analytical techniques, including microscopy, spectroscopy, and chromatography which provide important information about physical (such as size and shape) and chemical properties (including surface coatings and solubility) as shown in Table 1.1.

Three properties that dictate the nanomaterial's uniqueness are chemical composition, size, and shape. Depending on the composition of the nanomaterial, a specific function can be achieved; and depending on the size of the nanomaterial, the function can be varied. The structure defines the

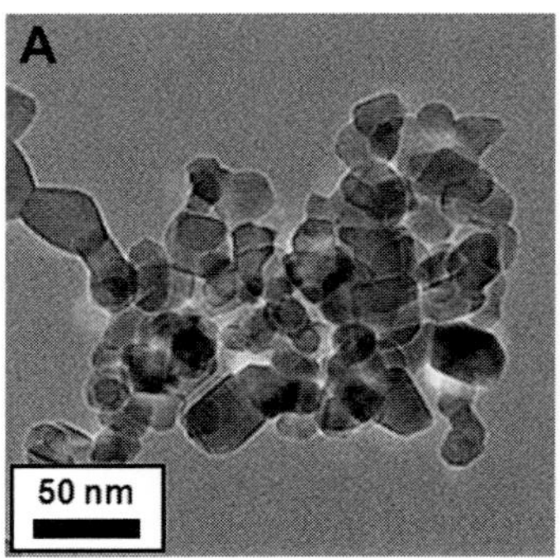

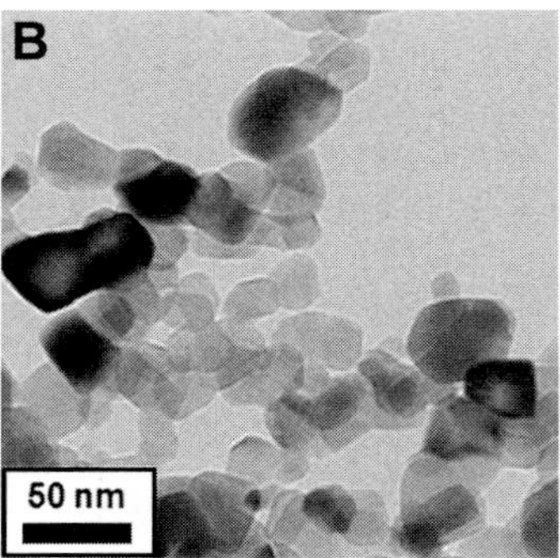

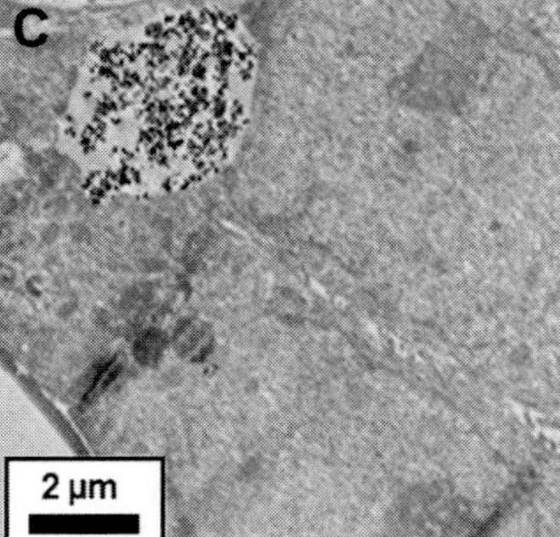

FIGURE 1.4 *Transmission electron micrographs of 25 nm TiO_2 particles: (A) dry-TEM; (B) cryo-TEM; (C) TEM of an exposed and fixed lung cell with TiO_2 nanoparticles inside.*

Table 1.1 Techniques for Evaluating Physicochemical Properties of Nanomaterials

Property	Definition	Technique
Chemical composition	■ Refers to the elements of which the material is composed ■ Includes both composition of the particle's core and its surface	Spectroscopy: X-ray photoemission (XPS), Raman, Inductively coupled plasma atomic emission (ICP-AES), Ultraviolet-visible (UV-Vis), Fourier-transform infrared (FTIR), Differential thermal analysis (DTA), X-ray diffraction (XRD); Energy Dispersive X-Ray (EDS)
Particle size distribution	■ Commonly referred to as PSD ■ The range of sizes of particles within a sample ■ Gives an indication of the aggregation/agglomeration state	■ Brunauer, Emmett, and Teller technique for specific surface area (SSA BET) ■ Dynamic light scattering (DLS) ■ Transmission electron microscopy (TEM) ■ Scanning electron microscopy (SEM)
Morphology	■ Information on aspect ratio for non-spherical particles ■ Crystal structure for crystalline materials ■ Allotropic forms for materials of similar chemical composition	■ X-ray diffraction (XRD) ■ Electron diffraction (ED) ■ X-ray photoemission spectroscopy (XPS)
Surface chemistry & reactivity	■ Chemical characteristics associated with surface of a material ■ Information about the interface of the solid particle and liquid solvent	■ Zeta potential ■ Isoelectric point (IEP) ■ Electron spin resonance (ESR)

This list is intended for establishing a relative metric of the physicochemical properties of materials.

material's function and activity and this activity can be exploited for use in biological, electronic, or industrial processes. Regardless of its chemical composition, manipulating its structure manipulates the function of the nanomaterial and there are many examples of this tunable phenomenon. For example, iron oxide (Fe_3O_4) nanocrystals exploit size-dependent magnetism, which is the premise behind magnetic separations or adsorption of a variety of materials. Emission properties are integral in biomedical research and in photothermal therapies (e.g., gold nanoshells and cadmium selenide quantum dots exhibit a size-dependent light absorption and emission phenomenon). These same properties that make nanoscience interesting are key to the development of nanomaterials and may also have an impact on their toxicological potential.

1.4.1 Primary phase

Primary phase physicochemical characterization refers to those nanoscale properties of the material in its dry or powder state. The primary phase properties related to toxicity testing of the nanomaterial include a wide range of particle features, including size, size distribution, and surface area; chemical composition and surface chemistry; and morphology.

1.4.1.1 Size, size distribution and surface area

The distribution of size within a nanoparticle sample is an example of a "nano" property. Particle size and size distributions are normally represented graphically as population versus size. Sizing data can be acquired using a variety of techniques and particle sizing in the wet phase involves different techniques than particle sizing in the dry state. There are numerous techniques for measuring particle size distributions based on a variety of physical principles, including laser diffraction, dynamic light scattering, differential mobility analysis, time of flight methods, impaction methods, microscopy, and surface area measurements (Powers et al., 2007). Due to the large number of instruments available from various manufacturers, significant effort has been directed toward global standardization of particle size analysis by International Standards Organization (ISO) Technical Committee 24 (TC24/SC4), "Particle sizing by methods other than sieving." Transmission Electron Microscopy (TEM) is one of the most common and informative methods used to size nanoparticles in the dry state. However, it is also one of the most time- and labor-intensive methods, as well. Other methods for dry phase nanoparticles include differential mobility analysis (DMA), time of flight mass spectroscopy (TOF-MS), and specific surface area measurements (SSA). DMA is used to evaluate aerosolized nanoparticle samples under a nitrogen purge or dry air and SSA using BET (Braunauer, Emmett, and Teller) methodologies to attain an area measurement that can then be converted (through stoichiometry) to a primary particle size.

In the model nanoparticle sample, a monodisperse population corresponds to a population of particles of the same size and is a highly desired form for most nanoparticles. Because there is such great control over the size and shape when producing an engineered nanoparticle sample, a small size distribution (typically <5 percent) can be easily achieved for many substances. As production techniques and sizing methods become more sophisticated, this size distribution will eventually be eliminated so that the nanoparticles all will be of a uniform size.

There is an inverse squared relationship between surface area and radius of a nanoparticle, so as the radius of the nanoparticle decreases, the surface area increases exponentially. The specific surface area for engineered nanomaterials is typically hundreds of square meters per gram (reported as m^2/g). As previously discussed, concerns have been raised regarding the effect of increasing surface area of particles on enhancing reactivity based on the greater number of reactive species (e.g., free oxygen radicals) on the particle surface and enhancing the rate of dissolution and solubility, which may impact bioavailability and toxicological potential. It is important to note that increasing particle surface area may also correspond to increasing risk of explosion for some energetic nanoparticles (for example, aluminum oxides).

For dry powders, the BET surface area technique is often used to estimate average size (based on a nonporous spherical model) and has the added advantage of providing a direct measurement of surface area (Powers et al., 2007). The BET theory is a common rule for the physical adsorption of gas molecules on a solid surface and was explored as a means of measuring surface area in 1938 by three scientists named Stephen Brunauer, Paul Emmett, and Edward Teller (Brunauer et al., 1938). After successfully measuring the surface area of particles in the dry state, they published an article about the "BET" theory in a journal for the first time (Braunauer et al., 1938). BET methodologies require a dry sample of material ($\sim$10 mg) and the accuracy of the measurements increases with increased sample size. Simply, nitrogen, argon, carbon dioxide, or krypton absorbs onto the surface of a few aerosolized particles from the powder sample. The instrument then applies the Langmuir theory and BET equations to this aerosolized monodispersed layer. The application of the Langmuir theory includes the following principles: for monolayer molecular adsorption to multilayer adsorption: (a) gas molecules physically adsorb on a solid in layers infinitely;

(b) there is no interaction between each adsorption layer; and (c) the Langmuir theory can be applied to each layer.

1.4.1.2 Chemical composition and surface chemistry

The composition of the nanomaterial may also define its function and toxicological potential. In nanoscale science and technology, nanomaterials are developed to have specific and unique applications. Spectroscopy, one of the most common analytical techniques in chemistry, is the science concerned with the production, measurement, and interpretation of electromagnetic spectra arising from either emission or absorption of radiant energy by various substances. It is commonly used to evaluate chemical composition of diverse substances and there are many different types of spectroscopic measurements that can be applied to each nanoparticle sample.

Surface chemistry is a function of the particle's molecular composition and structure of the surface. The concentration and types of surface modified functional groups on a nanomaterial increase as particle size decreases, which can also affect function and toxicological potential. Methods such as X-ray photoelectron spectroscopy (XPS) and electron spectroscopy for chemical analysis (ESCA) may be used to determine the chemical composition of a nanoparticle's surface (Ratner, 1996).

Raman spectroscopy has recently gained popularity for advanced chemical analysis of surfaces. In nanoscience, Raman spectroscopy is used to characterize surface properties of materials, measure temperature, and determine crystallinity. Raman spectroscopy is a spectroscopic technique used in material science to study vibrational and rotational frequencies in a system. The technique measures shifts in inelastic scattering, or Raman scattering, of light from a visible, near infrared or near ultraviolet light source and the shift in energy provides information about the material's surface characteristics. The Raman signal unit is a measurement of the ratio between the Stokes (down-shifted) intensity and anti-Stokes (up-shifted) intensity peaks.

1.4.1.3 Morphology

Typically, the size and shape of the nanoparticle sample is determined via microscopy. There are many microscopy methods that may be used to size nanoparticle solutions. Some include light/fluorescence microscopy, scanning electron microscopy (SEM), transmission electron microscopy of the dried sample (dried-TEM), and transmission electron microscopy of a cryogenically frozen sample (cryo-TEM). Dried-TEM is one of the methods in which the molecular structure of the sample can be identified. Cryo-TEM produces a more accurate micrograph of what the biological system will encounter when exposed to the nanoparticles or nanomaterial. The sample's molecular structure cannot be determined with Cryo-TEM, nor is the sizing resolution as precise as dried-TEM, but the potential for aggregation may be revealed and samples can be analyzed in the solvent of interest. Other techniques include atomic force microscopy (AFM) and laser-scanning confocal microscopy.

An analytical technique that characterizes both size and crystallinity is X-ray diffraction (XRD). An X-ray diffraction pattern does not exist in an amorphous sample, only in crystalline samples. Nanocrystals diffract X-rays in unique ways and their structure influences the nanoparticle's chemical and toxicological properties. In a crystalline sample, both the phase (lattice structure or molecular arrangements) and grain size (crystallite size or size of an individual crystal) can be elucidated. Because nanocrystals have such small grain sizes, a long collection time is necessary for the sample of interest. The diffraction peak widths of the nanoparticle correlate to the size of the nanocrystals and sizes will change depending on the chemical composition of the crystal. An ideal nanocrystalline sample is composed of nanoparticles that are highly uniform in size and shape.

1.4.2 Secondary phase

Secondary phase physicochemical characterization refers to those nanoscale properties of the material as a wet state. Secondary phase physical and chemical characterization relevant to toxicity testing includes concentration and purity; size and size distribution (including aggregation/agglomeration/coagulation state); surface activity/reactivity; and presence of reactive oxygen species in the solution/suspension.

1.4.2.1 Concentration and purity

The endproduct of a nanomaterial sample can be in the form of a solid powder or in solution/suspension. For a dried powder in solution, concentration is easily determined by dispersing a known amount of sample (in grams) into a known amount of solvent (in liters). For the best measurement of particles in solution, cryo-transmission electron microscopy should be used. Usually, a known volume of sample is used when preparing nanoparticles in suspension for cryo-TEM analysis. After images are taken from the sample, the nanoparticles in each micrograph are counted.

There are few techniques commonly used to test the purity of the nanoparticle sample and some methods, such as liquid chromatography and mass spectroscopy, require more nanomaterial sample than can be typically spared. For gravimetric tests, samples are not recovered, but do require less sample volume for analysis. X-ray diffraction can also distinguish crystalline phase and relative purities.

1.4.2.2 Size and size distribution

A commonly employed technique for evaluating the size distribution of the nanomaterial prior to toxicological evaluations is manually measuring particles from literally thousands of micrographs taken from either the transmission electron microscope (dried or cryogenic) or the scanning electron microscope. There is a variety of software (e.g., ImagePro, Media Cybernetics, Inc., Bethesda, Maryland, US or NanoSight, NanoSight Ltd., Salisbury, Wiltshire, UK) designed to aid in this time intensive task. Alternative to this method is dynamic light scattering (DLS). Although traditional methodologies are limited to the particle's size (data are less reliable as the size of the particle decreases), recent advances in the technique have improved light scattering measurements (Powers et al., 2006).

Measuring the size and size distribution of a nanoparticle sample in the wet phase is analogous to measuring its state of dispersion. The formation of agglomerates is partly driven by particle–particle interactions known as Van der Waals forces. Agglomerations can also be formed due to increasing the particle concentration in the solvent or changing the pH or ionic strength of the solvent. Because the potential for agglomerate formation increases once nanoparticles are introduced to a solvent, it may be necessary to disperse the agglomerated particles back into a mono-dispersed system.

1.4.2.3 Surface activity/reactivity

The most important parameter surrounding nanoparticle surface chemistry is the fraction of surface coated with a particular type of coating. On an average, a 100 mg nanoparticle sample could be coated up to 30 percent by weight with a surface coating. In biological media, protein sorption may compete for binding sites; therefore, biomolecules can potentially replace surfactant surface coating molecules. Absorbed species on the surface of a particle may also change the chemical nature of the particle. A secondary parameter is the stability of surface coatings. The activity (or reactivity) of the particle's surface can be measured using a variety of techniques and there is no single technique that can be used for all nanomaterials. Surface charge, a measure of the positive or negative charge on the surface of a particle in solution or in suspension, can aid in the determination of the particle's dispersion characteristics. Surface charge is also a measurement of a material's surface chemistry and the charge can be measured using zeta potential measurements. Further, information on the particle's absorbed species, such

as proteins or salts, can be obtained as well (Adamson and Gast, 1997). The generation of free oxygen radicals on the particle surfaces may be measured by electron paramagnetic resonance spectroscopy.

1.4.3 Tertiary phase

Tertiary phase physicochemical characterization refers to those nanoscale properties of the material under in vitro or in vivo conditions. Tertiary phase physical and chemical properties relevant to toxicological testing include surface reactivity, size and size distribution (including aggregation state), and particle translocation. While characterization in the tertiary phase is complex and non-trivial, it is the most relevant toxicological nanomaterial characterization parameter because nanomaterials may behave differently once they have been introduced into environmental or biological systems. The properties of a nanoparticle in non-polar solvents change when extracted into the aqueous phase; further, nanoparticles in biological fluids (buffered solutions, cell culture media, or blood) may behave differently as well. The nanoparticle surface is the part of the nanoparticle system that will have direct interactions with the biological entity; therefore, the surface of the nanoparticle may significantly influence the biological response.

1.4.3.1 Surface activity

There are a few sophisticated techniques utilizing biochemical analyses that can potentially determine particle reactivity under in vivo conditions. Some of these techniques include measuring hemolytic potential, which demonstrates the differential surface activity particles from non-reactive particles when incubated with red blood cells. Other techniques for measuring nanomaterial surface activity include electron spin resonance, electron microscopy, and mass spectroscopy.

1.4.3.2 Size and size distribution

Just as particle characteristics differ from the dry versus the wet state, particle size distributions can differ once the material is in the body of an experimental animal or in a human. For toxicity testing, the size distribution "as dosed" might be quite different than the same system "as-generated" or "as-received". Even if the size/agglomerate distribution is captured right at the point of exposure, changes in environmental conditions or physiological clearance mechanisms may continue to alter the state of the particles in vivo (Powers et al., 2007). The difficulty in measuring changes in particle size and size distribution in vivo is partly due to the information-limited and non-trivial analytical techniques. To circumvent these difficulties, scientists use simulated biological fluids to conduct sizing analyses of particles in the tertiary phase. Ultimately, post-mortem or histological examination of the cells, tissues and organs exposed to the test materials is perhaps the best way to ascertain what changes may have occurred to the particles during testing, and this is best accomplished through microscopy.

Information about the effects of nanoparticles on biological systems can also be obtained in cell-free environments. Characterization data and functionality information of nanoparticles suspended in serum, media, buffers, or other biological fluids may be different than data obtained from nanoparticles suspended in water or other vehicles. It is possible for biomolecules, such as peptides or proteins, to absorb onto the surface of the particle, thus increasing the hydrodynamic diameter of the nanoparticle and making it less or more bioavailable. Also, the biomolecules may provide an environment for enhanced generation of reactive oxygen species. In addition, the salts and sugars present in cell culture media and biological fluids may alter the pH and ionic strength of the nanoparticle solution, which has the potential to confound observed effects.

1.4.4 Summary of characterizing nanomaterials

Connecting the fields of nanoscience, chemistry, and toxicology is a collaborative effort. The purpose of this bridge is to determine the effects of nanomaterials in environmental and biological systems. When conducting toxicological studies of nanomaterials, researchers should be mindful of the nanomaterial synthesis techniques and characterization data. When reporting a study addressing potential environmental or human health effects of nanomaterials, the characterization data for the material being tested should be reported in as much detail as possible. It is imperative that specific parameters be included when reporting the results of a toxicological study with nanomaterials. Some common guidelines include the following: at the very least, report size, surface area, and structure; obtain TEM and/or SEM micrographs of the nanomaterial when possible; identify and quantify small molecular weight contaminants, such as residual solvents or metals intercalated within the nanomaterial's structure; report how the material was manufactured; describe any information about surface coatings; and investigate changes in the nanomaterial's physicochemical properties when moving from the sample preparation to sample administration to in vivo conditions (Figure 1.5).

Identifying the potential toxicity of a new material can be a difficult venture, especially for a nanomaterial. In many instances, it is difficult to produce nanomaterials on a large scale because the mass of material

Common Guidelines: the types of characterization information that should be included with toxicological studies of engineered nanomaterials

1. Size and size distribution
2. Surface coating and charge
3. Crystallinity and purity
4. Solubility and bioavailable metals

FIGURE 1.5 *Common Guidelines.*

produced is very small (for example, one gram of nanoparticles is approximately equivalent to at least one trillion particles). The immediate challenge of toxicological studies of nanomaterials is not only producing enough material for conducting in vivo studies, but also to produce enough material for physicochemical characterization purposes.

There are a few key points in the growing body of nanotoxicology literature. Morphological characterization, such as particle size, surface area, and shape, should be measured in the most dispersed state achievable. For example, data have shown that particles suspended in a "buffered" solution are more dispersed than particles suspended in ultrapure water, correlating with increased conductance, solubility, and ionic strength and decreased surface charge. Further, particle characterization data should be measured under conditions as close to the point of sample administration or application as possible. For instance, in whole animal toxicological evaluations, the nanomaterials should be measured in the vehicle or when dispersed in an inhalation chamber. When possible, it will be very important to obtain as much information about the nanomaterial in cells or tissues following administration and at various points during the study period. One important message is that no single technique can accurately describe all biologically relevant properties of a material and adequate physicochemical characterization of nanomaterials may require multiple analytical techniques at various stages of the study.

1.5 TOXICOLOGICAL TESTING FRAMEWORKS AND SCREENING STRATEGIES FOR NANOMATERIALS

Several groups have recommended frameworks and/or screening strategies that may be followed for the development of nanomaterials that may be used safely. Frameworks have been developed by groups such as the International Life Sciences Institute, the European Centre for Ecotoxicology and

Toxicology of Chemicals, and a collaborative partnership between Environmental Defense and DuPont (Oberdörster et al., 2005b; Warheit et al., 2007b; Environmental Defense and DuPont, 2007). These frameworks provide guidance for studies that may be necessary for conducting future hazard evaluations and risk assessments of nanomaterials.

a. International Life Sciences Institute

The International Life Sciences Institute Research Foundation/Risk Science Institute (ILSI) convened an expert working group to develop a screening strategy for the hazard identification of nanoparticles and engineered nanomaterials (Oberdörster et al., 2005b). The ILSI report presents elements of a screening strategy for obtaining data necessary for conducting hazard evaluations for nanomaterials. Several routes of exposure (oral, dermal, inhalation, and injection) are considered in this screening strategy, recognizing that, depending on use patterns, exposure to nanomaterials may occur by any of these routes. The three key elements of the toxicity screening strategy include: (1) physicochemical characterization, (2) in vitro assays (cellular and non-cellular), and (3) in vivo assays. Physicochemical properties that may be important to evaluate and may assist in the interpretation of any observed effects of the nanomaterials include particle size and size distribution, agglomeration state, shape, crystal structure, chemical composition, surface area, surface chemistry, surface charge, and porosity. Nanomaterial characterization of administered material and characterization of as-produced or supplied material are recommended. In addition, appropriate selection of dose metric is recommended for in vitro and in vivo studies. Appropriate selection of the dose metric will depend on the hypothesized parameter most closely associated with anticipated response or the metric which may be most accurately measured. It is strongly recommended that in all cases, sufficient information be collected to enable the future determination of nanomaterial dose by mass, surface area, and particle number. The dose metric may also vary depending on the shape and form of the nanomaterial (e.g., fibrous, particulate, spherical, tubular). In addition, it was recommended that "benchmark" particle controls, such as crystalline silica and respirable titanium dioxide be utilized in all studies. Requirements for in vitro and in vivo screening studies will differ according to the anticipated routes of exposure for the nanomaterials. In vitro techniques allow specific biological and mechanistic pathways to be isolated and tested under controlled conditions, in ways that are not feasible in in vivo tests. In vitro studies are suggested as part of the screening strategy to evaluate point-of-entry toxicity in cells from the lungs, skin, and the mucosal membranes, and target organ toxicity for endothelium, blood, spleen, liver, nervous system, heart, and kidney. It was recommended that as always, care should be taken in interpreting data obtained from in vitro systems because of the high doses normally used for in vitro studies, the impact of a bolus effect, and the difficulty in extrapolating results to in vivo. Non-cellular assessment of nanomaterial durability, protein interactions, complement activation, and pro-oxidant activity is also recommended in this screening strategy.

The ILSI screening strategy recommends that in vivo studies to evaluate nanomaterials should be conducted in two Tiers. Tier 1 assays are proposed for pulmonary, oral, skin, and injection exposures and additional Tier 2 evaluations for pulmonary exposures are also proposed. Tier 1 evaluations include markers of inflammation, oxidant stress, and cell proliferation in portal-of-entry and selected remote organs and tissues. Tier 2 studies include: (1) use of susceptible models, (2) effects of multiple exposures, (3) pulmonary deposition, translocation, and biopersistence studies (toxicokinetics), (4) evaluation of reproductive effects, and (5) mechanistic studies employing genomic and proteomic techniques. Tier 2 studies will provide additional information to either characterize further effects observed in Tier 1 studies or to obtain new data using specific models of susceptibility. The ILSI screening strategy provides detailed descriptions about the types and methods of in vitro and in vivo studies that may be implemented to evaluate the toxicity of nanomaterials.

b. European Centre for Ecotoxicology and Toxicology of Chemicals

The European Centre for Ecotoxicology and Toxicology of Chemicals (ECETOC) convened a workshop with 70 scientific experts in Barcelona, Spain, in November 2005 to develop testing strategies to establish the safety of nanomaterials (Warheit et al., 2007b). It was concluded that although many physical factors can influence toxicity, including nanoparticle composition, it is dissolution, surface area and characteristics, size, size distribution, and shape, that largely determine the functional, toxicological, and environmental impacts of nanomaterials. The working definition of nanoparticles established by the participants was defined as particles <100 nm in one dimension or <1000 nm to include aggregates or agglomerates. With respect to the assessment of external exposures and metrics appropriate for nanoparticles, the consensus was that it is currently not appropriate to select one form of dose metric (such as mass, surface area, or particle number) as the most appropriate measurement. As more studies are conducted on specific nanomaterials and data show which dose metric most closely correlates with observed responses, the most appropriate dose metric will become clearer.

In conducting human health hazard evaluations of nanoparticles, the participants suggested that a first step to determine potency should include a prioritization-related in vitro screening strategy to assess the possible reactivity, biomarkers of inflammation, and cellular uptake of nanoparticles, and reported observations should be validated using in vivo techniques. The Workshop concluded that the toxicity of nanoparticles could be evaluated by using a Tiered strategy. A Tier 1 in vivo testing strategy could include a short-term inhalation or intratracheal instillation of nanoparticles as the route of exposure in the lungs of rats or mice. The endpoints that should be assessed may include indices of lung inflammation, cytotoxicity, and cell proliferation, as well as histopathology of the respiratory tract and the major extrapulmonary organs. For Tier 2 in vivo testing, a longer-term inhalation study was recommended, including more substantive toxicokinetic and mechanistic endpoints (for example, determination of particle deposition, translocation, and disposition within the body). In addition, the Workshop participants concluded that it has to be determined whether nanoparticles are harmful to living cells and whether they penetrate through the skin barrier into the living tissue under actual exposure conditions. They recommended the use of several analytical methods to evaluate dermal penetration, including tape stripping, diffusion cell chambers, and microscopic techniques. Using the method of differential stripping, the penetration kinetics of nanoparticles in the stratum corneum and the hair follicles can be evaluated in vivo. Diffusion cell chamber experiments are an efficient method for evaluating in vitro penetration and laser-scanning microscopy is useful for evaluating dermal penetration kinetics, although it may require fluorescently labeled nanoparticles. With respect to evaluating ambient exposure levels of nanoparticles, the Workshop members concluded that there is a clear and immediate need to develop instruments which are smaller, more portable, and less expensive than the currently available state-of-the-art instrumentation for measuring nanoparticles in air, particularly for the workplace.

c. Environmental Defense and DuPont Framework

In June 2007, Environmental Defense and DuPont launched a risk management framework for nanomaterials entitled, "Nano Risk

Framework" (Environmental Defense and DuPont, 2007). This Framework is the result of a joint effort by the two organizations to establish a process for ensuring the responsible development of nanoscale materials that can be widely used by companies, researchers, and other organizations. The intent of the Framework is to define a systematic and disciplined process for identifying, managing, and reducing potential environmental, health, and safety risks of engineered nanomaterials across all stages of a product's "lifecycle," from initial sourcing through manufacture, use, disposal, and ultimate fate. It is intended that the primary users of the Framework will be organizations (such as companies and public and private research institutions) that are actively working with nanomaterials and developing associated products and applications. The Framework focuses on a series of organized steps, including the following:

1. describing the material and its use(s);
2. profiling the material's life cycle (material, hazard, exposure);
3. evaluating its risks;
4. assessing the risk management;
5. deciding, documenting, and acting on the risk; and
6. reviewing and adapting the assessments.

The goal of a Framework is to implement a methodical procedure for recognizing potential EHS risks related to exposures to novel nanomaterials. The Framework was released to the public for comments, suggestions, and critiques and the final version included three case studies to evaluate the comprehensiveness, practicality, and flexibility of the Framework. The nanomaterials in the case studies included DuPont™ Light Stabilizer 210, a surface-treated high-rutile phase titanium dioxide, carbon nanotubes, and nanoparticles of zero-valent iron. The inevitable commercialization of nanomaterials for use in manufacturing and industry, physicochemical research, and medical and diagnostic applications will pose a challenge for regulatory and corporate entities. The public will want assurance of the safety of products for workers exposed to nanomaterials, consumers using the products containing the nanomaterials, and the environment. The development of effective and safe products containing nanomaterials should be a fundamental component of the product stewardship process and this is an essential part of the collaborative practice of all stakeholders on EHS issues. The contributions to the public awareness, which leads to public confidence in consumer products, will aid in the successful development of products from the nanotechnology and engineering fields.

1.6 CHALLENGES ASSOCIATED WITH EVALUATING THE SAFETY OF NANOMATERIALS

There are several challenges associated with the evaluation of the potential human and environmental health risks from the development and use of novel nanomaterials, including the selection of appropriate toxicological studies for conducting hazard evaluations, a need for instruments that can measure nanomaterials in various media (air, soil, and water), information about nanomaterial levels in products, and the need for increased funding for EHS research.

a. **Appropriate Toxicological Studies for the Hazard Evaluation of Nanomaterials**

   Currently, there are several groups suggesting screening strategies and frameworks to standardize the methods used to characterize the physicochemical properties of nanomaterials, measure toxicity in vitro and in vivo and develop techniques for ecotoxicity testing and measuring environmental exposures. In addition, some have suggested the use of standard nanoscale reference materials incorporated into any toxicity testing of nanomaterials, although it is not clear what standard materials will be most appropriate for specific nanomaterials. There is, however, still debate and uncertainties in the scientific community about the most appropriate in vitro and in vivo study designs and what endpoints to measure when evaluating nanomaterials and developing toxicological profiles for use in future risk assessments. Three aspects to evaluating nanomaterial toxicity that may be important for generating high-quality research and preventing the unnecessary use of hazardous nanomaterials include: (1) validated screening tests, (2) developing viable alternatives to in vivo tests, and (3) determining the toxicity of fiber-shaped nanoparticles (Maynard et al. 2006). Because fiber-shaped nanomaterials possibly represent a unique inhalation hazard, their pulmonary toxicity should be evaluated as a priority (Maynard et al., 2006). Although it is not clear whether fiber-shaped nanoscale particles formed from carbon and other materials will behave like asbestos or not, some materials are sufficiently similar to cause concern and any failure to pick up asbestos-like behavior as early as possible would be potentially devastating to the health of exposed individuals and to the future of the nanotechnology industry (Maynard et al., 2006). Recent studies have reported that carbon nanotubes may elicit carcinogenic and pulmonary effects similar to asbestos (Poland et al., 2008; Takagi et al., 2008; Sakamoto et al., 2009), while others have reported a lack of carcinogenic response (Muller et al., 2009). However, there are several variables to consider when evaluating the rodent studies with carbon nanotubes and developing conclusions from the reported findings.

b. Measuring Exposure Levels of Nanomaterials

Individuals working with nanomaterials urgently need inexpensive personal aerosol samplers that are capable of measuring exposure in the workplace and environment. The current thrust of research to address this issue is focusing on developing instrumentation for measuring nanomaterials, in particular, developing a portable particle monitor that can detect very small concentrations of nanomaterials in the air, soil, and in water. Currently, scientists are developing instrumentation that can measure particles by mass, size, particle number, and/or surface area. However, as previously discussed, which parameter is most relevant in the workplace and in the environment is not known for most nanomaterials, but the general consensus is that it will be important to be able to detect very small quantities of nanomaterials and measure surface area of detected particles.

c. Characteristics of Nanomaterial-Containing Products

To conduct future risk assessments for nanomaterials, it will be important to have an understanding of the potential exposure levels resulting from the use of nanomaterial-containing products. This may require more transparency in the amounts of nanomaterial present in the product(s) of interest and a thorough understanding of exposure pathways and exposure levels.

d. Increased Funding for EHS Research and Opportunities for Collaborations

The real challenge in creating a safe technology is providing scientists, engineers, risk assessors, regulators, and policy-makers with the appropriate amount of funds to conduct their research and to provide opportunities for collaboration. There is a need for an increase in the amount of funding available for toxicological studies and conducting safety evaluation of nanomaterials. It will be critical to establish toxicity profiles and conduct exposure assessments for the development of safe nanomaterials, both of which will require significant amount of funding.

1.7 CONCLUSIONS

This review provides an overview of issues regarding the emerging field of nanotoxicology, the safety and risk assessment process for nanomaterials, characterizing nanomaterials for toxicological evaluations and toxicological testing frameworks and screening strategies for nanomaterials.

At this point, it appears that the research, development, and production of nanomaterials are greatly outpacing the speed by which toxicological and exposure information is being acquired on nanomaterials. An understanding of the mammalian and ecotoxicological profiles of nanomaterials will be necessary to prioritize those nanomaterials that are safe for use and to establish appropriate safety procedures for handling those nanomaterials that may pose potential health hazards if there is sufficient exposure in the workplace, to consumers, or in the environment. For newly developed nanomaterials, it may be necessary to conduct a broad range of in vitro and in vivo studies to evaluate potential toxicological effects following oral, dermal, or inhalation exposure, and toxicological study designs should include doses that most closely reflect the anticipated exposure levels for the nanomaterial. The hazard evaluation of nanomaterials will likely require both in vitro and in vivo toxicological studies, however, when possible, the use of in vitro assays to screen nanomaterials may reduce the need for extensive in vivo studies when appropriate endpoints and cell types are evaluated.

When conducting physicochemical characterization of nanomaterial properties, each material property should be measured using the most appropriate technique, and when possible, results should be confirmed with an additional analytical technique. No single technique can accurately describe the physicochemical properties of a nanomaterial. Methodological limitations, non-trivial sample preparation, and incorporation of the appropriate controls are all issues investigators should consider when analyzing nanomaterial samples. The physicochemical parameters of the nanomaterial that are found to be affected by solvent conditions, mode of administration, and behavior in vivo should also be reported in toxicological studies. The successful development of safe nanomaterials requires a strong collaborative effort between toxicologists, physical scientists, and engineers.

The development of a risk management framework for nanoscale materials requires a base set of hazard and exposure data, which are both critical elements for evaluating human and environmental risks. The lessons we have learned from the chemical and biotechnology industries pave the way for the successful and safe incorporation of materials developed from technologies such as nanotechnology into products that can improve the quality of life. It is important that nanomaterials are developed responsibly, with optimization of benefits and minimization of risks, and with international cooperation to identify and resolve gaps in knowledge. There is much research that needs to be completed to gather sufficient information for developing toxicological profiles and exposure assessments for most nanomaterials that are currently being developed, manufactured, and incorporated into products. Once sufficient information is available, the conduct of appropriate safety or risk assessments will be possible for nanomaterials. To maintain a high level of public health, occupational health, and environmental protection it will likely be necessary to conduct nanomaterial-specific assessments to evaluate any potential human and environmental health effects and to ensure the development of safe nanomaterial-containing consumer products.

REFERENCES

Adamson, A.W., Gast, A.P., 1997. Physical Chemistry of Surfaces. Wiley, New York.

Agarwal, A., Lariya, N., Saraogi, G., et al., 2009. Nanoparticles as novel carrier for brain delivery: a review. Current Pharmaceutical Design 15 (8), 917–925.

Aschner, M., Guilarte, T.R., Schneider, J.S., Zheng, W., 2007. Manganese: recent advances in understanding its transport and neurotoxicity. Toxicology and Applied Pharmacology 221 (2), 131–147.

Bai, S., Thomas, C., Rawat, A., Ahsan, F., 2006. Recent progress in dendrimer-based nanocarriers. Critical Reviews in Therapeutic Drug Carrier Systems 23 (6), 437–495.

Baker, G.L., Gupta, A., Clark, M.L., et al., 2008. Inhalation Toxicity and Lung Toxicokinetics of C60 Fullerene Nanoparticles and Microparticles. Toxicology Science 101 (1), 122–131.

Bockmann, J., Lahl, H., Eckert, T., Unterhalt, B., 2005. Titanium blood levels of dialysis patients compared to healthy volunteers. Pharmazie 55 (6), 468.

Borm, P., Robbins, D., Haubold, S., et al., 2006. The potential risks of nanomaterials: a review carried out for ECETOC. Particle and Fibre Toxicology 3, 1–35.

Bucher, J., S. Masten, B. Moudgil, et al., 2004. Developing Experimental Approaches for the Evaluation of Toxicological Interactions of Nanoscale Materials. Final Workshop Report 3–4 November 2004, University of Florida, Gainesville, FL. Available at: www.nanotoxicology.ufl.edu/workshop/images/NanoToxWorkshop.pdf

Braydich-Stolle, L., Hussain, S., Schlager, J.J., Hofmann, M.C., 2005. In vitro cytotoxicity of nanoparticles in mammalian germline stem cells. Toxicological Sciences 88, 412–419.

Brook, R.D., 2008. Cardiovascular effects of air pollution. Clinical Science 115 (6), 175–187.

Brunauer, S., Emmett, P.H., Teller, E., 1938. Adsorption of gases in multimolecular layers. Journal of the American Chemical Society 60, 309–319.

Christenson, E.M., Anseth, K.S., van den Beucken, J.J., et al., 2007. Nanobiomaterial applications in orthopedics. Journal of Orthopedic Research 25 (1), 11–22.

des Rieux, A., Fievez, V., Garinot, M., et al., 2006. Nanoparticles as potential oral delivery systems of proteins and vaccines: a mechanistic approach. Journal of Control Release 1, 1–27.

Doull, J., Borzelleca, J.F., Becker, R., et al., 2007. Framework for use of toxicity screening tools in context-based decision-making. Food and Chemical Toxicology 45 (5), 759–796.

Environmental Defense and DuPont, 2007. Nano Risk Framework. EDF, New York.

Galindo-Rodriguez, S.A., Allemann, E., Fessi, H., Doelker, E., 2005. Polymeric nanoparticles for oral delivery of drugs and vaccines: a critical evaluation of in vivo studies. Critical Reviews in Therapeutic Drug Carrier Systems 22 (5), 419–464.

Gamer, A.O., Leibold, E., van Ravenzwaay, B., 2006. The in vitro absorption of microfine zinc oxide and titanium dioxide through porcine skin,. Toxicology in Vitro 20 (3), 301–307.

Gopee, N.V., Roberts, D.W., Webb, P., et al., 2007. Migration of intradermally injected quantum dots to sentinel organs in mice. Toxicological Sciences 98 (1), 249–257.

Guo, B., Zebda, R., Drake, S.J., Sayes, C.M., 2009. Synergistic effect of co-exposure to carbon black and Fe_2O_3 nanoparticles on oxidative stress in cultured lung epithelial cells. Particle and Fibre Toxicology 9 (6), 4.

Hadgraft, J., Lane, M.E., 2005. Skin permeation: the years of enlightenment. International Journal of Pharmaceutics 305 (1–2), 2–12.

Hagens, W.I., Oomen, A.G., de Jong, W.H., et al., 2007. What do we (need to) know about the kinetic properties of nanoparticles in the body? Regulatory Toxicology and Pharmacology 49 (3), 217–229.

Hardman, R., 2006. A toxicologic review of quantum dots: toxicity depends on physicochemical and environmental factors,. Environmental Health Perspectives 114 (2), 165–172.

Haws, L., Harris, M., Su, S., et al., 2004. Development of a refined database of relative potency estimates to facilitate better characterization of variability and uncertainty in the current mammalian TEFs for PCDDs, PDCFs, and dioxin-like PCBs. Organohalogen Compounds 66, 3426–3432.

Helland, A., Wick, P., Koehler, A., et al., 2007. Reviewing the environmental and human health knowledge base of carbon nanotubes. Environmental Health Perspectives 115 (8), 1125–1131.

Hussain, S.M., Hess, K.L., Gearhart, J.M., et al., 2005. In vitro toxicity of nanoparticles in BRL 3A rat liver cells. Toxicology in Vitro 19, 975–983.

Isakovic, A., Markovic, Z., Todorovic-Markovic, B., et al., 2006. Distinct cytotoxic mechanisms of pristine versus hydroxylated fullerene. Toxicological Sciences 91 (1), 173–183.

Ji, J.H., Jung, J.H., Kim, S.S., et al., 2007. Twenty-eight-day inhalation toxicity study of silver nanoparticles in Sprague–Dawley rats. Inhalation Toxicology 19 (10), 857–871.

Juillerat-Jeanneret, L., 2008. The targeted delivery of cancer drugs across the blood–brain barrier: chemical modifications of drugs or drug–nanoparticles? Drug Discovery Today 13 (23–24), 1099–1106.

Kanikkannan, N., Kandimalla, K., Lamba, S.S., Singh, M., 2000. Structure-activity relationship of chemical penetration enhancers in transdermal drug delivery. Current Medicinal Chemistry 7 (6), 593–608.

Kogan, A., Garti, N., 2006. Microemulsions as transdermal drug delivery vehicles. Advances in Colloid and Interface Sciences 123–126, 369–385.

Kreuter, J., 2004. Influence of the surface properties on nanoparticle-mediated transport of drugs to the brain. Journal of Nanoscience and Nanotechnology 4 (5), 484–488.

Lam, C.-W., James, J.T., McCluskey, R., Hunter, R.L., 2004. Pulmonary toxicity of single-wall carbon nanotubes in mice 7 and 90 days after intratracheal instillation. Toxicological Sciences 77, 126–134.

Levin, J., Maibach, H., 2005. The correlation between transepidermal water loss and percutaneous absorption: an overview,. Journal of Control Release 103 (2), 291–299.

Lockman, P.R., Koziara, J.M., Mumper, R.J., Allen, D.D., 2004. Nanoparticle surface charges alter blood–brain barrier integrity and permeability. Journal of Drug Targeting 12, 635–641.

Malik, D.K., Baboota, S., Ahuja, A., Hasan, S., Ali, J., 2007. Recent advances in protein and peptide drug delivery systems. Current Drug Delivery 2, 141–151.

Mavon, A., Miquel, C., Lejeune, O., Payre, P., Moretto, P., 2007. In vitro percutaneous absorption and in vivo stratum corneum distribution of an organic and a mineral sunscreen. Skin Pharmacology and Physiology 20 (1) m, 10–20.

Maynard, A.D., Aitken, R., Tilman, B., et al., 2006. Safe Handling of Nanotechnology. Nature 444 (16), 267–269.

Monteiro-Riviere, N.A., Nemanich, R.J., Inman, A.O., et al., 2005. Multi-walled carbon nanotube interactions with human epidermal keratinocytes. Toxicology Letters 155 (3), 377–384.

Monteiro-Riviere, N.A., Inman, A.O., Zhang, L.W., 2008. Limitations and relative utility of screening assays to assess engineered nanoparticle toxicity in a human cell line. Toxicology and Applied Pharmacology.

Muller, J., Delos, M., Panin, N., et al., 2009. Absence of carcinogenic response to multi-wall carbon nanotubes in a 2-year bioassay in the peritoneal cavity of the rat. Toxicological Sciences 8 May.

Murray, A.R., Kisin, E., Leonard, S.S., et al., 2009. Oxidative stress and inflammatory response in dermal toxicity of single-walled carbon nanotubes. Toxicology 257 (3), 161–171.

Nanoderm, 2007. Quality of Skin as a Barrier to ultra-fine Particles: Final Report. Nanoderm, Brussels.

National Research Council, 1983. Risk Assessment in the Federal Government: Managing the Process. National Academy Press, Washington, DC.

National Research Council, 1994. Science and judgment in risk assessment. Committee on Risk Assessment of Hazardous Air Pollutants. National Academy Press, Washington, DC.

Nel, A., Xia, T., Madler, L., Li, N., 2006. Toxic potential of materials at the nanolevel. Science 311, 622–627.

Nohynek, G.J., Lademann, J., Ribaud, C., Roberts, M.S., 2007. Grey Goo on the Skin? Nanotechnology, Cosmetic and Sunscreen Safety. Critical Reviews in Toxicology 37 (3), 251–277.

Nohynek, G.J., Dufour, E.K., Roberts, M.S., 2008. Nanotechnology, cosmetics and the skin: is there a health risk? Skin Pharmacology and Physiology 21 (3), 136–149.

Nygaard, U.C., Hansen, J.S., Samuelsen, M., et al., 2009. Single-walled and multi-walled carbon nanotubes promote allergic immune responses in mice. Toxicological Sciences 109 (1), 113–123.

Oberdörster, E., 2004. Manufactured nanomaterials (fullerenes, C60) induce oxidative stress in the brain of juvenile largemouth bass. Environmental Health Perspective 112 (10), 1058–1062.

Oberdörster, G., Oberdörster, E., and Oberdörster, J., 2005a. Nanotoxicology: An emerging discipline evolving from studies of ultrafine particles, Environmental Health Perspective 113, 823–839.

Oberdörster, G., Maynard, A.D., Donaldson, K., et al. 2005b. Principles for characterizing the potential human health effects from exposure to nanomaterials: elements of a screening strategy, Particle and Fibre Toxicology 2(8).

Park, B., Donaldson, K., Duffin, R., et al., 2008. Hazard and risk assessment of a nanoparticulate cerium oxide-based diesel fuel additive – a case study. Inhalation Toxicology 20 (6), 547–566.

Park, S., Lee, Y.K., Jung, M., et al., 2007. Cellular toxicity of various inhalable metal nanoparticles on human alveolar epithelial cells. Inhalation Toxicology 19 (1), 59–65.

Petry, T., Schmid, P., Schlatter, C., 1996. The use of toxic equivalency factors in assessing occupational and environmental health risk associated with exposure to airborne mixtures of polycyclic aromatic hydrocarbons (PAHs). Chemosphere 32 (4), 639–648.

Poland, C.A., Duffin, R., Kinloch, I., et al., 2008. Carbon nanotubes introduced into the abdominal cavity of mice show asbestos-like pathogenicity in a pilot study. Nature Nanotechnology 3 (7), 423–428.

Powers, K.W., Brown, S.C., Krishna, V.B., et al., 2006. Research strategies for safety evaluation of nanomaterials. Part VI. Characterization of nanoscale particles for toxicological evaluation. Toxicological Sciences 90, 296–303.

Powers, K.W., Palazuelos, M., Moudgil, B.M., Roberts, S.M., 2007. Characterization of the size, shape, and state of dispersion of nanoparticles for toxicological studies. Nanotoxicology 1 (1), 42–51.

Purchase, I.F.H., 2000. Risk assessment. Principles and consequences. Pure and Applied Chemistry 72 (6), 1051–1056.

Ratner, B.D., 1996. Biomaterials Science: An Introduction to Materials in Medicine. Academic Press, San Diego.

Rouse, J.G., Yang, J., Ryman-Rasmussen, J.P., et al., 2007. Effects of mechanical flexion on the penetration of fullerene amino acid-derivatized peptide nanoparticles through skin. Nano Letters 7 (1), 155–160.

Ryman-Rasmussen, J.P., Riviere, J.E., Monteiro-Riviere, N.A., 2006. Penetration of intact skin by quantum dots with diverse physicochemical properties. Toxicological Sciences 91 (1), 159–165.

Sakamoto, Y., Nakae, D., Fukumori, N., et al., 2009. Induction of mesothelioma by a single intrascrotal administration of multi-wall carbon nanotube in intact male Fischer 344 rats. Journal of Toxicological Sciences 34 (1), 65–76.

Sayes, C.M., Fortner, J., Wehn, G., et al., 2004. The differential cytotoxicity of water soluble fullerenes. Nano Letters 4 (10), 1881–1887.

Sayes, C.M., Liang, F., Hudson, J.L., et al., 2006. Functionalization density dependence of single-walled carbon nanotubes cytotoxicity in vitro. Toxicological Letters 161 (2), 135–142.

Sayes, C.M., Reed, K.L., Warheit, D.B., 2007. Assessing toxicity of fine and nanoparticles: Comparing in vitro measurements to in vivo pulmonary toxicity profiles. Toxicological Sciences 97 (1), 163–180.

Scientific Committee on Emerging and Newly Identified Health Risks, 2006. Modified Opinion (after public consultation) on the appropriateness of existing methodologies to assess the potential risks associated with engineered and adventitious products of nanotechnologies. Health and Consumer Protection Directorate-General. European Commission, Brussels.

Scientific Committee on Emerging and Newly Identified Health Risks, 2007. Opinion on the appropriateness of the risk assessment methodology in accordance with the technical guidance documents for new and existing substances for assessing the risks of nanomaterials. Health and Consumer Protection Directorate-General. European Commission, Brussels.

Shvedova, A.A., Castranova, V., Kisin, E.R., et al., 2003. Exposure to carbon nanotube material: Assessment of nanotube cytotoxicity using human keratinocyte cells. Journal of Toxicology and Environmental Health A66, 1909–1926.

Shvedova, A.A., Kisin, E., Murray, A.R., et al., 2008. Inhalation vs. aspiration of single-walled carbon nanotubes in C57BL/6 mice: inflammation, fibrosis, oxidative stress, and mutagenesis. American Journal of Physiology – Lung Cellular and Molecular Physiology 295 (4), L552–L565.

Shvedova, A.A., Kisin, E.R., D Porter, et al., 2009. Mechanisms of pulmonary toxicity and medical applications of carbon nanotubes: Two faces of Janus? Pharmacology and Therapeutics 121 (2), 192–204.

Silva, G.A., 2007. Nanotechnology approaches for drug and small molecule delivery across the blood brain barrier. Surgical Neurology 2, 113–116.

Sint, T., Donohue, J.F., Ghio, A.J., 2008. Ambient air pollution particles and the acute exacerbation of chronic obstructive pulmonary disease. Inhalation Toxicology 20 (1), 25–29.

Stern, S.T., McNeil, S.E., 2008. Nanotechnology Safety Concerns Revisited. Toxicology Science 101 (1), 4–21.

Stone, V., Johnston, H., Clift, M.J., 2007. Air pollution, ultrafine and nanoparticle toxicology: cellular and molecular interactions. IEEE Trans Nanobioscience 6 (4), 331–340.

Takagi, A., Hirose, A., Nishimura, T., et al., 2008. Induction of mesothelioma in p53+/− mouse by intraperitoneal application of multi-wall carbon nanotubes. Journal of Toxicological Science 33 (1), 105–116.

Teeguarden, J.G., Hinderliter, P.M., Orr, G., et al., 2007. Particokinetics in vitro: Dosimetry Considerations for in vitro Nanoparticle Toxicity Assessments. Toxicological Sciences 95 (2), 300–312.

Tsuji, J.S., Maynard, A.D., Howard, P.C., et al., 2006. Research Strategies for Safety Evaluation of Nanomaterials, Part IV: Risk Assessment of Nanoparticles. Toxicology Sciences 89 (1), 42–50.

Tran, C.L., Buchanan, D., Cullen, R.T., et al., 2000. Inhalation of poorly soluble particles. II. Influence of particle surface area on inflammation and clearance. Inhalation Toxicology 12, 1113–1126.

Tran, C.L., Donaldson, K., Stone, V., et al., 2005. A scoping study to identify hazard data needs for addressing the risks presented by nanoparticles and nanotubes. Institute of Occupational Medicine, Edinburgh.

Van den Berg, M., Birnbaum, L.S., Denison, M., et al., 2006. The 2005 World Health Organization reevaluation of human and mammalian toxic equivalency factors for dioxins and dioxin-like compounds. Toxicology Sciences 93 (2), 223–241.

Wang, J., Chen, C., Liu, Y., et al. 2008a. Potential neurological lesion after nasal instillation of TiO2 nanoparticles in the anatase and rutile crystal phases, Toxicology Letters 183(1–3), 72–80.

Wang, J., Liu, Y., Jiao, F., et al., 2008b. Time-dependent translocation and potential impairment on central nervous system by intranasally instilled TiO(2) nanoparticles, Toxicology 254(1–2), 82–90.

Wang, M.D., Shin, D.M., Simons, J.W., Nie, S., 2007. Nanotechnology for targeted cancer therapy. Expert Review of Anticancer Therapy 7 (6), 833–837.

Warheit, D.B, Hoke, R.A., Finlay, C., et al., 2007a. Development of a base set of toxicity tests using ultrafine TiO_2 particles as a component of nanoparticle risk management, Toxicology Letters 171, 99–110.

Warheit, D.B., Borm, P.J., Hennes, C., and Lademann, J., 2007b. Testing strategies to establish the safety of nanomaterials: conclusions of an ECETOC workshop, Inhalation Toxicology 19(8), 631–643.

Warheit, D.B, Webb, T.R., Reed, K.L., et al., 2007c. Pulmonary toxicity study in rats with three forms of ultrafine-TiO_2 particles: differential responses related to surface properties, Toxicology 230(1), 90–104.

Warheit, D.B., Laurence, B.R., Reed, K.L., et al., 2004. Comparative pulmonary toxicity assessment of single-wall carbon nanotubes in rats. Toxicology Science 77 (1), 117–125.

Williams, D., 2007. Carbon nanotubes in medical technology. Medical Device Technology 8 (2), 8–10.

Yang, X., 2007. Nano- and microparticle-based imaging of cardiovascular interventions: overview. Radiology 243 (2), 340–347.

Zhang, L.W., Monteiro-Riviere, N.A., 2008. Assessment of quantum dot penetration into intact, tape-stripped, abraded and flexed rat skin. Skin Pharmacology and Physiology 21 (3), 166–180.

CHAPTER 2

Are We Willing to Heed the Lessons of the Past? Nanomaterials and Australia's Asbestos Legacy

Steve Mullins

CONTENTS

2.1 INTRODUCTION

Australian trade unions have been campaigning since the 1960s (Wragg, 1995, p. 32–33) against the use of asbestos and for the rights of workers who have been affected by asbestos to just compensation, with the most high profile case being the James Hardie Industries asbestos tragedy (Australian Council of Trade Unions (ACTU), 2008, p. 383–390). We have witnessed the devastating fallout of an approach to safety and technology that put profits and technological gains ahead of worker safety. Have we learnt from the reckless approach to safety exhibited in the past? Has the approach of governments and business to worker safety and new technology changed? Could nanomaterials prove to be as devastating to workers in years to come as asbestos has been?

This chapter draws from the asbestos legacy and in it I argue that it is imperative that a rigorous health and safety framework be applied to the use of nanomaterials. Without specific regulation and in the absence of conclusive research we will be exposing thousands of workers to an uncertain future.

While the trade union movement has a long history of campaigning to eliminate workplace exposure to toxic dust, the potential health and safety impacts of nanotechnology are a relatively recent cause for concern.

I first turned my mind to the issue of nanotechnology midway through 2005 when preparing the ACTU's submission to the *Senate Community Affairs Committee: Inquiry into Workplace Exposure to Toxic Dust*. It came as a bit of a surprise that the last in a long list of issues to be dealt with under the Inquiry's terms of reference was to address the potential for emerging technologies, including nanoparticles, to result in workplace-related harm (Senate Community Affairs Committee, 2005).

Working through the available evidence, it became clear to me that there were a number of health, safety, and regulatory concerns and challenges that were not being addressed within Australia's existing federal regulatory framework. In light of growing concerns about the potential health effects of nanomaterials, and the increasing number of workers potentially exposed, the ACTU recommended, as a matter of urgency, the introduction of laws to regulate importers and manufacturers who were utilizing the unique properties of nanomaterials in their products. The ACTU also recommended the development of appropriate nanoparticle exposure levels (ACTU, 2005).

Almost 4 years have passed since that submission and not one piece of nano-specific regulation addressing health and safety concerns has passed through any Australian parliament.

2.2 LESSONS OF THE PAST

While writing this chapter, I attended a Workers' Memorial Day service in Melbourne. Workers' Memorial Day is a trade union event held annually on 28 April to commemorate the lives lost to industrial injury and illness. It is an occasion for family members who have lost loved ones to workplace incidents to remember and mourn. Not surprisingly, the tragedy caused by asbestos continues to be a theme each year. One speaker movingly recounted the pain of losing her husband to an asbestos-related disease and the bitterness she feels toward those who caused her husband's death. Trade unions have become custodians of many similar tragic stories. We continue to campaign for not only just compensation but we are also obliged to ensure that these lost lives are not forgotten, and that their pain is not repeated.

Australia is recognized as having the worst record for asbestos-related diseases in the world. Since records of asbestos-related deaths began in the early 1980s, lives lost to mesothelioma have already reached around 10,000 and is predicted to reach 25,000 in Australia over the next 40 years (Peto, 2008).

Notwithstanding these disturbing statistics, almost everyone in our society has been exposed to asbestos fibers (National Institute of Health, 2009). For workers in occupations where there is the potential for daily exposure, such as plumbers and electricians, there are acute risks. The peak use of asbestos in Australia was in 1983, when 700,000 tons was used—much of it in houses. Any house built before 1987 is likely to contain some asbestos. In Australia 40,000 tons of asbestos waste continues to be generated each year (Asbestos Diseases Society of Victoria, 2008).

When asbestos is disturbed it forms a dust of tiny fibers which can be inhaled. Some asbestos fibers can split into smaller needle-like pieces and travel deep into the body's respiratory system, where they pierce the lining of the lungs and become permanently lodged. Asbestos-related diseases are caused by the inhalation or ingestion of these particles of asbestos. The diseases caused by exposure include asbestosis, pleural plaques, lung cancer, mesothelioma, and cancer of the intestinal tract (Asbestos Diseases Society of Victoria, 2008). Despite decades of knowledge about the toxicity of asbestos, chrysotile asbestos was not prohibited until 31 December 2003 and adopted simultaneously under regulations in each Australian Occupational Health and Safety (OHS) jurisdiction, as well as in Australian Customs. Unions had been fighting and lobbying the Australian government to prohibit this deadly fiber for over a generation.

So in a few short paragraphs I have detailed the devastating fallout, the illnesses caused, the lives lost, and the ongoing blight of this thing called asbestos. However, in times past we were told that asbestos was a cutting-edge technology with thousands of uses and business was quick to commercialize its properties, sometimes in unusual ways.

While we generally associate asbestos with mining and building materials, it was commercialized in other ways too. You do not generally think of asbestos when considering the latest fashions coming off the catwalks of Paris or London. In 1936, however, asbestos clothing was très chic when (Chillicothe Constitution-Tribune, 1936, p. 9):

> *[p]ink asbestos aprons for careless ladies who lean on stoves sizzled into the International Fashion Market today from Great Britain.*

Further, for those who were a little lazy or simply careless with fire, there were

> *...striped asbestos table cloths for folks who don't like ash trays, and lavender asbestos mittens for pickers of hot potatoes. London manufacturers also produce red asbestos rugs, on which bonfires may be built, and lacy asbestos window curtains guaranteed to defy a blow torch.*

And it was also used in children's clothing:

For little girls anything is good that even has a suggestion of the Shirley Temple styles. Fine broadcloths and silk prints are the most popular materials. For little boys there are [two]-piece knits and for boys just a little older there are worsteds in a tailored coat and short trousers. (Chillicothe Constitution-Tribune, 1936, p. 9)

We might assume that if they had the benefit of hindsight they might have acted differently. In fact by 1936, when this article was published there was, as illustrated by Figure 2.1, a substantial accumulation of scientific knowledge concerning asbestos-related disease (Asbestos Diseases Foundation of Australia, 2009; Wragg, 1995). Business and governments chose to ignore the warnings as it jeopardized a thriving industry. Are we willing to heed the lessons of the past when it comes to nanomaterials?

In the field of nanotechnology, there is growing evidence about the potential toxicity, health effects, and invasive nature of nanomaterials and although there are still many uncertainties, all the research to date has simply increased the need for caution (Lam et al., 2004, 2006; Shvedova et al., 2005, 2008; Takagi et al., 2008; Poland et al., 2008; Radomski et al., 2005; Donaldson et al., 2006; Li et al., 2007; Oberdörster et al., 2002, 2005; Elder et al., 2006). In a recently released report by the European Agency for Health and Safety at Work (2009), nanoparticles were put at the top of the list of risks to workers; and research by Flinders Consulting commissioned by the Australian Safety and Compensation Council (ASCC, 2006, p. 11) stated that:

The occupational health and safety effects of engineered nanoscale particles are mostly unknown. This can be attributed to the relatively recent development of the nanotechnology sector and, as a result, the lack of available information on human exposures and working conditions. As a consequence our abilities to accurately predict the impact of nanoparticle exposures on worker health are limited at this time. In particular our abilities to measure nanoparticles in the workplace (or more generally) are limited by current technologies. Nanotechnology presents us with new challenges as the properties of nanoparticles now depend on size and shape as much as the more conventional factors of chemical structure and composition. The measurement of these additional attributes will be necessary to accurately assess nanoparticle concentrations in the workplace. In addition, the capability of the human body to recognise and appropriately respond to these tiny entities is essentially unknown at the moment.

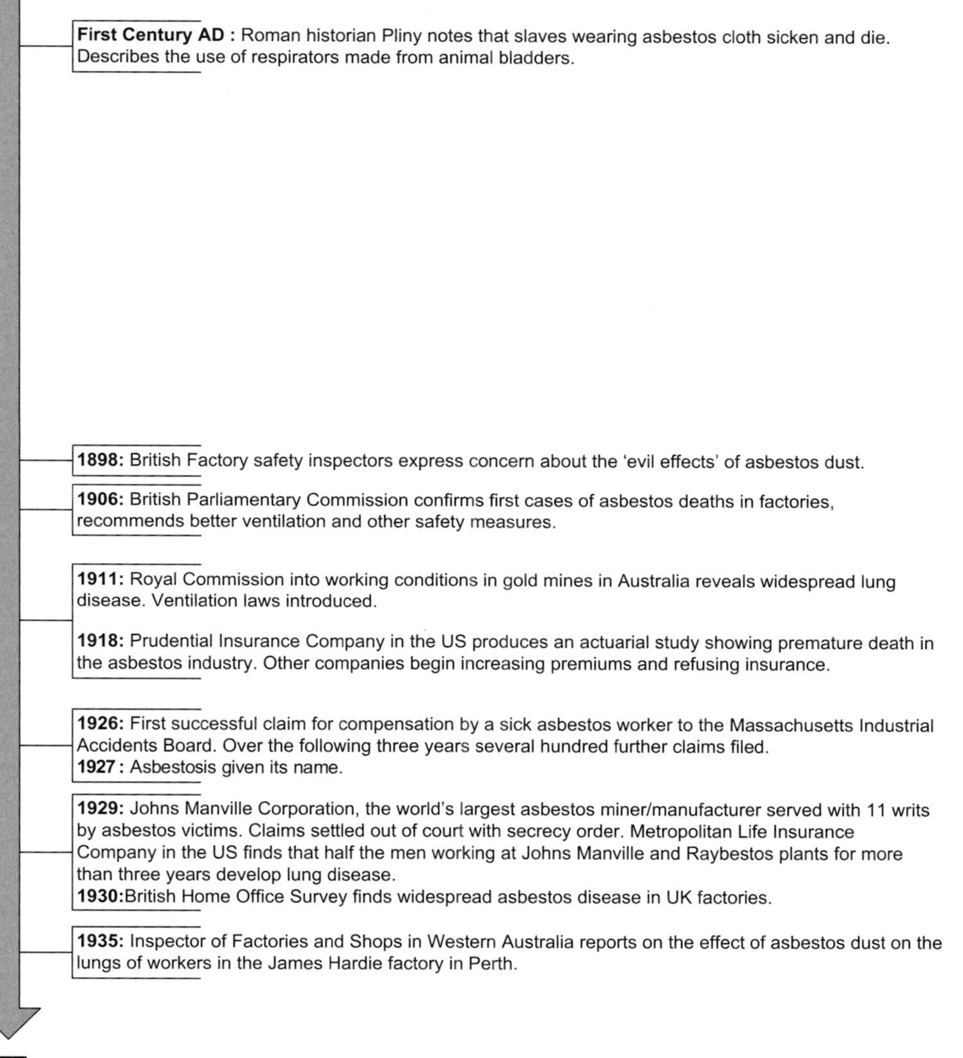

First Century AD : Roman historian Pliny notes that slaves wearing asbestos cloth sicken and die. Describes the use of respirators made from animal bladders.
1898: British Factory safety inspectors express concern about the 'evil effects' of asbestos dust.
1906: British Parliamentary Commission confirms first cases of asbestos deaths in factories, recommends better ventilation and other safety measures.
1911: Royal Commission into working conditions in gold mines in Australia reveals widespread lung disease. Ventilation laws introduced.
1918: Prudential Insurance Company in the US produces an actuarial study showing premature death in the asbestos industry. Other companies begin increasing premiums and refusing insurance.
1926: First successful claim for compensation by a sick asbestos worker to the Massachusetts Industrial Accidents Board. Over the following three years several hundred further claims filed.
1927 : Asbestosis given its name.
1929: Johns Manville Corporation, the world's largest asbestos miner/manufacturer served with 11 writs by asbestos victims. Claims settled out of court with secrecy order. Metropolitan Life Insurance Company in the US finds that half the men working at Johns Manville and Raybestos plants for more than three years develop lung disease.
1930: British Home Office Survey finds widespread asbestos disease in UK factories.
1935: Inspector of Factories and Shops in Western Australia reports on the effect of asbestos dust on the lungs of workers in the James Hardie factory in Perth.

FIGURE 2.1 *A Brief History of Asbestos.*
Adapted from Asbestos Diseases Foundation of Australia (2009)

These uncertainties raise a number of questions about how regulators should respond. Is it acceptable to say we do not know enough so we should wait until more evidence emerges? Where is the tipping point, the imperative to act, when weighing up the evidence? If history has taught us anything, it is that we can ill afford to be complacent.

Acting strongly to protect workers' health only to find out later that there was little cause for concern is a morally acceptable position to take, but acting slowly or responding ineffectively only to find out later that our worst fears were confirmed is morally bankrupt.

In 2008, the ACTU joined a broad coalition of civil society, public interest, environmental and labor organizations concerned about various aspects of nanotechnology's human health, environmental, social, ethical, and other impacts by signing an international declaration called the *Principles for the Oversight of Nanotechnologies and Nanomaterials* (NanoAction, 2007). By signing the declaration the ACTU committed to eight principles.

I. A Precautionary Foundation

Simply put, the precautionary principle means "no health and safety data, no market." Such an approach requires preventative action in the face of uncertainty, assigns the burden of protection to those responsible for the potentially harmful activities, considers all alternatives to new activities and processes, and insists on public participation in decision-making. This would include prohibiting the marketing of untested or unsafe uses of nanomaterials and requiring product manufacturers and distributors to bear the burden of proof.

II. Mandatory Nano-specific Regulations

A nano-specific regulatory regime must be an integral aspect of the development of nanotechnologies. Voluntary initiatives are wholly inadequate to oversee nanotechnology.

III. Health and Safety of the Public and Workers

Any regulatory regime designed to protect workers from the health effects of nanomaterials requires written, comprehensive safety and health programs addressing workplace nanotechnology issues. Employers should use the precautionary principle as the basis for implementing protective measures for assuring the health and safety of workers. The hierarchy of exposure controls—elimination, substitution, engineering controls, work practice/administrative approaches, and personal protective equipment—should be employed. Exposure monitoring, medical surveillance, and worker training are necessary to ensure that workers receive the most up-to-date information on nanomaterials. Workers and their representatives should be involved in all aspects of workplace nanotechnology safety and health issues without fear of retaliation or discrimination. Finally, existing occupational, safety and health standards must be scrutinized for their applicability to nanomaterials.

IV. Environmental Protection

Full lifecycle environmental, health and safety effects must be assessed prior to commercialization.

V. Transparency

"A Right to Know"—assessment and oversight of nanomaterials require mechanisms ensuring transparency, including labeling of consumer products that contain nanomaterials, installing workplace right to know laws and protective measures, and developing a publicly accessible inventory of health and safety information.

VI. Public Participation

The public must be enabled to fully participate in the deliberative and decision-making processes.

VII. Inclusion of Broader Impacts

Consideration of nanotechnology's wide-ranging effects, including ethical and social impacts or the disruption of markets for existing commodities.

VIII. Manufacturer Liability

All who market nanoproducts, including nanomaterial developers, handlers, and commercial users, the makers of products containing nanomaterials, and retailers who sell nano-containing products to the public, must be held accountable for liabilities incurred from their products.

These principles now underpin the ACTU's approach to nanotechnology and I contend that the full implementation of this approach would eliminate the risk of a human health disaster potentially greater than that of asbestos.

The link to the asbestos tragedy is pertinent not only as a precautionary tale. There is disturbing evidence emerging of the potential for asbestos-like diseases to be caused by carbon nanotubes. A recent laboratory study has shed new light on the possibility of a nexus between carbon nanotube exposure and asbestos-like health effects (Poland et al., 2008). The study, which involved laboratory mice, indicated that upon introduction into the lower abdomen, multi-walled carbon nanotubes had virtually identical effects as asbestos fibers. While more research is required to state definitively that carbon nanotubes cause mesothelioma or other asbestos-like diseases in humans, this research is a clear trigger for governments and regulators to enact the precautionary foundation. As yet, this has not occurred and to be blunt, not only will history condemn those who ignored the opportunity to prevent a health disaster, but I can also guarantee that trade unions will hold them accountable.

2.3 BIG PROBLEMS WITH SMALL MATERIALS

While there is growing evidence of potential health effects and invasive nature of nanoparticles, the nanotechnology industry is booming with the support and encouragement of many governments around the world, our own included. The global value of revenues related to nanotechnology is expected to increase from US$ 32 billion to US$ 3.1 trillion over the next decade (Lux Research, 2008) and it is predicted to potentially extend into almost every industry sector (Victorian Nanotechnology Statement, 2008).

It is difficult to know what commercially available products contain nanomaterials, because there is no mandatory registry of companies using engineered nanomaterials. However, the Woodrow Wilson Project on Emerging Nanotechnologies (PEN) (2008) has published a limited inventory listing over 800 nanoproducts currently on the market worldwide.

The Australian Nanotechnology Business Forum (ANBF), the peak industry body in Australia, is not shy in promoting the "bright future" in store for Australia's nanotechnology industry (Keenihan and Bolton, 2009, p. 28) and has provided a "snapshot" of Australian companies currently utilizing nanotechnology (Keenihan and Bolton, 2009, p. 27). A number of these companies are highlighted in Figure 2.2.

At the same time as industry is ploughing ahead, regulators are paralyzed by indecision and apathy, using lack of knowledge about the health impacts and the need for more research as reasons why they cannot or will not create new nano-specific regulation or even amend our current regulation to capture chemicals in their nanoform. Interestingly, the peak business lobbyists agree that regulations should be introduced (Power, 2009) and support the ACTU's approach (ANBF, 2009). Instead, it is the governments who are blocking the way for the introduction of new regulations. Governments nervously turn their minds to the implications of regulating in this area on free trade agreements and industry development. These issues are manageable and certainly should not be prioritized over workers' health.

Government safety regulators have failed to act to protect workers and instead endorse applying existing, but unproven, measures and continue to monitor health and safety implications (WorkSafe Victoria, undated). It is particularly troubling that there is neither the will, nor a sense of urgency that this is an issue needing to be addressed.

Gaps in existing regulations were identified back in 2004 in a report from the UK Royal Society and Royal Academy of Engineering (RS-RAE, 2004). Professor Ann Dowling from the Academy pointed out that nanoparticles have different properties from the same chemical in larger form, but that at

INDUSTRY SECTOR	COMPANY	COMMERCIAL PRODUCT/PROCESS
Materials science	Antaria	Nanopowder manufacturing technology
	Tenasi Tech	Nanocoatings for sporting goods
	PolyNovo	Biomaterials for medical use
	Micronisers	Advanced milling and chemical processes
Biotechnology & life sciences	pSivida	Biosilicates for drug delivery and diagnosis
	Starpharma	Dendrimers for drug delivery
	Universal BioSensors	Blood sensor
	Nanosonics	Biocide 'Nanonebulant' for sterilisation
	Sirtex Medical	Biocompatible radioactive microspheres to target liver cancer
	miniFAB	Polymer micro- and nano-engineered systems
Energy	Dyesol	Dye-sensitised solar cells
	CAP-XX	Production of supercapacitators using nanostructured carbon
	BluGlass	Production of low-cost, high brightness LEDs
	Very Small Particle Company	Production of cost-effective catalytic converters for cars and compact, long-life mobile batteries
	Ceramic Fuel Cells	Solid oxide fuel cells
Building & construction	G James Glass	Nanocoated, insulating self-cleaning glass
	Viridian	
	Ceram Polymerik	Polymer composites for passive fire protection
	iGlass	Film technology
Corporate	Orica	Nanotechnology-based polymers and additives
	Rio Tinto	Nanotechnology research activities
	BHP Billiton	Nanotechnology research activities
	Cadbury-Schweppes	Nanostructured dental product 'Recaldent'
	Ansell	Nanostructured scaffolds in industrial gloves
	Cochlear	Nanoscale biomaterial interface in bionic ear implant technology

FIGURE 2.2 *Selection of Australian Companies Currently Utilizing Nanotechnology (2009).*

that time there was no trigger to exercise additional testing. Dowling (2004) concluded that regulations had to be tightened up so that nanoparticles would be assessed, and labeled, as new chemicals.

It has been suggested by the Australian Department of Innovation, Industry, Science and Research (DIISR) that existing federal regulatory regimes are capable of being adapted to meet the specific challenges of nanomaterials (DIISR, 2008). Even if this were true, none of the regimes have actually been adapted. Governments and regulators reacting slowly to the development and implementation of new technologies is not a problem unique to Australia (Davies, 2009). However in the case of Australia, recent research commissioned by the Commonwealth government into the regulatory impacts of nanotechnology had identified six areas of concern with existing regulatory frameworks that can and ought to be fixed as a matter of urgency (Ludlow et al., 2007).

First, the most significant potential concern is whether new nanoforms of conventional products will be considered as "different" to traditional products. Under our current system, they are not, in the vast majority of cases, considered "different."

Second, many regulatory triggers currently exist on the basis of a threshold weight or volume. These measures may not be meaningful when applied to nanoparticles and need to be reviewed.

Third, appropriate regulation requires particular knowledge of the presence of and the risks posed by the presence of nanomaterials for regulatory triggers to take effect. Current public awareness and scientific knowledge are such that these triggers are unlikely to be met. It is particularly the case that awareness of employers and workers in workplaces is unlikely, and so again nothing will be triggered.

Fourth, it is uncertain whether current risk assessment methodologies, on which Australia's current regulatory regimes rely, are suitable for products that contain nanomaterials.

Fifth, exemptions for research and development, while commonplace for conventional materials, take on a greater significance for potentially hazardous nanomaterials and their products. Safety guidelines for research using nanomaterials are required.

Sixth, further potential regulatory gaps may be exposed if international documents or other non-regulatory advice referred to in our regulatory framework do not adequately address health, safety, and environmental concerns raised by nanomaterials.

Is it not then hypocritical that, on the one hand, industry and governments are lauding nanoparticles for their unique properties set to revolutionize all industries (Victorian Nanotechnology Statement, 2008; Keenihan and Bolton, 2009) and are actively encouraging and investing in the development of industry in Australia (Victorian Nanotechnology Statement, 2008; Australian Government Budget, 2009/2010). Yet they are reluctant to accept that it is that very uniqueness that opens gaps in the current regulatory standards and exposes workers to potential hazards?[1]

2.4 CONTROLS AND RISK ASSESSMENT

Not long ago, I was invited to tour the department of a leading Australian university researching nanotechnology. We were proudly given the tour of the facility by the Professor of the department.

[1] The Australian Office of Nanotechnology (2008, p. 1) released a report on Australian Government Approach to the Responsible Management of Nanotechnology stating "There are established and robust regulatory arrangements already in place to address human health and environmental safety issues associated with these materials and products, as well as manufacturers' and suppliers' liability obligations."

The department is performing groundbreaking research into the development and application of nanomaterials and also uses its research and million dollar technology for commercial applications. They grow high-quality carbon nanotubes and sell them to business and research centers around the world.

The facility and work undertaken are impressive but, at the same time, I was deeply disturbed by what I saw. The Professor raised concerns about possible exposure to nanoparticles and knew of the potential health risks. He said he always used personal protective equipment (PPE) such as gloves when handling nanomaterials, unlike some of his colleagues from other research centers who have been known to dip their exposed fingers into a Petri dish full of nanoparticles.

When pushed a little further on the topic, it soon became apparent that he was relying on protective equipment not specifically designed for handling nanomaterials (because it does not exist) and a lot of "make do with what you've got" risk management.

There were two vacuum boxes with in-built gloves used to handle the nanotubes. When asked if and how the Professor monitors whether nanoparticles penetrate the gloves and then potentially his skin, he simply pointed out that he has been working with nanotechnology for 10 years and was still standing. One of the clear lessons learnt from worker exposure to asbestos is the long latency period before the health impacts emerge leading to death.

The Professor then went on to say that it is possible for the nanomaterials to penetrate the gloves but there was, in fact, no way to monitor this exposure. In other words, he was operating on a wing and a prayer.

And that this is where we are at this particular moment in time. The top nanotechnology research lab in Australia, arguably the world, at the cutting edge of the technology and working with nanomaterials everyday has no way of knowing whether their staff are being exposed. Spare a thought for the maintenance and cleaning staff who, in the execution of their daily duties, may also be exposed. What, if any, risk management systems are in place for them? What PPE will they be using?

Workers around the world, including those within Australia, are handling products containing nanoparticles.

The United States National Institute for Occupational Safety and Health (NIOSH) has reported that workers performing any of the following activities may be at risk (NIOHS, 2006, p. vii):

- Working with nanomaterials in liquid media without adequate protection (e.g., gloves) will increase the risk of skin exposure.

- Working with nanomaterials in liquid during pouring or mixing operations or where a high degree of agitation is involved will lead to an increased likelihood of inhalable and respirable droplets being formed.
- Generating nanoparticles in the gas phase in non-enclosed systems will increase the chances of aerosol release to the workplace.
- Handling nanostructured powders will lead to the possibility of aerosolization.
- Maintenance of equipment and processes used to produce or fabricate nanomaterials or the clean-up of spills or waste material will pose a potential for exposure to workers performing these tasks.
- Cleaning of dust collection systems used to capture nanoparticles can pose a potential for both skin and inhalation exposure.
- Machining, sanding, drilling, or other mechanical disruptions of materials containing nanoparticles can potentially lead to aerosolization of nanomaterials.
- Depending on their composition and structure, some nanomaterials may initiate catalytic reactions and increase their fire and explosion potential that would not otherwise be anticipated from their chemical composition alone.

A significant proportion of these workers will have no idea that they are handling nanoparticles, let alone what nanoparticles are or what potential harm they could cause. Furthermore, a significant proportion of employers, importers, manufactures, and suppliers will not know either.

How are then businesses advised to respond to the issue of worker exposure to nanomaterials? A final draft of a report by RMIT commissioned by Safe Work Australia (SWA) noted the plethora of potential disease outcomes identified in research and stated (SWA, 2009a, p. 9):

> *It is important therefore that there are effective risk management systems and exposure control systems in place in order to negate or reduce worker exposure to engineered nanomaterials.*

But concluded (SWA, 2009a, p. 1)

> *The review has determined that there is evidence to suggest that* control *and* risk management *methodologies which are already known* can *protect workers from exposure to engineered nanomaterials in the occupational environment.*

It is important to cite this report because it represents the latest in thinking and examples of the effectiveness of existing controls to protect workers potentially exposed to nanomaterials.

The report acknowledged that there is a lack of data to adequately inform a rigorous risk management process to deal with nanomaterials and as a result risk management processes are based on "considerable professional judgement" (SWA, 2009a, p. 18).

A 2008 International Standards Organization (ISO) report is of the same mind (ISO, 2008, Chapter 6):

> *Presently, quantitative health hazard and exposure data are not available for most nanomaterials. Therefore, health risk evaluation for the workplace currently relies to a great degree on professional judgments for hazard identification, potential exposures and the application of appropriate safety measures.*

But to whose judgement does it refer? What is the measure of "considerable"? With all due respect to those in the field trying to establish risk management procedures to deal with nanomaterials in their workplaces, this is simply not evidence of an effective approach—it is in fact the very opposite. It is evidence of an ad hoc, uncoordinated and unregulated approach.

The ACTU accepts that the risk management methodology, that is, identifying, assessing, controlling and monitoring, and using the hierarchy of controls is, broadly speaking, an accepted approach to managing health and safety risks in the workplace. It is then logical that such an approach is applied to the issue of nanomaterials in the workplace. However, it is a dangerous leap of faith to suggest that there is evidence that existing controls can protect workers, when in fact there is significant evidence to suggest the opposite.

The hierarchy of controls is, as its name states, a hierarchy. Employers are directed to work their way down the hierarchy via the following steps:

1. Eliminate;
2. Substitute;
3. Engineering controls;
4. Administrative controls; and
5. Personal protective equipment.

Due to the fact that nanomaterials are being intentionally manufactured specifically due to their unique properties, the first two controls normally applied to hazardous materials are not relevant—they cannot be eliminated or substituted with other materials. So how can it be claimed that existing controls are effective when the two controls at the top of the hierarchy are not even considered?

The risk management measure promoted by regulators and governments of nanomaterials is the "As Low As Reasonably Practical" (ALARP) approach (Workcover NSW, 2008; SWA, 2009a). There is a fundamental problem with this approach. ALARP is based on balancing the risk of exposure against the cost to lower the risk further to, what is commonly referred to as, a "tolerable risk." Effectively, ALARP defines risk as an economic decision—do I spend the money or not? Regrettably, experience shows us, too often, that the answer is not.

Unfortunately, the one group of people who have been forgotten in the "risk" equation are the workers. Is it a "tolerable risk" for them to suffer poor health due to exposure to a toxic substance? Is the "sacrifice required" (SWA, 2009a, p. 22), ultimately, their health or life?

Add to this the suggestion that (SWA, 2009a, p. 1):

> *...consideration should be given with respect to whether the increased risk of exposure to a particular nanomaterial is justified by the level of improved properties that are achieved in the product.*

As a note of caution about promoting "improved properties" as a counterpoint to risks to health and safety—asbestos was once considered a wonder substance because it was hardy, flexible, wearable and fire resistant with any number of commercial uses, it just turned out to be a killer. It took thousands of deaths before governments were finally convinced that the risks indeed outweighed the "improved properties."

Predictably, there is more research into controls further down the hierarchy, such as engineering, administration, and PPE controls. While some interesting work is being done on PPE and engineering controls, little of it amounts to evidence of effective workplace controls.

There are a number of reasons why this is the case.

First, while there are specific regulations for workplace chemicals, which include engineered nanomaterials, these regulations do not specifically mention nanomaterials and only apply to chemicals in their "bulk" form. Employers (or importers/manufacturers/suppliers) do not have a specific legal obligation to evaluate and manage nano-specific OHS risks in their workplace.

Until such time those nanomaterials are classified as unique materials taking into account the size, shape, catalytic potential, coating, charge, surface structure, and presence or absence of other chemicals. The nanoform of a chemical remains a dangerous but ultimately unassessed feature of the chemical. Employers (as well as importers, manufacturers, and suppliers) will continue to treat the substance as if it were in a bulk form. In fact, without information about the nanocontent of a substance, it may be difficult for employers to properly exercise their general duty of care with regard to employees, and others, in relation to substances in the workplace.

Fundamentally, unless employers and workers are provided with information about the use and presence of nanomaterials at work, controls cannot be implemented.

Second, there is a lack of evidence that these controls have been used or could practicably be used in commercial business settings, which are quite different to lab conditions, especially given the divergent industrial settings in which nanomaterials could be used. For example, it is not realistic (or for that matter healthy or safe) to compel a factory worker handling nano-containing products to wear a filter-based facemask respirator N95 efficiency or above, a self-contained breathing apparatus (SCBA), or double gloving using glove materials that are resistant to penetration by engineered nanomaterials, together with other protective garments that are made of non-woven fiber, for 8–12 h a day.

Finally, as alluded to earlier, the evidence actually shows that engineering controls and PPE controls are either ineffective or lack sufficient testing or data to ensure their effectiveness. Most tests on the effectiveness of PPE are done within the controlled environment of a lab setting. Will these be effective in a commercial setting?

Drawing on a few examples referenced in the SWA draft report, we can see that there are significant gaps in the evidence that highlight the ineffectiveness of existing controls:

- On the use of electrostatic filters: "information has not been found relating to issues associated with managing parameters such as lifetime (how often to change), preventing nanomaterial release at changeover and safe disposal" (SWA, 2009a, p. 32);
- On facemasks: "A significant amount of evidence has been found on the efficiency of filter materials in capturing nanoparticles, and this is presented in this section. However, no data specific to nanomaterials was found relating to the critical issue of mask fitting" (SWA, 2009a, p. 34);
- On clothing and gloves: "It was noted by Huang et al. (2007) that there are currently no accepted practical methods of determining the barrier protective properties of protective clothing media to aerosol penetration" (SWA, 2009a, p. 40);
- On workplace monitoring: "The effective monitoring for engineered nanomaterial in the workplace is problematic at present" (SWA, 2009a, p. 41);

- On medical surveillance: "The major barrier to specific health surveillance for workers is reported to be the lack of actual epidemiological data for worker exposure" (SWA, 2009a, p. 45); and
- On data: "Overall, there is limited data on actual workplace measurements taken before/after a nanomaterial process commences, and before/after control measures have been employed, that would provide accurate comparisons of the levels of both engineered and incidental particulates between each situation. There is an absence of data on controlling and detecting nanomaterial types that are more commonly produced by Australian nanotechnology industries, such as silicon, metal/metal oxide and carbon nanotube-based nanomaterials" (SWA, 2009a, p. 54).

Using as an example the facemasks (rapid palatal expansion [RPE]), the capture efficiency of the filter material used is rendered entirely ineffective if the mask is not properly fitted. Despite the fact that no available filter material is 100% effective and even the best filter material becomes less efficient below 50 nm, if the RPE is incorrectly fitted, the worker will continue working with a false sense of security. This is because where the RPE is used as a component in a "control banding" approach (utilizing more than one control at one time), the failure of that component will contaminate the whole banding system. Individually the failure of these control measures is of significant concern; collectively they represent a failure in occupational health and safety. The improvement of any one of these measures alone will not sufficiently address the problem.

Add to that the prohibitive cost and the experimental nature of some of the controls and it becomes a question of how suitable these controls are for use in commercial settings. The Safe Work Australia Nanotechnology OHS Program (SWA, 2009b) recognizes that this is an issue and is undertaking research into the effectiveness of existing nanocontrols and the development of cost-effective monitoring equipment. The results of these inquiries could be years away.

2.5 WHAT NEEDS TO BE DONE?

Unions agree that nanotechnology has important potential in the fields of medicine and the environment, but argue that nano-specific regulation is needed to protect workers.

There is an incorrect assumption that existing regulations and information about nanomaterials in substances (or substances in nano-form) are sufficient to trigger the introduction of controls and processes in workplaces. The ACTU is concerned that without an acknowledgment that new regulatory triggers are required that address the unique properties of nanomaterials, there will not be any obligations on importers, manufacturers, or suppliers to provide information or on employers to either provide information to workers or implement nano-specific controls and processes.

Despite the years of warnings that nanoparticles may be unsafe and calls by unions for nano-specific safety regulations, Australia still lacks:

- a regulatory acceptance or acknowledgment that nanomaterials are different and potentially hazardous in their own right;
- nano-specific regulatory triggers to assess and test;
- nano-specific risk assessment or controls required;
- mandatory registry of products;
- nano-specific monitoring required;
- nano-specific Material Safety Data Sheets;
- nano-specific exposure levels;
- nano-specific labels;
- requirements to inform workers they are potentially exposed to nano-sized particles;
- nano-specific health surveillance required;
- nano-specific training; and
- nano-specific PPE required.

The ACTU is calling for the introduction of the following regulatory mechanisms by the end of 2009:

- That there be a mandatory requirement that all commercial products containing nanomaterials be labeled and that all substances or goods containing nanomaterials have an accompanying Material Safety Data Sheet;
- That a publically accessible federal registry be established of all companies and organizations manufacturing, importing, and supplying products containing nanomaterials. Registration must be mandatory and should include the organization's name and their products/substances containing nanomaterials and the quantities; and

- That a tripartite body be established to oversee the implementation of a regulatory framework.

December 2009 is a sufficient timeframe given the pace of industry development. This would also coincide with the introduction of Australia's new nationally harmonized health and safety laws that are scheduled for release around the same time.

Also, work must immediately begin to fix the following regulatory gaps:

- Nano-sized chemicals are classified as new chemicals under Australia's National Industrial Chemicals and Notification and Assessment Scheme (NICNAS); and
- The current "regulatory triggers" based on threshold weight and volume are not relevant to nanomaterials. A new set of triggers and risk assessment protocols based on nano-specific characteristics and hazardous potential be introduced for nanomaterials.

Furthermore, the ACTU is calling on the Australian federal, state, and territory governments to urgently:

- Adopt the "Precautionary Foundation" when dealing with nanomaterials;
- Develop and improve hazard identification, assessment, and control mechanisms for nanomaterials;
- Develop and implement exposure standards for nanomaterials;
- Enforce the exposure standards through an active inspectorate;
- Monitor the health impacts on Australian workers and invest in medical research; and
- Raise awareness in workplaces and the community about the potential risks of exposure.

Under the dark shadow of the Australia's asbestos legacy, there is a moral and political imperative on the Australian government to act quickly and strongly to regulate and protect the next generation of Australian workers against another health disaster.

2.6 ACKNOWLEDGMENTS

I would like to acknowledge and thank Kate Lappin and Renata Musolino for their invaluable contributions and proofing skills in the preparation of this chapter.

REFERENCES

Asbestos Diseases Foundation of Australia, 2009. Asbestos safety. <http://www.adfa.org.au>.

Asbestos Diseases Society of Victoria, 2008. Advocacy domestic asbestos campaign. <http://www.adsvic.org.au/cms/templates/tmp_advocacy.aspx?articleid=24&>.

Australian Council of Trade Unions, 2005. ACTU submission to the Senate Community Affairs Committee: inquiry into workplace exposure to toxic dust. <http://www.aph.gov.au/senate/committee/clac_ctte/completed_inquiries/2004-07/toxic_dust/submissions/sub28.pdf>.

Australian Council of Trade Unions, 2008. James Hardie asbestos victims compensation summary. New Solutions: A Journal of Environmental and Health Policy 18 (3), 383–390.

Australian Nanotechnology Business Forum, 17 April 2009. Press Release: Workplace Safety with Nanoparticles. ANBF, Canberra.

Australian Safety and Compensation Council, July 2006. A Review of the Potential Occupational Health & Safety Implications of Nanotechnology. ASCC, Canberra.

Chillicothe Constitution-Tribune, 17 September 1936. Asbestos into Fashion Picture. Chillicothe, Missouri.

Commonwealth Government, 2009. Australian Government Budget 2009–10. Australian Government, Canberra.

Commission for Occupational Safety and Health, 2007. Annual Report 2006/07. Department of Commerce, Perth.

Davies, J.C., 2009. Oversight of Next Generation Nanotechnology. Project on Emerging Nanotechnologies. Washington, DC.

Department of Innovation, Industry, Science and Research, 2008. Australian Government approach to the responsible management of nanotechnology. <http://www.innovation.gov.au/Industry/Nanotechnology/Documents/ObjectivesPaper.pdf>.

Donaldson, K., Aitken, R., Tran, L., et al., 2006. Carbon nano-tubes: a review of their properties in relation to pulmonary toxicology and workplace safety. Toxicological Sciences 92 (1), 5–22.

Dowling, A., 29 July 2004. Quoted in The Royal Society and The Royal Academy of Engineering press releases. Nanotechnologies Bring Great Potential and Need for Responsible Development. RS-RAE, London.

Elder, A., Gelein, R., Silva, V., et al., 2006. Translocation of inhaled ultrafine manganese oxide particles to the central nervous system. Environmental Health Perspectives 114 (8), 1172–1178.

European Agency for Health and Safety at Work, 2009. Expert Forecast on Emerging Chemical Risks. European Commission, Brussels. <http://osha.europa.eu/en/press/press-releases/european_workers_face_new_increasing_health_risks_hazardous_substances_01.11032009>.

International Organization for Standardization, 2008. Health and Safety Practices in Occupational Settings Relevant to Nanotechnologies, ISO/TR 12885:2008. ISO, Geneva.

Keenihan, S., Bolton, L., February 2009. Australian Nanotechnology—Ensuring an Appropriate Environment for Commercialisation. ANBF, Canberra. <http://www.anbf.com.au/PDF/MateralsAust_feb09_CommcercialisingNano_5MB.pdf>.

Lam, C.W., James, J.T., McCluskey, R., et al., 2006. A review of carbon nanotube toxicity and assessment of potential occupational and environmental risks. Critical Reviews in Toxicology 36, 189–217.

Lam, C.W., James, J.T., McCluskey, R., Hunter, R.L., 2004. Pulmonary toxicity of single-wall carbon nanotubes in mice 7 and 90 days after intratracheal instillation. Toxicological Sciences 77 (1), 126–134.

Li, Z., Hulderman, T., Salmen, R., et al., 2007. Cardiovascular effects of pulmonary exposure to single-wall carbon nanotubes. Environmental Health Perspectives 115, 377–382.

Lux Research, 2008. Nanomaterials State of the Market Q3 2008: Stealth Success, Broad Impact. Lux Research, New York.

Ludlow, K., Bowman, D.M., Hodge, G.A., 2007. A Review of Possible Impacts of Nanotechnology on Australia's Regulatory Framework. Monash Centre for Regulatory Studies, Melbourne.

NanoAction, 31 July 2007. A Project of the International Center for Technology Assessment. Principles for the Oversight of Nanotechnologies and Nanomaterials. Consumer Coalition, Washington, DC. <http://www.nanoaction.org/nanoaction/index.cfm>.

National Institute for Occupational Safety and Health, 2006. Approaches to Safe Nanotechnology: An Information Exchange with NIOSH. NIOSH, Washington, DC.

National Institute of Health, 2009. National Cancer Institute Fact Sheet—Asbestos Exposure and Cancer Risk. US Government, Washington, DC. <http://www.cancer.gov/images/documents/5ac7d2fc-27df-4ecc-839f-dc5bc1909e01/FS3_21.pdf>.

Oberdörster, G., Oberdörster, E., Oberdörster, J., 2005. Nanotoxicology—an emerging discipline involving studies of ultrafine particles. Environmental Health Perspectives 113 (7), 823–839.

Oberdörster, G., Sharp, Z., Atudorei, V., et al., 2002. Extrapulmonary translocation of ultrafine carbon particles following whole-body inhalation exposure of rats. Journal of Toxicology and Environmental Health 65 (20), 1531–1543.

Peto, J., 2008. Quoted in The University of Melbourne Voice, Issues, Views, Debate. University News and Events 3 (2).

Poland, C.A., Duffin, R., Kinloch, I., et al., 2008. Carbon nanotubes introduced into the abdominal cavity of mice show asbestos-like pathogenicity in a pilot study. Nature Nanotechnology 3, 423–428.

Power, B., 18 March 2009. Quoted in Science meets parliament—nanotechnology and safety. <http://www.aussmc.org.au/ScienceMeetsParliament2009.php>.

Project on Emerging Nanotechnologies, 2008. Nano-product inventory—analysis of on-line inventory. <http://www.nanotechproject.org/inventories/consumer/>.

Radomski, A., Juraz, P., Alonso-Escolano, D., et al., 2005. Nanoparticle-induced platelet aggregation and vascular thrombosis. British Journal of Pharmacology 146 (6), 882–893.

Royal Society and The Royal Academy of Engineering, 2004. Nanoscience and Nanotechnologies: Opportunities and Uncertainties. RS-RAE, London.

Safe Work Australia, 2009a. Evidence on the Effectiveness of Workplace Controls to Prevent Exposure to Engineered Nanomaterials. Draft for Final Comment. SWA, Melbourne.

Safe Work Australia, 2009b. Nanotechnology OHS Program to Support the National Nanotechnology Strategy. SWA, Melbourne. <http://www.Safeworkaustralia.Gov.Au/Swa/Healthsafety/Emergingissues/Nanotechnology/Nanotechnologyohsprogram.Htm>.

Senate Community Affairs Committee, 2005. Community Affairs Reference Committee—Workplace Exposure to Toxic Dust—Terms of Reference. Commonwealth Government, Canberra.

Shvedova, A.A., Kisin, E., Murray, A.R., et al., 2008. Inhalation of carbon nanotubes induces oxidative stress and cytokine response causing respiratory impairment and pulmonary fibrosis in mice. The Toxicologist 102, A1497.

Shvedova, A.A., Kisin, E.R., Mercer, R., et al., 2005. Unusual inflammatory and fibrogenic pulmonary responses to single-walled carbon nanotubes in mice. Lung Cellular and Molecular Physiology 289, L698–L708.

Takagi, A., Hirose, A., Nishimura, T., et al., 2008. Induction of mesothelioma in p53+/− mouse by intraperitoneal application of multi-wall carbon nanotube. The Journal of Toxicological Sciences 33 (1), 105–116.

Victorian Nanotechnology Statement, February 2008. Taking Leadership in Innovations in Technology.

WorkSafe Victoria, undated. Nanotechnology Online Fact Sheet. Victorian Government, Melbourne. <http://www.worksafe.vic.gov.au/wps/wcm/connect/WorkSafe/Home/Safety+and+Prevention/Health+And+Safety+Topics/Nanotechnology/>.

WorkCover New South Wales, 12 September 2008. WorkCover Response to Additional Questions on Notice, NSW Parliamentary Inquiry into Nanotechnology in New South Wales. WorkCover NSW, Sydney. <http://www.parliament.nsw.gov.au/prod/PARLMENT/committee.nsf/0/a452d8666bde54c9ca2574f000064893/$FILE/080912%20Response%20to%20QoN%20-%20WorkCover%20Stephen%20Higham.pdf>.

Wragg, G., 1995. The Asbestos Time Bomb. Catalyst Press, New York.

SECTION 2

Regulation

CHAPTER 3

Global Perspectives on the Oversight of Nanotechnologies

Diana M. Bowman

CONTENTS

Fifty years have now passed since Professor Richard Feynman presented his now legendary lecture, *There's Plenty of Room at the Bottom: An Invitation to Enter a New Field of Physics*, to the 1959 annual meeting of the American Physical Society. During the course of his evening address, the Nobel Prize winning physicist eloquently presented his vision for "manoeuvring things atom by atom." He articulated a "top–down" approach for manipulating matter for the purpose of exploiting the novel properties of materials that exist at this scale. In doing so, the scientist challenged his colleagues to think beyond the traditional boundaries of physics and chemistry in order to work within the "very, very small world" (Feynman, 1960). While the lecture is just one of the many events or contributions that has helped to shape the field of scientific endeavor which has now been labeled as "nanotechnologies" (Toumey, 2005, in press), Feynman's message to think beyond the conventional borders would appear to be equally relevant when considering how to govern such a dynamic and multi-faceted area of technology.

As the chapters of this book highlight, the nascent field of nanotechnologies has evolved to the stage where an increasingly large volume of engineered nanoparticles, including, for example, nanotubes, metal oxides, quantum dots, and fullerenes, have being manufactured and incorporated into a broad array of products. The often cited Project on Emerging Nanotechnologies (PEN) Consumer Product Inventory (2008) lists over 800 self-identified, commercially available, nanotechnology-based products (nanoproducts), with products ranging from electronic equipment, personal care products, foods and food contact materials, and sporting equipment. While many of these nanoproducts may be superior to their conventional counterparts, it is envisaged that in the next few years nanotechnologies will offer more than simply invisible sunscreen- and stain (and wrinkle)-resistant clothing. The Royal Society and Royal Academy of Engineers (RS-RAE) (2004) anticipate that nanotechnologies will enable the creation of more energy-efficient membranes for water purification, advanced safety and security sensors, multi-functional materials, personalized medicines, and scaffolding materials for human tissues and bones. Salamanca-Buentello et al. (2005, p. 97) have suggested that while nanotechnologies will not by themselves be a "silver bullet" to the current challenges facing governments, the technology could "be harnessed to address some of the world's most critical development problems," through the commercialization of, for example, cheap and efficient energy cells and air and water remediation technologies.

Despite the anticipated benefits associated with the technology, there can be little doubt that over the past few years there has been increasing concern among some members of society over the potential risks posed by the technology to human and environmental health and safety (see, for example, Aitken et al., 2004; Thomas and Sayre, 2005; Maynard, 2006; Maynard et al., 2006; Friends of the Earth [FoE] Australia, 2006; Royal Commission on Environmental Pollution, 2008). This has in turn resulted in an increasing number of commentators, including those within the government, industry, and civil society, engaging in debates over the effectiveness of current regulatory regimes for managing any potential risks posed by the technology. With the maturation of nanotechnology itself and the increasing number of nano products in the market place, the debate has shifted to consider both the need for, and the possible form(s) of, nano-specific product regulation. This includes discussion concerning the point during the technology's development trajectory, or at which stage, that regulatory controls should and could be applied. As with earlier technologies and applications, concerns have also been raised by some commentators over the ability of industry to adequately protect their workers (see, for example, Australian Council of Trade Unions, 2005, 2009).

With the European Parliament having recently passed a resolution which has the potential to be the first national or supranational piece of legislation which expressly incorporates nano-specific provisions (European Parliament, 2009)—it adapted by the European Council—and, for example, Australia's New South Wales Government (2009, p. 6) stating that it supports "the development of a national mandatory labelling scheme for engineered nanomaterials used in the workplace," questions relating to risk management and the governance of nanotechnologies are unlikely to disappear. Indeed, as noted by Marchant et al. (2008, p. 43) "nanotechnology presents both an unprecedented challenge and an unparalleled opportunity for risk management." With this in mind, the aim of this chapter is to outline how the regulatory and governance challenges posed by nanotechnologies are currently being confronted and met by governments and other relevant stakeholders (see also Monica and van Calster, 2009). In doing so, the chapter begins by defining what is meant by regulation, its objectives, and the strengths and weaknesses adopted by different regulatory approaches. With the regulation of nanotechnologies having largely occurred under a range of existing state-based regulations, Section 3.2 of the chapter will provide an overview of a number of regulatory reviews undertaken to date within jurisdictions such as Australia, the European Union (EU), and the United States of America (US), and the key findings and implications for the governance of nanotechnologies. Multi-lateral and multi-party activities aimed at ensuring the benefits of the technology and minimizing potential risks are considered in Section 3.3 of the chapter. Finally, key challenges, common issues, and conclusions are brought together in Section 3.4.

3.1 SHAPING BEHAVIOR THROUGH REGULATION: SUBTLE AND NOT SO SUBTLE APPROACHES

The concept of regulation is often discussed but not necessarily well defined. Regulation has of course been a fundamental way in which risks—scientific and societal—associated with certain activities or actions have been traditionally managed or controlled by governments (Little, 2004). This will be no different with respect to nanotechnologies.

While the notion of regulation has traditionally referred to legislative instruments enacted by bodies such as Parliaments or Congress through formal processes as well as developments in the common law (Brownsword, in press), regulation today is considered to be much broader than simply "command and control" or "black letter law." Black (2002, p. 19) has eloquently defined this contemporary view of regulation as:

> *the sustained and focused attempt to alter the behaviour of others according to defined standards or purposes with the intention of producing a broadly identified outcome or outcomes.*

According to this view, regulation is primarily interested in influencing behavior. As noted by Brownsword (in press) "'regulation' refers [therefore] to any instrument (legal or non-legal in its character, governmental or non-governmental in its source, direct or indirect in its operation)...that is designed to channel behaviour." Regulation may therefore be undertaken by a range of different actors, not just government, in order to elicit or shape a range of outcomes, albeit positive or negative. While regulation may often be perceived as a way to minimize or manage risk of, for example, a particular type of harm, it may also be used as a way to encourage behavior, for example, by advancing a particular type of activity in order to promote economic interests or innovation.

3.1.1 State-based regulation

As noted, products and applications incorporating nanotechnologies have largely been regulated under the regulatory framework established by Acts, Regulations, Directives, and Government Guidelines. These traditional state-based "command and control" forms of regulation have considerable legitimacy with the public despite their perceived imperfections. Their compulsory nature, the appearance of strong accountability, and higher certainty are all characteristics that appeal to voters. Moreover, Ludlow et al. (2009) have suggested that:

> *clear and consistent state-based regulation provides many advantages compared with no regulation. In many instances industry prefers this form of regulation because it provides a level playing field, as well as providing protection against short-cutting competitors. It also provides certainty, assisting in securing capital finance and insurance.*

However, in order to achieve these objectives, Ludlow et al. (2009) have argued in the context of regulating nanotechnologies that the instruments employed must also be appropriate for the subject matter being regulated. "Appropriate" is, however, an ambiguous term, and one which is open to interpretation. How one determines whether or not the form of regulation is appropriate will, as Ludlow et al. (2009) note, depend on past experiences, different views on risk, benefits, innovation, and broader societal considerations, and the degree to which the instruments favorably or unfavorably impact upon your behavior or that of others.

So, while state-based regulation may provide clarity to those with products being the focus of the regulation, as well as providing guidance more generally, this traditional form of regulation suffers from a number of shortcomings (see, for example, Gunningham and Rees, 1997; Aalders and Wilthagen, 1997; Vogel, 2006). State-based regulation is often perceived as being slow, cumbersome, rigid, and involving high transaction costs (Moran, 1995; Sinclair, 1997). These perceived limitations can often be amplified in the context of rapidly evolving fields or areas where the regulatory requirements are more dynamic and the information required to craft the framework is imperfect.

Given these general limitations it is unsurprising that some commentators have suggested that in the short-term nano-specific state-based regulation may not be the most appropriate or effective way to regulate specific areas of the technology. Renn and Roco (2006) have for instance already noted that the development of state-based regulatory instruments for nanotechnologies would take substantially longer than alternative regulatory mechanisms. A case in point is that while BASF, one of the world's largest chemical companies, introduced their own in-house code of conduct for nanotechnology in 2004, it was not until March 2009 that the first piece of legislation specifically incorporating nanotechnology-specific provisions was introduced by Parliament at the national or supranational level (European Parliament, 2009). While the recast of, in this instance, the European Union's Cosmetic Directive was not initiated for the purposes of specifically regulating cosmetic products incorporating nanotechnologies, the fact that it took approximately 2 years to negotiate and develop the text of the Parliament's resolution underscores the complexities and challenges associated with formulating and introducing new legislative instruments.

3.1.2 Civil-based regulation

In light of the broadly accepted limitations associated with command and control regulation, there has been increasing interest among scholars and other stakeholders to develop alternative tools and other mechanisms that can be employed instead of traditional state-based regulation in order to effectively regulate certain activities (Sinclair, 1997). Many of these approaches are considered to be "soft law" approaches that sit at the opposite end of the regulatory continuum from state-based legislation due to the limited role of government in their development and operation. "Soft law" or civil law regulatory mechanisms are part of a regulatory continuum and include various forms of self-regulation, voluntary regulation, and third-party regulation (Gunningham and Rees, 1997; Vogel, 2006; Levi-Faur and Comaneshter, 2007). Importantly, "civil regulation extends regulatory authority 'sideways' beyond the state to civil society and to nonstate actors," thereby removing the potential for legally binding standards (Vogel, 2006, p. 3). Although under these mechanisms government no longer functions as the regulatory authority, the very broad nature of this regulatory category may enable the state to have some level of involvement in the broader governance framework (Gunningham and Rees, 1997).

It is not surprising that the term "governance" is often employed when discussing these non-legislative-based activities (Brownsword, in press). While traditionally associated with the activities of government (Stoker 1998, p. 17), the use of the term today has suggested that governance now "refers to the development of governing styles in which boundaries between and within public and private sectors have become blurred. The essence of governance is its focus on governing mechanisms which do not rest on recourse to the authority and sanctions of government."

The use of different types of civil regulation, such as voluntary codes of conduct, risk management frameworks, and industry codes, has steadily increased. High-profile activities have included the chemical industry's Responsible Care Program (see, for example, Rees, 1997; King and Lenox, 2000). It has been argued that these voluntary forms of regulation are less resource intensive to develop and administer and have the ability to evolve and respond to the changing environment quicker than state-based regulation (Braithwaite, 1982; Sinclair, 1997). It has also been suggested that this regulatory approach provides breathing space for innovation and creativity to occur. Arguably it is these perceived strengths that have inspired a number of different organizations, including government, industry, and non-governmental organizations, across different sectors and jurisdictions to develop and implement voluntary codes of conduct and risk management frameworks. These have included, for example, the ambitious principle-based "Responsible NanoCode," the "NanoSafe" Five-point Program, the "NanoRisk Framework," and the "Principles for the Oversight of Nanotechnology" (Royal Society et al., 2007; Hull, 2009; Environmental Defense and DuPont, 2007; Coalition of Non-Governmental Organizations, 2007). Many of these programs draw upon and incorporate to varying degrees traditional risk management principles including "(a) acceptable risk, (b) cost-benefit analysis, and (c) feasibility (or best available technology)" (Marchant et al., 2008, p. 44). These programs operate within the shadow of formal regulatory obligations and do not seek to "roll back the state" or replace the regulatory frameworks in which they operate. This is done by, for example, incorporating a precautionary approach to the manufacturing of nanoscale materials, by implementing innovative processes and state-of-the-art scientific knowledge into current practices, or through the data gathering processes which can then be used to develop risk appropriate management practices for nanomaterials. These approaches therefore work in combination with other forms of regulation in order to govern the safe and responsible development of nanotechnologies.

Gilligan and Bowman (2008, p. 241) have suggested that this investment by industry is due, in part, to their need to "be at the forefront of risk management in an increasingly technology-based economy." Webb (2004, p. 4) has also suggested that civil regulation is also driven in some instances by the desire to "harness market, peer and community energies to influence behaviour and draw on the infrastructure of intermediaries such as industry associations, standards organisations and non-governmental organisations for rule development and implementation." This contention sits comfortably with Black's (1996) broad notion of regulation in that it views regulation as something more than merely government enacted legislation.

While Black (1996, p. 25) has sought to remind us that "self-regulation is neither a new phenomenon, nor one which is likely to disappear," the increasing use of this form of soft law instruments across different sectors has not been without controversy. All forms of civil regulation have the potential to suffer from a range of perceived limitations. Self-regulation in particular has been accused of serving the interests of industry above that of society by, for example, circumventing market forces, having variable standards of enforcement, and lacking the accountability and legitimacy of government regulation (see, for example, Braithwaite, 1993; Webb and Morrison, 1996). Gunningham and Rees (1997, p. 370) also note that in relation to self-regulation "the effectiveness (or ineffectiveness) of self-regulation [can] var[y] enormously among industries..."

3.1.3 Co-regulation

State-based and civil regulation sit at the two ends of the continuum, with co-regulation straddling the middle. This form of regulation may be defined, for example, as the "use of a panoply of tools and actors, formal and informal, governmental and nongovernmental, national and international" (National Research Council, 2001, p. 200). Sitting therefore at the interface of state-based and civil regulation, this third type of regulation has the ability to draw upon the strengths of these other approaches, while avoiding a number of their perceived weaknesses. Given the flexibility of this regulatory approach it is therefore not surprising that governments have viewed this third approach as a fertile and productive area for regulatory innovation (Ayres and Braithwaite, 1992; Utting, 2005). For Sinclair (1997, p. 544), this approach enables industry to "shape regulatory outcomes, with government still retaining general design oversight."

Evidence of co-regulation has already emerged in relation to managing the challenges presented by nanotechnologies with a number of governments having developed, in consultation with industry and other stakeholders, and implemented voluntary reporting schemes or data stewardship programs (Department of Environment Food and Rural Affairs [Defra], 2006; National Industrial Chemical Notification and Assessment Scheme, 2007, 2008; Environmental Protection Agency [EPA], 2008; Californian Department of Toxic Substances Control, 2009). The UK's voluntary scheme was implemented in order to assist the government to "develop appropriate controls in respect of any risks to the environment and human health from free engineered nanoscale materials... in the shortest time giving a predictable regulatory environment for all" (Defra, 2006, p. 3). The development of the European Commission's (2007) voluntary "Code of Conduct for Responsible Nanosciences and Nanotechnologies Research" provides a further example of how government may work with industry and civil society to shape behavior.

With each regulatory approach having both its strengths and weaknesses, it is not surprising therefore that regulatory scholars such as Gunningham and Sinclair (1999, p. 50) have sought to remind us that the approaches are complementary and not mutually exclusive, and that "such 'single instrument' or 'single strategy' approaches are misguided, because all instruments have strengths and weaknesses, and because none are sufficiently flexible and resilient to be able to address all environmental problems in all context[s]." As noted by Ludlow et al. (2009, p. 3) in relation to the regulation of nanotechnologies, "the ongoing challenge for stakeholders will [therefore] be finding the acceptable balance between the different approaches." This is likely to be dependent in part on, for example, the evolving state of scientific knowledge, the degree of legitimacy attached to any one approach, the jurisdiction in which it is employed, and the way in which benefits and risks of particular areas are perceived within those jurisdictions (Ludlow et al., 2009).

There will be no "magic bullet" or single approach that will solve the regulatory challenges currently posed by the different dimensions of nanotechnologies. And even when government, industry, or other stakeholders have found what they believe to be a suitable solution, it is inevitable that the proposed response will not be acceptable to all those likely to be affected by its implementation. Finding a workable and effective balance, which has the necessary legitimacy with the public, will be an ongoing and evolving task which will require each area on the regulatory continuum to be represented.

3.2 KEY LESSONS AND RECOMMENDATIONS OF REGULATORY REVIEWS TO DATE

Despite the increasing manufacture of engineered nanoparticles and the commercialization of products containing nanoparticles, there is—as highlighted by a number of chapters in this book (see, for example, Mullins, 2009; Blaunstain and Linkov, 2009)—significant uncertainty as to the potential risks posed by some types of nanoparticles under certain conditions (Oberdörster et al., 2005; Nel et al., 2006; Maynard, 2006; Poland et al., 2008). This is in part not only due to the current lack of quantitative scientific data on the risks posed by nanoscale substances, including basic toxicity data and epidemiological studies, but it is also due to a lack of consensus over which physiochemical parameters must be evaluated as part of the risk assessments as well as the publication of contradictory findings. It would appear that these uncertainties present enormous challenges for regulators responsible for ensuring the safety of the work environment and the protection of the public interest.

Faced with these uncertainties and increasing scrutiny over the adequacy of existing regulatory arrangements—in terms of not only the statutory instruments, but also their operation, including implementation—governments in a number of jurisdictions have initiated reviews of their regulatory frameworks in order to examine their appropriateness for dealing with the current challenges. Reviews have, for instance, been undertaken in Australia, the European Union, the UK, and the US (see, for example, RS-RAE, 2004; Chaudhry et al., 2006; Health and Safety Executive, 2006; FDA, 2007; Ludlow et al., 2007; Food Safety Authority of Ireland, 2008; European Commission, 2008a, 2008b). These reviews have varied in their scope and focus. One of the earliest reviews undertaken in relation to the UK and EU focused specifically on the "appropriateness of existing regulatory frameworks for environmental regulation" (Chaudhry et al., 2006, p. 10). In contrast, Ludlow et al. (2007) were required to, pursuant to the request for tender, "...assess Australia's existing regulatory frameworks to determine if, and under what conditions, nanotechnology-based materials, products and applications, and their manufacture, use and handling, are covered by the existing regulatory frameworks;..." (Australian Government, 2006, p. 5). The European Commission's (2008a, p. 2) in-house review examined EU legislation most relevant to "nanomaterials currently in production and/or placed on the market."

Despite their differences, including the statutory instruments analyzed, the principles incorporated into the regimes, and the enforcement thereof, these reviews are important to the broader risk management framework. This is because they both define the regulatory landscape by which all parties must operate and hence obey, as well as the associated limitations of the landscape itself. Armed with this knowledge, regulatory and research efforts may be prioritized in order to address the knowledge gaps. Moreover, industry can use the finding to help shape their own proactive responses to best manage the potential challenges and risks posed by nanotechnology within the confines of the broader regulatory framework.

Bearing this in mind, what have been the key lessons and recommendations to come out of the various reviews undertaken to date? There are several, many of which are horizontal in nature as they are likely to be common across jurisdictions. For instance, despite some concerns that

Table 3.1 Four Common Misconceptions about the Regulation of Nanotechnologies

Belief	Response
1. Nanotechnologies are unregulated	Current nanotechnology products and processes fall within existing regulatory frameworks; it is the adequacy of the frameworks (i.e., their implementation) for effectively regulating nanotechnologies that is in question
2. Including nano-specific provisions in regulations will address many of the existing regulatory challenges	While such action may be a first step in refining current frameworks, the inclusion of nano-specific language in legislation will not by itself ensure the safety of products and processes. A greater understanding of the potential hazards and suitability of conventional risk assessment regimes is needed
3. Scientific uncertainty regarding the potential risks of some nanoparticles does not mean that governments and other parties cannot act at this time so as to minimize any potential risks	Uncertainty and the need for more scientifically sound data should not in itself give rise to paralysis in relation to the broader governance framework. However, any action taken, must be flexible and adaptive, so that it can evolve in line with new scientific information
4. The only way to effectively regulate nanotechnology products and processes is through state-based regulation	There are a number of different regulatory models that can be employed to regulate nanotechnologies, each of which have their own strengths and weaknesses and will have varying degrees of governmental involvement. Effective regulation, especially in relation to complex and dynamic regulatory questions, requires harnessing the strengths of these different models and finding a range of different regulatory solutions

nanotechnologies are "essentially unregulated" (see, for example, ETC Group, 2004; Salleh, 2007), each of the reviews showed that the nanotechnology-based products and processes fall within the ambit of the statutory instruments analyzed, and as such, were "regulated." This is despite the earlier misconception of some that the technology was "unregulated" (see Table 3.1 for several other important misconceptions associated with the regulation of nanotechnologies). The reviews found that instruments were sufficiently broad in their application and were considered to be technology-neutral.

Authors such as Chaudhry et al. (2006) and Ludlow et al. (2007), however, went on to suggest that the implementation of the instruments, and the principles underpinning them, was potentially problematic. These two reviews highlighted how current scientific uncertainties had the capacity to impact upon the operation and effectiveness of the broader regulatory frameworks. Chaudhry et al. (2006) identified a number of gaps in the broader regulatory framework including, but not limited to, those relating to definition, thresholds and/or exemptions, the effect or impacts, and specific substances. In their view (2006, p. 8), for example:

> *The regulatory gaps identified in this study derive either from exemptions (on tonnage basis) under legislative frameworks, or from the lack of information, or uncertainties over:*
>
> - *clear definition(s) encompassing the novel (or distinct) properties of nanotechnologies and [nanomaterials]; i.e. whether an [nanomaterial] should be considered a new or an existing material;*
> - *current scientific knowledge and understanding of hazards, and risks arising from exposure to [nanomaterials];*
> - *agreed dose units that can be used in hazard and exposure assessments;*
> - *reliable and validated methods for measurement and characterisation that can be used in monitoring potential exposure to [nanomaterials];*
> - *potential impacts of [nanomaterials] on human and environmental health.*

Discussion of the significant scientific and technical issues posed by these uncertainties in relation to the operation and implementation of the statutory frameworks was common to each of the reviews. This challenge was arguably best summarized by the European Commission (2008b, p. 9) when they stated that:

> [w]*hilst the Community legislative framework generally covers nanomaterials, implementation of legislation needs further elaboration. Important elements are the test methods and the risk assessment methods that serve as a basis for implementing legislation, administrative decisions, manufacturer's obligations or employer's obligations. The scientific basis to fully understand all properties and risks of nanomaterials is not sufficiently available at this point in time.*

Governments, regulators, and risk assessors around the world will have to continue to grapple with these uncertainties for the short-to-medium term, but so too will employers who wish to implement additional risk management measures in order to minimize any potential risks, such as those associated with worker exposure to certain free nanoparticles (see also Monica and van Calster, 2009).

These government-initiated reports have been complemented by a large number of regulatory and policy assessments by members of the research community, non-governmental organizations, and other interested stakeholders (see, for example, Pinson, 2004; Taylor, 2006, 2008; Davies, 2006, 2009; Ludlow, 2007, in press; Fuhr et al., 2006; Bowman and van Calster, 2007; Marchant et al., 2008; Miller and Senjen, 2008; Gergely et al., 2009). Against this backdrop, a number of Royal Commissions and Parliamentary Inquiries have now been initiated (see, for example, Royal Commission on Environmental Pollution, 2008; New South Wales Legislative Council Standing Committee on State Development, 2008; House of Lords Science and Technology Committee, 2009). At the same time a number of scientific opinions concerning the potential risks associated with nanotechnologies have also been published (see, for example, Aitken et al., 2004; Scientific Committee on Emerging and Newly Identified Health Risks, 2006, 2009; Scientific Committee on Consumer Products, 2007; European Food and Safety Authority, 2009).

While the findings and recommendations of these publications and inquiries vary significantly they nonetheless highlight the need for, as eloquently stated by Maynard et al. (2006, p. 267), "risk-focused research" in order to address the knowledge gaps currently challenging regulators and risk managers. Moreover, the increasing number of such reviews, inquiries, and opinions suggests that concerns over the adequacy of current regulatory arrangements for governing different facets of nanotechnology, including worker safety and food safety, are unlikely to be resolved soon.

With a number of these reports highlighting the need for coordination between not only jurisdictions, but also other key stakeholders (including industry, members of the research community, and non-governmental organizations), a number of multi-lateral and multi-party activities aimed at ensuring the safety of nanotechnologies have been initiated. The following section provides an overview of a number of activities that have been undertaken to date.

3.3 MULTI-LATERAL AND MULTI-PARTY INITIATIVES: THE STORY SO FAR

There can be little doubt that dialogue at the international level has gathered pace in relation to addressing the scientific, policy and regulatory challenges posed by nanotechnologies, with inter-governmental bodies, such as the Organization for Economic Cooperation and Development (OECD), the United Nations (UN), and the World Health Organization (WHO) in partnership with the Food and Agricultural Organization (FAO), having turned their attention to these issues. The International Organization for Standardization (ISO), a voluntary standards development body, is also supporting governments and industry around the globe through the development of definitions, common nomenclature, and standards for classification and testing of nanotechnology and nanomaterials (Miles, 2007). The activities and initiatives of these organizations have not been designed to develop regulatory instruments for dealing with nanotechnologies. Rather, they have instead largely focused on the safety aspects of nanotechnologies and in identifying the challenges faced by, for example, safety regulators. Ethical and social dimensions have also been considered within the context of, for example, the United Nations Educational, Scientific and Cultural Organization (2006). Also of importance, industry and civil society have been key players within many of these discussions and have assisted in shaping their outcomes.

Looking first at the activities of the OECD, the inter-governmental body has established two Working Parties to consider different aspects of nanotechnologies: the Working Party on Manufactured Nanomaterials (WPMN) and the Working Party on Nanotechnology (WPN). The first of these, WPMN, has been charged with a mandate "to promote international cooperation in human health and environmental safety related aspects of manufactured nanomaterials (MN), in order to assist in the development of rigorous safety evaluation of nanomaterials" (OECD, 2008, p. 3). The focus of the WPMN is on finding globally oriented solutions for the challenges posed by engineered nanomaterials, and has implemented eight projects in order to help achieve this overarching goal. Projects include, for example, the creation of a database on human health and environmental safety research (publically launched April 2009[1]), safety testing of a representative set of manufactured nanomaterials, including, for example, fullerenes, single-walled carbon nanotubes, and titanium dioxide, to which a number of countries and private sector participants have contributed to, and cooperation on risk assessment schemes in order to determine their suitability for nanomaterials (OECD, 2008).

The role of the WPN is to "advise on emerging policy-relevant issues in science, technology and innovation related to the responsible development of nanotechnology" (OECD, 2008, p. 7) and to do so within a global context (OECD, 2007). This has been achieved by focusing on six specific project areas, which include public outreach activities, documenting the ways in

---

1 Available at: <http://webnet.oecd.org/NanoMaterials/Pagelet/Front/Default.aspx?>.

which nanotechnologies may be employed to assist in addressing global challenges such as climate change and access to clean water, and acting as a facilitator for international cooperation and collaboration on research activities (OCED, 2007, 2008). While the objectives of the WPN are clearly ambitious, the proposed outputs should provide governments with well-informed insights into the potential impacts—both positive and negative—of nanotechnologies across a range of areas and provide them with fundamental knowledge and tools to move forward with policy development.

The inter-governmental cooperation on the promotion and implementation of these projects illustrates the fact that the challenges posed by nanotechnologies are not bound by jurisdictional borders or industry sectors. Moreover, it shows that a coordinated and strategic approach to the most pressing research requirements will assist in addressing the current knowledge deficits in the shortest possible timeframe. The findings and outcomes of these projects will arguably not only inform government activities, but also provide industry with fundamental knowledge that can be used to inform risk management activities.

Committees and agencies of the UN have similarly been engaged in discussions about nanotechnologies on the international stage, as outlined by the work agenda of UNESCO (2006, 2007), and more recently the FAO—in partnership with the WHO (2008)—and the United Nations Committee of Experts on the Transport of Dangerous Goods and on the Globally Harmonized System of Classification and Labelling of Chemicals (2009). UNESCO, has focused their efforts on "ethical reflection… to address the potential benefits and harms of nanotechnologies but even more important is assessing and publicly discussing the goals for which these technologies will be used" (UNESCO, 2007, p. 3). It has recognized the scientific challenges and current knowledge deficit associated with nanotechnologies. In order to address the numerous scientific and social challenges posed by the technology, UNESCO has advocated for voluntary ethical guidelines. In their words, "[t]he guidelines would represent a first attempt by UNESCO to propose a harmonization of ethical principles related to nanotechnologies and to recommend actions to be undertaken for research and applications in this field" (2007, p. 11). While aspirational in nature, the principles and approach advocated by UNESCO highlight how longer-term regulatory instruments within this area may solely not only focus on the scientific risks, but may also address a range of societal risks.

The recognition of the increasing commercialization of food and feed products processed with nanotechnology, or incorporating engineered nanomaterials, and the potential safety implications thereof prompted the FAO and WHO to convene an "Expert Meeting" for June 2009. The aim of this high-level meeting has, as the FAO and WHO (2008, p. 1) have explained, "to identify knowledge gaps including issues on food safety, review current risk assessment procedures, consequently support further food safety research and *develop global guidance on adequate and accurate methodologies to assess potential food safety risks that may arise from nanoparticles*" (emphasis added). Issue identification and capacity building of national food safety regulators to meet the potential challenges posed by the use of nanotechnologies in the agri-food sector appear to be paramount considerations for the FAO and WHO. While not designed specifically to do so, the outcomes of the joint meeting may have the capacity to influence or shape regulatory activities at the national level in the short-to-medium term.

The work agenda of the United Nations Committee of Experts on the Transport of Dangerous Goods and on the Globally Harmonized System of Classification and Labelling of Chemicals in relation to nanomaterials appears to be somewhat less advanced than those being pursued by UNESCO and the FAO. However, it is clear that the issues of health and safety and international harmonization are likely to be of increasing interest to this Committee moving forward.

Against this backdrop of high-profile and formal activities, a number of multi-party initiatives focused on the responsible development and governance of nanotechnologies have been occurring. These have included, the International Dialogue on Responsible Research and Development of Nanotechnology (Meridian Institute and National Science Foundation, 2004), the establishment of the International Council on Nanotechnology (ICON) (2005), and the International Risk Governance Council's (IRGC) project on risk governance of nanotechnology (see, for example, IRGC, 2006, 2007, 2008). The high-level nature of these initiatives, which draw together not only government representatives, but also industry, academics, and civil society, serves to highlight the many interests at play in relation to policy development for nanotechnologies, including the regulation thereof.

Moving forward, it is clear that some sectors or actors will be better positioned to influence the development of policies for nanotechnologies at the international level than others, especially those with representation at multiple forums. Given the diverse interests and economic value involved, it is argued that this sphere is likely to become increasingly populated by parties with vested interests pushing their own policy and regulatory agendas. The uncertainty here lies in the ultimate impact that these activities will have at the national level and the policy and regulatory frameworks that will be fashioned as a result.

3.4 MOVING FORWARD AMIDST UNCERTAINTY

There can be little doubt now that Marchant and Sylvester (2006, p. 714) were correct when they wrote that:

> *[m]any other questions continue to nip at nanotechnology's heels, not the least of which are debates about what is and is not technically feasible. Despite these uncertainties, we can have complete confidence in one aspect of nanotechnology's future—it will be subject to a host of regulations.*

At the time Marchant and Sylvester (2006) foreshadowed the enactment of nano-specific provisions and/or new statutory instruments, significant inertia on the part of government(s) existed with respect to future regulatory pathways for different facets of nanotechnologies. While uncertainty persists in relation to the development trajectories and the potential health and safety risks posed by particular engineered nanoparticles there appears to be some consensus that change is needed under the broader regulatory matrix. This is in part due to the need to ensure that the benefits of nanotechnologies are realized while at the same time ensuring consumer acceptance of the products and processes.

While the text of the final resolution recast of the European Union's Cosmetics Directive may have been the first national or supranational instrument to be passed by a Parliament with nano-specific provisions within its text, it will certainly not be the last. The European Parliament and Council is still to vote on the inclusion of nano-specific provisions in the recast of its Novel Food Regulation and nano-specific amendments to the Registration, Evaluation, Authorization, and Restriction of Chemicals (REACH) Regulation (Regulation (EC) No 1907/2006) appear inevitable. While such measures are jurisdiction specific, their impact—it passed—will be felt more widely: non-European parties wishing to place products onto the European Community market will be required to comply with such instruments. As such, regulatory action within any one jurisdiction will have an impact beyond their territorial boundaries.

At present, there is growing speculation that existing voluntary reporting or data collection activities may be hardened (see also the discussion of Monica and van Calster, 2009), while other countries, such as France, have proposed the adoption of their own nano-specific regulations (Mayer Brown, 2009). Such actions, if they transpire are still atypical of the overarching approach being taken by governments around the world: they do, however, suggest that some governments are willing to enact regulations despite the many uncertainties and the challenges thereof. Such action will have wide ranging implications for regulators, not least that they will be required to stay on top of the changes within a dynamic regulatory environment.

In moving forward, a number of key challenges and issues must be addressed to ensure that the predicted benefits of the technology are fully realized. Arguably, the most pressing of these is the need to tackle the known scientific uncertainties in a systematic way. In doing so, the continuation and expansion of the current multi-party and multi-jurisdiction collaborations will be most beneficial in identifying and managing potential risks. However, uncertainty and the need for more scientifically sound data should not in itself give rise to paralysis in relation to the broader governance framework. While there is little consensus as to the nature and form that regulatory frameworks for nanotechnologies should take, there have been a number of early attempts to develop largely voluntary, governance regimes. While such voluntary codes of conduct, risk management frameworks, and certification schemes may not be perfect, they nevertheless provide a foundational framework for managing risks. In this sense, these initiatives illustrate that innovative, consent-based governance regimes can be developed and implemented by institutions despite the fast moving pace of the technologies. Frameworks of this type can be easily refined over time in order to reflect the evolving scientific state. Importantly though, these types of regulatory approaches will only be part of the broader regulatory environment.

Moving forward, nanotechnologies are destined to play a significant role in driving innovation across sectors and jurisdictions. But without doubt, all stakeholders—ranging from government to industry and civil society—are faced with significant challenges in ensuring that the as yet unknown risks do not compromise human and environmental health and safety or the longer-term potential of the technology. This represents a difficult and ongoing challenge, and as with the science itself, there are likely to be many events, contributions, and players within the international and national spheres that will shape the regulatory environment. Moreover, in an area in which the pace of evolution is so rapid, the message to think beyond conventional boundaries would appear to be equally relevant to considering how to govern such a dynamic and multi-faceted technology. This will not be an easy task, but it is pivotal to ensuring safety and success of nanotechnologies.

REFERENCES

Aalders, M., Wilthagen, T., 1997. Moving beyond command-and-control: reflexivity in the regulation of occupational safety and health and the environment. Law & Policy 19 (4), 415–443.

Aitken, R.J., Creely, K.S., Tran, L., 2004. Nanoparticles: An Occupational Hygiene Review. Prepared by the Institute of Occupational Medicine for the Health and Safety Executive, Edinburgh.

Australian Council of Trade Unions, 2005. Submission to the Senate Community Affairs Committee: Inquiry into Workplace Exposure to Toxic Dust. ACTU, Melbourne.

Australian Council of Trade Unions, 14 April 2009. Media Release: Nanotech Poses Possible Health and Safety Risk to Workers and Needs Regulation. ACTU, Melbourne.

Australian Government, 2006. Request for Tender: Review of Possible Impacts of Nanotechnology on Australia's Regulatory Frameworks. Department of Industry, Tourism and Resources (Innovation Division), Canberra.

Ayres, I., Braithwaite, J., 1992. Responsive Regulation: Transcending the Deregulation Debate. Oxford University Press, New York.

Black, J., 2002. Critical reflections on regulation. The Australian Journal of Legal Philosophy 27, 1–36.

Black, J., 1996. Constitutionalising self-regulation. The Modern Law Review 59 (1), 24–55.

Blaunstain, R., Linkov, I., 2009. Risk management: an insurance industry's perspective. In: Hull, Matthew, Bowman, Diana M. (Eds.), Nanotechnology Risk Management. Springer, London, pp. 143–179.

Bowman, D., van Calster, G., 2007. Does REACH go too far? Nature Nanotechnology 1, 525–526.

Braithwaite, J., 1982. Enforced self-regulation: a new strategy for corporate crime control. Michigan Law Review 80 (7), 1466–1507.

Braithwaite, J., 1993. Responsive regulation for Australia. In: Grabosky, Peter N., Braithwaite, John (Eds.), Business Regulation and Australia's Future. Australian Institute of Criminology, Canberra, pp. 81–96.

Brownsword, R., in press. The age of regulatory governance and nanotechnologies. In: Hodge, Graeme, Bowman, Diana, Maynard, Andrew (Eds.), International Handbook on Regulating Nanotechnologies. Edward Elgar, Cheltenham.

Californian Department of Toxic Substances Control, 22 January 2009. Chemical Information Call-In: Carbon Nanotubes. DTSC, Sacramento.

Chaudhry, Q., Blackburn, J., Floyd, P., et al., 2006. Final Report: A Scoping Study to Identify Gaps in Environmental Regulation for the Products and Applications of Nanotechnologies. Defra, London.

Coalition of Non-Governmental Organizations, 31 July 2007. Principles for the Oversight of Nanotechnologies and Nanomaterials. <http://www.foeeurope.org/activities/nanotechnology/Documents/Principles_Oversight_Nano.pdf>.

Davies, J.C., 2006. Managing the Effects of Nanotechnology. Project on Emerging Nanotechnologies. Washington, DC.

Davies, J.C., 2009. Nanotechnology Oversight: An Agenda for the New Administration. Project on Emerging Nanotechnologies. Washington, DC.

Department of Environment Food and Rural Affairs, 2006. UK Voluntary Reporting Scheme for Engineered Nanoscale Materials. Defra, London.

Environmental Defense and DuPont, 2007. Nano Risk Framework. EDF, New York.

Environmental Protection Agency, 2008. Notice: nanoscale materials stewardship program. Federal Register 73 (18), 4861–4866.

ETC Group, 2004. News Release—Nanotech: Unpredictable and Un-Regulated: New Report from the ETC Group. ETC Group, Ottawa.

European Commission, 2007. Towards a Code of Conduct for Responsible Nanosciences and Nanotechnologies Research—Consultation Paper. EC, Brussels.

European Commission, 2008a. Regulatory Aspects of Nanomaterials: Summary of Legislation in Relation to Health, Safety and Environment Aspects of Nanomaterials, Regulatory Research Needs and Related Measures. EC, Brussels.

European Commission, 2008b. Regulatory Aspects of Nanomaterials. EC, Brussels.

European Food and Safety Authority, 2009. Scientific Opinion: The Potential Risks Arising from Nanoscience and Nanotechnologies on Food and Feed Safety—Scientific Opinion of the Scientific Committee (Question No EFSA-Q-2007-124a). EFSA, Brussels.

European Parliament, 24 March 2009. Press Release: MEPs Approve New Rules on Safer Cosmetics. European Parliament, Brussels.

Feynman, R.P., February 1960. There's plenty of room at the bottom. Engineering and Science, 22–36.

Food and Agriculture Organization and World Health Organization, 2008. Joint FAO/WHO Expert Meeting on the Application of Nanotechnologies in the Food and Agriculture Sectors: Potential Food Safety Implications. FAO and WHO, Rome.

Food and Drug Administration, 2007. Nanotechnology—A Report of the U.S. Food and Drug Administration Nanotechnology Task Force. Washington DC, FDA. FDA, Washington, DC.

Food Safety Authority of Ireland, 2008. The Relevance for Food Safety of Applications of Nanotechnology in the Food and Feed Industries. FSAI, Dublin.

Friends of the Earth Australia, 2006. Nanomaterials, Sunscreens and Cosmetics: Small Ingredients, Big Risks. Friends of the Earth Australia and Friends of the Earth United States, Sydney.

Fuhr, M., Hermann, A., Merenyi, S., Moch, K., Moller, M., 2006. Legal Appraisal of Nanotechnology: Existing Legal Frameworks, the Need for Regulation and Regulative Options at a European and National Level. Society for Institutional Analysis, Darmstadt.

Gergely, A., Bowman, D.M., Chaudhry, Q., 2009. Small ingredients in a big picture: regulatory perspectives on nanotechnologies in foods and food contact materials. In: Chaudhry, Qasim, Castle, Lawrence, Watkins, Richard (Eds.), Nanotechnologies in Food. The Royal Society of Chemistry, London.

Gilligan, G., Bowman, D., 2008. 'Netting Nano': regulatory challenges of the Internet and nanotechnologies. International Review of Law Computer & Technology 22 (3), 231–246.

Gunningham, N., Rees, J., 1997. Industry self-regulation: an institutional perspective. Law & Policy 19 (4), 363–414.

Gunningham, N., Sinclair, D., 1999. Regulatory pluralism: designing policy mixes for environmental protection. Law & Policy 21 (1), 49–76.

Health and Safety Executive, 2006. Review of the Adequacy of Current Regulatory Regimes to Secure Effective Regulation of Nanoparticles Created by Nanotechnology: The Regulations Covered by HSE. HSE, London.

House of Lords Science and Technology Committee, 2009. Call for Evidence: Nanotechnologies and Food. United Kingdom Parliament, London.

Hull, M., 2009. Nanotechnology environmental, health and safety: a guide for small business. In: Hull, Matthew, Bowman, Diana, M. (Eds.), Nanotechnology Risk Management. Springer, London, pp. 247–293.

International Council on Nanotechnology, 2005. About. <www.icon.rice.edu.about.cfm?doc_id4383>.

International Risk Governance Council, 2006. White Paper on Nanotechnology Risk Governance—Towards an Integrative Approach. IRGC, Geneva.

International Risk Governance Council, 2007. Policy Brief: Nanotechnology Risk Governance—Recommendations for a Global, Coordinated Approach to the Governance of Potential Risks. IRGC, Geneva.

International Risk Governance Council, 2008. Risk Governance of Nanotechnology Applications in Food and Cosmetics. IRGC, Geneva.

King, A.A., Lenox, M.J., 2000. Industry self-regulation without sanctions: the chemical industry's responsible care program. The Academy of Management Journal 43 (4), 698–716.

Levi-Faur, D., Comaneshter, H., 2007. The risks of regulation and the regulation of risks. The governance of nanotechnology. In: Hodge, Graeme, A., Bowman, Diana, M., LudlowKarinne (Eds.), New Global Regulatory Frontiers in Regulation: The Age of Nanotechnology. Edward Elgar, Cheltenham, pp. 149–165.

Little, G., 2004. BSE and the Regulation of Risk. The Modern Law Review 64 (5), 730–756.

Ludlow, K., 2007. One size fits all? Australian regulation of nanoparticle exposure in the workplace. Journal of Law and Medicine 15, 136–152.

Ludlow, K., in press. The readiness of Australian food regulations for the use of nanotechnology in food and food packaging. Tasmania Law Review.

Ludlow, K., Bowman, D.M., Hodge, G.A., 2007. A Review of Possible Impacts of Nanotechnology on Australia's Regulatory Framework. Monash Centre for Regulatory Studies, Melbourne.

Ludlow, K., Bowman, D.M., Kirk, D., 2009. Hitting the mark or falling short with nanotechnology regulation? Trends in Biotechnology 27 (11).

Marchant, G.E., Sylvester, D.J., 2006. Transnational models for regulation of nanotechnology. The Journal of Law, Medicine & Ethics 34 (4), 714–725.

Marchant, G.E., Sylvester, D.J., Abbott, K.W., 2008. Risk management principles for nanotechnology. NanoEthics 2 (1), 43–60.

Maynard, A.D., 2006. Nanotechnology: A Research Strategy for Addressing Risk. Project on Emerging Technologies. Washington, DC.

Maynard, A.D., Aitken, R., Butz, T., et al., 2006. Safe handling of nanotechnology. Nature 444, 267–269.

5 March 2009. EU Competition—Brussels Client Alert: France Might Take the Lead on Nanotechnology Regulation. Mayer Brown Brussels.

Meridian Institute and National Science Foundation, 2004. International Dialogue on Responsible Research and Development of Nanotechnology. Meridian Institute and NSF, Alexandria, VA.

Miles, J., 2007. Metrology and standards for nanotechnology. In: Hodge, Graeme, A., Bowman, Diana M., Ludlow, Karinne (Eds.), New Global Regulatory Frontiers in Regulation: The Age of Nanotechnology. Edward Elgar, Cheltenham, pp. 333–352.

Miller, G., Senjen, R., 2008. Out of the Laboratory and on to Our Plates: Nanotechnology in Food & Agriculture. FoE Australia, Europe and US, Melbourne.

Monica, J.C., van Calster, G., 2009. A nanotechnology legal framework. In: Hull, Matthew, Bowman, Diana M. (Eds.), Nanotechnology Risk Management. Springer, London, pp. 97–140.

Moran, A., 1995. Tools of environmental policy: market instruments versus command-and-control. In: Eckersley, R. (Ed.), Markets, the State and the Environment: Towards Integration. Macmillan Education, South Melbourne.

Mullins, S., 2009. Are we willing to heed the lessons of the past? Nanomaterials and Australia's asbestos legacy. In: Hull, Matthew, Bowman, Diana M. (Eds.), Nanotechnology Risk Management. Springer, London, pp. 49–69.

National Research Council, 2001. Global Networks and Local Vales—A Comparative Look at Germany and the United States. National Academy Press, Washington, DC.

Nel, A., Xia, T., Madler, L., Li, N., 2006. Toxic potential of materials at the nanolevel. Science 311, 622–627.

New South Wales Government, 2009. NSW Government Response to the Legislative Council Standing Committee on State Development Inquiry into Nanotechnology in NSW. NSW Government, Sydney.

New South Wales Legislative Council Standing Committee on State Development, 2008. Nanotechnology in NSW. NSW Legislative Council, Sydney.

National Industrial Chemical Notification and Assessment Scheme, 2007. Summary of Call for Information and the Use of Nanomaterials. Australian Government, Canberra.

National Industrial Chemical Notification and Assessment Scheme, 2008. Industrial nanomaterials: voluntary call for information. Australian Government Gazette C 10 (7 October), 25–38.

Oberdörster, G., Maynard, A.D., Donaldson, K., et al., 2005. Review: principles for characterizing the potential human health effects from exposure to nanomaterials: elements of a screening strategy. Particle and Fibre Toxicology 2 (8), 1–35.

Organization for Economic Cooperation and Development, 2007. OECD Working Party on Nanotechnology (WPN): Vision Statement. OECD, Paris.

Organization for Economic Cooperation and Development, 2008. Nanotechnologies at the OECD. OECD, Paris.

Pinson, R., 2004. Is nanotechnology prohibited by the biological and chemical weapons conventions? Berkeley Journal of International Law 22 (2), 279–309.

Poland, C.A., Duffin, R., Kinlock, I., et al., 2008. Carbon nanotubes introduced into the abdominal cavity of mice show asbestos like pathogenicity in a pilot study. Nature Nanotechnology 3, 423–428.

Project on Emerging Nanotechnologies, 2008. Nano-product inventory—analysis of on-line inventory. <http://www.nanotechproject.org/inventories/consumer/>.

Renn, O., Roco, M.C., 2006. Nanotechnology and the need for risk governance. Journal of Nanoparticle Research 8, 153–191.

Rees, J., 1997. Development of Communitarian Regulation in the Chemical Industry. Law & Policy 19 (4), 477–528.

Royal Commission on Environmental Pollution, 2008. Novel Materials in the Environment: The Case of Nanotechnology. UK Parliament, London.

Royal Society and Royal Academy of Engineering, 2004. Nanoscience and Nanotechnologies: Opportunities and Uncertainties. RS-RAE, London.

Royal Society, Insight Investment, Nanotechnology Industries Association, Nanotechnology Knowledge Transfer Network, 2007. Responsible Nanotechnologies Code: Consultation Draft—17 September 2007 (Version 5). Responsible NanoCode Working Group, London.

Salamanca-Buentello, F., Persad, D.L., Martin, D.K., Daar, A.S., Singer, P.A., 2005. Nanotechnology and the developing world. Public Library of Science Medicine 2 (5), 97–103.

Salleh, A., 12 July 2007. Nanotech regulation under the spotlight. ABC News. <http://www.abc.net.au/news/stories/2008/07/12/2301936.htm>.

Scientific Committee on Emerging and Newly Identified Health Risks, 2006. Modified Opinion (After Public Consultation) on the Appropriateness of Existing Methodologies to Assess the Potential Risks Associated with Engineered and Adventitious Products of Nanotechnologies. Directorate General for Health and Consumers, EC, Brussels.

Scientific Committee on Emerging and Newly Identified Health Risks, 2009. Risk Assessment of Products of Nanotechnologies. Directorate General for Health and Consumers, EC, Brussels.

Scientific Committee on Consumer Products, December 2007. Opinion on Safety of Nanomaterials in Cosmetic Products. Health and Consumer Protection Directorate-General, EC, Brussels.

Sinclair, D., 1997. Self-regulation versus command and control? Beyond false dichotomies. Law & Policy 19 (4), 529–559.

Stoker, G., 1998. Governance as theory: five propositions. International Social Science Journal 17–28.

Taylor, M.R., 2006. Regulating the Products of Nanotechnology: Does FDA Have the Tools It Needs? Project on Emerging Nanotechnologies, Washington, DC.

Taylor, M.R., 2008. Assuring the Safety of Nanomaterials in Food Packaging: The Regulatory Process and Key Issues. Project on Emerging Nanotechnologies, Washington, DC.

Thomas, K., Sayre, P., 2005. Research strategies for safety evaluation of nanomaterials, part I: evaluating the human health implications of exposure to nanoscale materials. Toxicological Science 87 (2), 316–321.

Toumey, C., 2005. Apostolic succession. Engineering & Science 1 (2), 16–23.

Toumey, C., in press. Tracing and disputing the story of nanotechnology. In: Hodge, Graeme, Bowman, Diana, Maynard, Andrew (Eds.), International Handbook on Regulating Nanotechnologies. Edward Elgar, Cheltenham.

United Nations Committee of Experts on the Transport of Dangerous Goods and on the Globally Harmonized System of Classification and Labelling of Chemicals, 2009. Ongoing Work on the Safety of Nanomaterials. UN, Geneva.

United Nations Educational, Scientific and Cultural Organization, 2006. The Ethics and Politics of Nanotechnology. UNESCO, Paris.

United Nations Educational, Scientific and Cultural Organization, 2007. Nanotechnology and Ethics: Policies and Actions—COMEST Policy Recommendations. World Commission on the Ethics of Scientific Knowledge and Technology, Paris.

Utting, P., 2005. Rethinking Business Regulation—From Self-Regulation to Social Control. United Nations Research Institute for Social Development, Geneva.

Vogel, D., 2006. The Private Regulation of Global Corporate Conduct. Centre for Responsible Business Working Paper Series. University of California, Berkeley.

Webb, K., 2004. Understanding the voluntary code phenomenon. In: Webb, K. (Ed.), Voluntary Codes: Private Governance, the Public Interest, and Innovation. Carleton University, Ottawa, pp. 3–32.

Webb, K., Morrison, A., 12–13 September 1996. The legal aspects of voluntary codes. Paper presented at the Exploring Voluntary Codes in the Marketplace Symposium, Ottawa.

CHAPTER 4

A Nanotechnology Legal Framework

John C. Monica Jr. and Geert van Calster

CONTENTS

Other authors in this book have provided an excellent review of the potential environmental, health, and safety (EHS) concerns accompanying the manufacturing and/or use of select nanoscale materials which may occur under certain conditions. These potential concerns include exposure through dermal penetration and/or inhalation, possible translocation through the bloodstream, accumulation in various organs, and theoretical penetration through cell membranes and the blood–brain barrier (see, for example, Oberdörster et al., 2005; Gwinn and Vallyathan, 2006). There is also concern that engineered nanoscale materials may adversely affect the environment in the event of unintended releases. Simply put, there is a worry that because engineered nanoscale materials are so small and often have unique properties, they may be able to infiltrate the human body and the environment in ways which larger particles cannot, and once there, may cause unique adverse EHS consequences (Maysinger et al., 2006).

While the science is currently inconclusive, some initial studies support theoretical cause for concern (see, for example, Maynard et al., 2006). In this modern legal age of successful tort lawsuits over spilled hot coffee,[1] these potential EHS concerns produce liability and regulatory anxiety for businesses venturing into the field of nanotechnology, as well as their investors, insurers, and customers. While many of these concerns are not unique to nanotechnology, it is rare that so many novel legal issues are arrayed all at once. Legal issues intersecting with nanotechnology research, development,

[1] *Liebeck V. McDonald's Restaurants, P.T.S., Inc.*, No. D-202 VS-93-02419, 1995 WL 36039 (N.M. Dist. Ct. 1994), *but see, McMahon v. Bunn-O-Matic Corp.*, et al., 150 F.3d 651 (7th Cir. 1997).

and commercialization include intellectual property; workplace and occupational liability; commercial/contractual liability; environmental regulation; food and drug regulation; consumer product safety; tort and product liability; and end-of-life disposal issues. It can be a daunting legal web to untangle unless analyzed piece-by-piece, one step at a time.

At the same time, nanotechnology businesses must take a holistic view of the interrelated legal issues they may confront over their lives. A single legal issue cannot be viewed in isolation, as it often implicates additional areas of commerce which can impact predicable outcomes. Depending upon where they fit into the life cycle of a nano-enabled product, businesses will experience varying types and amounts of potential legal exposure which must be managed proactively. The alternative is to cross one's fingers and hope for the best or attempt to solve legal problems after the fact which is often time-consuming, nerve racking, and expensive. Moreover, in Europe there is a well-documented example of how regulatory uncertainty coupled with public anxiety, may nearly kill-off an industry, seriously hindering it to reach its full potential. That of course is the example of the European regulatory framework for genetically modified organisms.

4.1 NANO-PRODUCT LEGAL LIFE CYCLE

For conceptual purposes, the legal life cycle of a nanotechnology product has five distinct stages:

- **a.** Supply;
- **b.** Manufacturing;
- **c.** Intermediate use;
- **d.** Consumer; and
- **e.** End-of-life disposal.

A business involved in making, selling, or distributing a product incorporating engineered nanoscale materials may be involved in any, several, or all of these five stages. While each stage may have multiple subparts in any given scenario, the five basic stages provide a useful backdrop for discussion. Once the five stages are explained, a basic legal framework can be superimposed which provides any nanotechnology-based business with a basic guide on how to spot and manage potential legal and regulatory needs. Of course, these five stages are only a starting point. Real life businesses involved in nanotechnology will undoubtedly face more complicated life cycles which reflect their

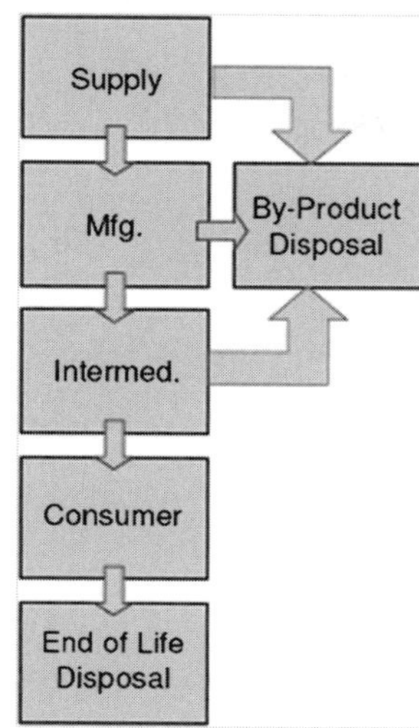

FIGURE 4.1 *Nanotechnology Product Legal Life Cycle.*

individual facts and circumstances. This framework is flexible enough, however, to be modified to embrace such changes (Figure 4.1).

4.1.1 Supply stage

The first stage in the conceptual nanotechnology product legal life cycle is the "supply stage." A supplier is a company that does not make a final nanotechnology-based product (nano-product), but rather creates a precursor which it then sells to others. A supplier can make any number of precursors and sell them to a variety of other suppliers and/or manufacturers. Take, for example, a carbon nanotube manufacturer which makes single-walled carbon nanotubes (SWCNTs) and then sells them as raw material to third parties who in turn use them to make new, innovative products. The SWCNTs may be made to a particular customer's specifications or they may be generic in the sense that the supplier makes only one type and purchasers are free to buy them or not. For our purposes, if all a company does is make and sell SWCNTs to other companies, it is considered a supplier. Suppliers may also develop and commercialize traditional chemical substances as well as equipment and intellectual property used by nano-manufacturers in their own internal processes. Additionally, there may be several hierarchies of suppliers, each supplying the next with a subcomponent or submaterial necessary to advance the whole through completion. On the other hand, suppliers may not always form a direct chain, with several suppliers acting in parallel to supply a single, master supplier or manufacturer with precursor materials. In such instances, the analogy is a wheel, with the main supplier or manufacturer representing the hub and the unrelated suppliers representing spokes. Finally, when a material leaves a supplier's hands it is considered to be that company's "product" for legal purposes.

4.1.2 Manufacturing stage

The second stage in the nanotechnology product legal life cycle—manufacturing—most often comes to mind when someone explains that their company is making a new nanotechnology product—some type of end product that can be held and/or seen. A company may make and supply its own raw nanomaterial—in our example SWCNTs—but what makes it a manufacturer for the purposes of our legal framework is that the company actually creates a finished product using the material. For example, a sporting goods' manufacturer may purchase SWCNTs or other precursor chemical substances from a supplier and then mix them in a resin in its own manufacturing facility which is then pressed and heated to form an extremely light and strong piece of sports equipment. This, of course, is an over simplification of the process. For conceptual purposes, picture a loading dock at the back of a manufacturing facility. An inspector opening one of the boxes being shipped out will find an actual product that typical consumers will recognize; the sports equipment in our example. Again, when the item leaves a manufacturer's hands it is considered to be that company's "product" for legal purposes. As noted above, the "supply" and "manufacturing" stages may overlap and may be hard to distinguish from each other at times. The main distinction for purposes of our framework is the degree of finish exhibited by the product.

4.1.3 Intermediate use stage

The third stage in the nanotechnology product legal life cycle—intermediate use—occurs when a business takes a completed product of another company and then incorporates it into its own product. An example is an automobile company that purchases fully made car batteries which use carbon nanotubes as energy storage media and then incorporates these batteries into its new electric hybrid vehicles. The ultimate product sold to the consumer—the car, incorporates the completed intermediate product—the battery, creating a linking distribution chain before ultimate purchase and use by a consumer. In modern commerce, it is not unusual for a product to pass through several intermediate use stages before it is ultimately sold to the consuming public. Beyond merely incorporating other companies' products into their own, an intermediate user may also be a distributor—a company that purchases a finished product from another company and then sells it to customers or relabels and sells it as its own.

4.1.4 Consumer stage

The fourth stage in our nanotechnology legal product life cycle is the "consumer" stage. This stage is reached when an ultimate product is sold into the hands of "Joe and Jane Public" who then use the product for its intended (and sometime unintended) purpose. The Project on Emerging Nanotechnologies (2008) at the Woodrow Wilson International Center for Scholars publishes a useful online inventory of existing consumer products claiming to contain engineered nanoscale materials. As of May 2009, there were over 800 consumer products on the inventory ranging from appliances, automotive applications, electronics, and computers, food and beverage containers, dietary supplements, health and fitness items, cosmetics, personal care products, and home and garden products. While not claiming to be comprehensive, the inventory is currently the best available. Users of the inventory, however, should realize that the label "nano" is sometimes used as a marketing tool, and any given product on the inventory may not truly be considered a nanotechnology product. Additionally, many products on the inventory may have never been actually sold or marketed in the real world. So, use the inventory, but take it with a grain of salt.

4.1.5 Disposal stage

The fifth and last stage of the conceptual nanotechnology legal product life cycle is the "disposal" stage. "Joe and Jane Public" are done using the product after its intended useful life and then get rid of it—usually by throwing it in the trash where it ultimately ends up in a landfill or less often in an unregulated dump. For our purposes, this stage also includes more than just traditional disposal. For example, a shampoo containing a nanoscale material is considered "disposed of" in our scheme when it is washed down the bathtub drain after cleaning the user's hair. Thus, it is not "thrown away" in a traditional sense, but it nonetheless enters the disposal chain for framework purposes. The supply, manufacturing, and intermediate use stages also present disposal issues for by-products of the manufacturing process and for unused materials. These present disposal scenarios are typically covered by federal, state, and local environmental regulations.

While this five-stage nanotechnology legal product life cycle is very basic and must be modified in any real life scenario, it provides a useful construct for discussing potential legal and liability issues facing businesses involved in nanotechnology.

4.2 LEGAL ISSUES

Superimposed on our five-stage nanotechnology legal product life cycle are five categories of primary legal issues:

1. Intellectual property;
2. Workplace and occupational liability;
3. Commercial and contractual liability;
4. Government regulation; and
5. Product and tort liability.

As we work our way through these legal issues as they specifically pertain to engineered nanoscale materials, the overarching "take away points" for nanotechnology companies are that they should have a full understanding of the potential EHS issues at each stage of the product life cycle, and this full understanding should be accompanied by full and complete written disclosures which should be adequately documented. Additionally, retaining counsel fully versed in nanotechnology will reduce risk of unforeseen legal problems with commercial relationships and contracts.

4.2.1 Intellectual property

Intellectual property (IP) legal issues confronting nanotechnology commercialization primarily accompany the supply stage and/or design and engineering phases of the manufacturing stage. It is in the early manufacturing stage before the first nano-product is ever stamped, pressed, molded, or otherwise created that a business must take all steps necessary to protect the value of its invention. Without protection from potential misappropriation, there can be no successful commercialization of new ideas (Smith and Parr, 2005).[2] For the purposes of our framework, IP includes patents, trademarks, and trade secrets (Figure 4.2).

4.2.1.1 Patents

Patents are granted by governments and are the legal right to exclude others from using an invention for a fixed period of time in exchange for publication of a complete explanation of what the invention is, what it does, and

[2] See also Bawa (2004), who has stated that, "[i]ntellectual property, a product or creation of the human mind, is an intangible asset representing humankind's only truly inexhaustible resource."

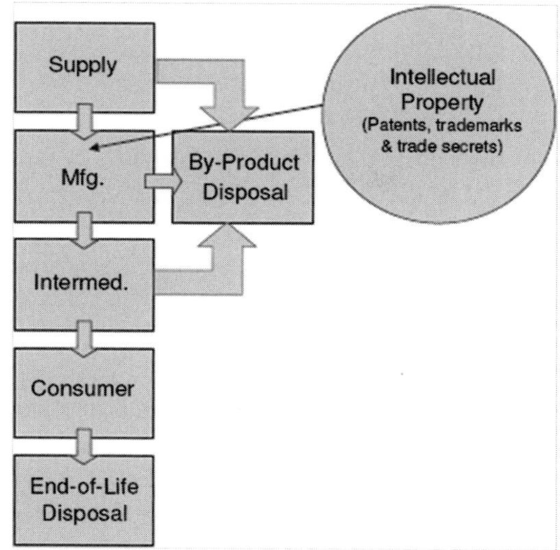

FIGURE 4.2 *Intellectual Property Rights as Part of the Product Legal Life Cycle.*

how it can best be recreated (United States Patent and Trademark Office, 2008). In the United States (US), patent rights are constitutional in nature and were designed to encourage innovation. Article I of the US Constitution provides that: "[t]he Congress shall have power…[t]o promote the progress of science and useful arts, by securing for limited times to authors and inventors the exclusive right to their respective writings and discoveries."[3] In the European Union (EU), patents by and large follow a similar path to the US system, with the additional challenge of making sure one can secure a European-wide patent, to avoid having to go through 27 different legal systems.

Patents have been described as "monopoly" rights because they totally exclude others from unlicensed use of the idea or invention during the patent period.[4] They are unusual because in most other areas of the law, the federal government seeks to limit or eliminate monopolies. However, the main objective of patent law is to provide an incentive to reward innovation and

---

[3] US Const. art. I, § 8, cl. 8, *available at* http://www.law.cornell.edu/constitution/constitution.articlei.html; *see also Graham v. John Deere Co. of Kansas City*, 383 US 1 (1996), *available at* http://supreme.justia.com/us/383/1/case.html.

[4] *Zenith Radio Corp. v. Hazeltine Research, Inc.*, 395 US 100, 135 (1969), *available at* http://supreme.justia.com/us/395/100/case.html (citing *Bement v. National Harrow Co.*, 186 US 70 (1902)).

facilitate its prompt use. Thus, in exchange for publicly explaining an invention, a period of exclusivity is granted (Smith and Parr, 2005).[5]

The multidisciplinary nature of nanotechnology often makes patenting issues difficult to manage. The science of nanotechnology encompasses everything from pharmaceuticals and medical devices to polymer additives to electronics. Over the past decade, there has been an explosion of patents employing nanotechnology, leading to what is called a "patent thicket." One commentator found that 264 nanotechnology patents were granted in the US in 1998 and that number had increased to 1577 in 2004 (Matsuura, 2006). Another expert estimated that there were approximately 4000 nanotechnology patents in the US by 2004 (Miller et al., 2005).[6] One thing is for certain, lawyers recognize the big business opportunities presented by nanotechnology. Currently, 65 US attorneys on Martindale–Hubbell list nanotechnology IP as a specialty. The number is sure to grow.

The three requirements for patentability are novelty (see, for example, Matsuura, 2006),[7] utility (see Miller et al., 2005; Matsuura, 2006),[8] and nonobviousness (see Matssura, 2006).[9] Traditionally, "obviousness" has focused on differences between the claimed invention and what the prior art/literature reveals.[10] A patent cannot be granted if "the subject matter as a whole would have been obvious at the time the invention was made to a person having ordinary skill in the art."[11] Reducing the size of something—with no other improvement—has traditionally been found to be

---

[5] *Woodbridge v. United States,* 263 US 50 (1923), *available at* http://supreme.justia.com/us/263/50/case.html; *see also* Smith and Part (2005) (quoting Burge (1984)): "While the right of ownership in most personally property is a positive right, the right of ownership in a patent is a negative right. It is the negative right to exclude others form making, using or selling the patented invention."

[6] Regarding search terms, Miller et al. (2005) reported that using different terms "can lead to numbers anywhere from 1100 to 17 000—depending on the search terms used."

[7] 35 U.S.C. §102 requires novelty as a condition for patentability. This largely requires the invention to be unknown, unused, unpublished, and/or unpatented and without prior patent applications.

[8] 35 U.S.C. §103 (2002). "The basic *quid pro quo* contemplated by the federal Constitution and Congress for granting a patent monopoly is the benefit derived by the public from an invention with substantial utility." *Brenner v. Manson,* 383 US 519 (1966).

[9] 35 U.S.C. §103. *Ramirez v. Perez,* 457 F. 2d 267 (5th Cir. 1972), *available at* http://bulk.resource.org/courts.gov/c/F2/457/457.F2d.267.71-2073.html; *Graham v. John Deere Co., 383* US 1 (1966), *available at* http://supreme.justia.com/us/383/1/case.html.

[10] *Graham v. John Deere Co. of Kansas City,* 383 US 1 (1996), *available at* http://supreme.justia.com/us/383/1/case.html.

[11] 35 U.S.C. §103.

nonobvious. Accordingly, nanoscale inventions must show some novel or new property in order to be patentable. Simply shrinking something to the nanoscale is insufficient (Miller et al., 2005; Troilo, 2005).

Additionally, naturally occurring materials are not patentable (Dunens et al., 2008). Several IP law commentators have questioned whether and to what extent this general rule is applicable to nanoscale materials (Dunens et al., 2008).[12] The key question is whether something new is being created by nanotechnology or whether the increasing sophistication and magnification of scanning and tunneling microscopes is simply allowing scientists to see what was already there in new and greater detail. Certain crude fullerenes and nanotubes have been found to occur naturally. Nanoparticles appear in clay and soil and are mined/harvested for use because of lower cost. Are some or all nanoscale materials naturally occurring, and hence unpatentable?

Because the area of nanotechnology patents is growing so quickly and presents unique intellectual property issues, many have questioned whether private IP attorneys, and more importantly examiners inside the US Patent and Trademark Office (USPTO), have sufficient knowledge and expertise to make and/or evaluate patent applications (Bawa, 2004; O'Neill, 2007). The USPTO took some steps to address this issue when it created its "Class 977—Nanotechnology" cross-reference art collection in 2005. Similarly, the European Patent Office in 2003 set up a nanotechnology working group and started using "Y01N" tags to label nanotechnology in EPO databases.

Class 977 is a cross-reference collection; patents are first placed in other categories and then provided a secondary nanotechnology classification. The Class only includes engineered nanoscale materials, not incidental or natural ones. By June 2006, there were 4800 patents in Class 977. The Class employs examiners from many different backgrounds. One estimate places the number of USPTO examiners used to assist with Class 977 at approximately 300 (Mouttet, 2005). The Class is designed to help examiners and attorneys search the prior art/literature for nanotechnology patents which would be otherwise scattered through numerous classes.

Once a company has protected its invention by obtaining a patent, it can proceed to commercialize its concept. Some companies—fewer and fewer these days—take an idea from inception completely through the manufacturing stage and into the marketplace itself. More likely is that

---

[12] Dunens et al. (2008, p. 31), citing *Diamond v. Chakrabarty*, 447 US 303, 309 (1980), have stated that "[t]he laws of nature, physical phenomena, and abstract ideas have been held not patentable."

a company will sell its patented ideas to another company outright or perhaps sell it the right to use the patent for some specified duration and/or specific purpose. The right to use the patent to the exclusion of all others is known as an "exclusive license."[13] The right to use the patent for a limited time or purpose at the same time as others use it is a "non-exclusive license."[14]

While technology licensing is not unique to nanotechnology, it does present some novel issues. Counsel retained for licensing purposes must not only know the ins-and-outs of the commercial law upon which the license itself is based (which is essentially a form of contract), he or she must also be intimately familiar with the specific subfield of nanotechnology covered by the patent in question. Without such specialized knowledge, it is virtually impossible to prepare a license that adequately protects the licensee's interests. For example, counsel must be fully versed in nanotechnology terminology and nomenclature in order to make sure the license is not overly broad or ambiguous in any respect. Additionally, incorporating standards developed by International Standards Organizations where appropriate is another valuable service that a skilled legal practitioner can provide to a client seeking to license nanotechnology intellectual property.

4.2.1.2 Trademarks

A trademark is "any word, name, symbol or device or any combination thereof [used to] identify and distinguish…goods, including a unique product, from those manufactured or sold by others and to indicate the source of the goods" (Smith and Parr, 2005, p. 38). If they are distinctive and are not easily confused with a previously registered mark, trademarks can be registered with the USPTO in order to help protect their unique commercial value (Miller et al., 2005). Not all trademarks are considered distinctive. A trademark that is generic or merely descriptive cannot be registered with the USPTO under normal circumstances. Trademarks that are considered "arbitrary and fanciful" or "suggestive," on the other hand, can be successfully registered which puts the world on formal notice of their ownership.

Once a trademark is registered by the USPTO it must be maintained by ensuring that it is used in a proper manner by the holder and that potential trespassers are kept at bay. If not properly maintained, a trademark can lose its USPTO protected status (Miller et al., 2005).

Because the word "nano" is a catchy metric prefix, many companies have placed the word "nano" with some other descriptive term and then claimed

---

[13] *Textile Prods., Inc. v. Mead Corp,* 134 F. 3d 1481, 1484 (Fed. Cir. 1998).

[14] *US Philips Corp. v. International Trade Comm.,* 424 F. 3d 1179, 1189 (Fed. Cir. 2005).

that the result is a brand or trademark. These types of "nano-marks" are ubiquitous, but businesses must understand that they are often unprotected by federal trademark law and indeed EU law because they are viewed as merely descriptive and are not truly distinctive (Du Mont, 2008). For example, the name "Nano Legal News" used for a legal journal could not be trademarked because it is merely descriptive. Adding the word "nano" in front of "legal news" does not make it distinctive; it only describes the type of legal news provided. The touchstone in these instances is that where the term "nano" is a primary term used in the proposed trademark, an examiner at the USPTO is likely to focus on the descriptive nature of the trademark and may reject its registration.[15]

4.2.1.3 Trade secrets

A trade secret is most commonly considered as "any information that can be used in the operation of a business or other enterprise and that is sufficiently valuable and secret to afford an actual or potential economic advantage over others."[16] Most nanotechnology companies have information which they believe is trade secret and would be ruinous if released to their competitors. Trade secrets should be protected from disclosure by making anyone who has access to the information sign a confidentiality and non-disclosure agreement.[17] This is not unique to the field of nanotechnology.

Once information is made a trade secret, its secrecy must be vigilantly maintained otherwise it loses its legal protection. Evidence that information is indeed a protected trade secret includes "restrictive covenants with

---

[15] *See, e.g., Holmes Prods. Corp. v. Honeywell Consumer Prods.,* Serial No. 74/236, 945, 1999 TTAB LEXIS 597 (Trademark Trial and Appeal Board 1992); *Cummins Engine Co. v. Continental Motors Corp.,* 359 F. 2d 892 (US Ct. Cust. & Pat. App. 1966); *In re: Fruit of the Earth, Inc.,* Serial No. 75/443, 437, 2001 TTAB LEXIS 391 (Trademark Trial and Appeal Board 2001); *In re: Manhattan Scientific, Inc.,* Serial No. 75/447, 259, 2001 TTAB LEXIS 779 (Trademark Trial and Appeal Board 2001); and *In re: Winfield Locks, Inc.,* Serial No. 75/357, 114, 2000 TTAB LEXIS 446 (Trademark Trial and Appeal Board 2000). *In re Microcell Corp.;* Serial No. 75931410, 2005 TTAB LEXIS 295 (Trademark Trust and Appeal Board 2005) ("The test for determining whether a term or phrase is merely descriptive is whether the term or phrase immediately conveys information concerning a significant quality, characteristic, function, ingredient, attribute, or feature of the product or service in connection with which it is used or is intended to be used." (citations omitted)).

[16] Restatement of the Law (Third), Unfair Competition §39 (1995), *available at* http://www.law.uconn.edu/homes/swilf/ip/statutes/restatement38.htm.

[17] *See, e.g., Intera Corporation v. Henderson,* 428 F. 3d 605, 609–610 (6th Cir. 2005), *available at* http://bulk.resource.org/courts.gov/c/F3/428/428.F3d.605.04-6081.html.

employees;" "control on a need-to-know basis;" "segmentation of knowledge;" "control of speeches, and technical articles;" "physical plant security;" "secure handling of visitors, vendors, suppliers;" "file and document controls;" "careful control when all or portion of knowledge must be divulged to vendors or customers;" "use of trade secret legends on documents;" and existence of a "security 'culture' in which employees are aware of the need to protect intellectual property" (Smith and Parr, 2005, pp. 24–25; see also Cummings, 2008). It is important to maintain these indicia in order to keep trade secret status.

4.2.2 Workplace and occupational liability

Workplace and occupational liability is most prevalent at the manufacturing stage, but can occur at any time prior to the consumer stage. Occupational liability of some sort typically occurs when an employer, researcher, or a worker is injured in the workplace during the course of his or her employment. Fortunately, there is already a good base of existing information available to attorneys and EHS professionals attempting to limit a nanotechnology company's potential workplace and occupational liability and protect its workers (Figure 4.3).

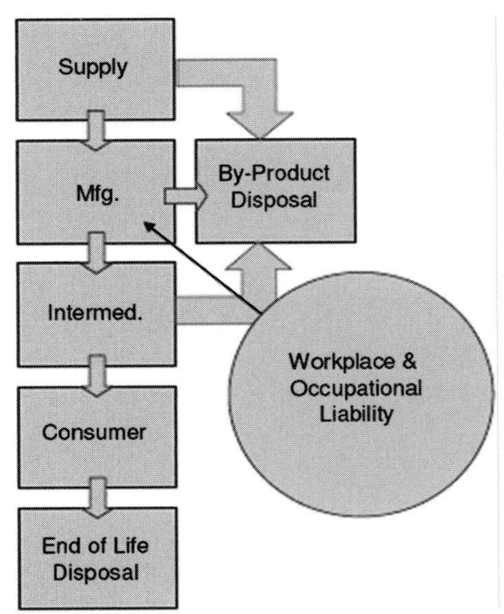

FIGURE 4.3 *Workplace and Occupational Liability.*

4.2.2.1 NIOSH, OSHA, and EU equivalents

Since 2004, the National Institute for Occupational Safety and Health (NIOSH) has given a considerable amount of attention to nanotechnology workplace safety issues. NIOSH has published three primary nano-related documents: "Approaches to Safe Nanotechnology: An Information Exchange with NIOSH;" "Progress Towards Safe Nanotechnology in the Workplace: A Report from the NIOSH Nanotechnology Research Center;" and "Strategic Plan for NIOSH Nanotechnology Research and Guidance, Filling the Knowledge Gaps."

By way of background, NIOSH theorizes that it is possible that an inordinate number of inhaled nanoparticles may deposit in deeper areas of the human respiratory tract when compared to their larger counterparts. If these nanoparticles are deposited deep in the lung, NIOSH is concerned that they may be able to translocate throughout the body via the bloodstream. Once in the bloodstream, NIOSH is also concerned that engineered nanoparticles may be able to cross cell membranes and the blood–brain barrier (Centers for Disease Control and Prevention, 2006). NIOSH recognizes that airborne or "free" nanoparticles present the greatest exposure risks. On the other hand, nanoparticles confined in a solid matrix or finished component are unlikely to present significant exposures unless those substances are somehow degraded.

According to NIOSH, engineered nanoscale materials present a unique workplace balancing act. Specifically, the scientific data and information available regarding the potential EHS risks of engineered nanoscale materials are new and relatively limited. Additionally, scientific data on the possible health effects in exposed workers are largely unavailable. These new, limited, and unavailable data present NIOSH and nanotechnology manufacturers with the dilemma of how to best protect workers when the full extent of risk is unknown (Centers for Disease Control and Prevention, 2006).

At the same time, NIOSH recognizes that the same novel characteristics of engineered nanoscale materials that make them attractive for research and development purposes may also mean that their fundamental toxicity characteristics differ from their bulk counterparts. Thus, commercialization must be balanced against preventing reasonably foreseeable injuries which might accompany any exposure to engineered nanoscale materials in the workplace.

While acknowledging that more research is necessary in almost every aspect touching workplace safety, NIOSH has published some general guidelines for companies working with nanoscale materials (Centers for Disease Control and Prevention, 2006). These recommendations should be of prime concern to attorneys and EHS specialists advising their clients in the area. NIOSH's specific recommendations include

- Employing interim occupational exposure measures until the risks presented by engineered nanoscale materials are better understood;
- Limiting exposure to nanoscale materials in gaseous phases or powders;
- Monitoring the amount of material being used, the duration of use, and particle size;
- Wearing adequate skin and inhalation protection devices when handling engineered nanoscale materials;
- Completely enclosing any pouring or mixing operations involving engineered nanoscale materials;
- Using traditional environmental engineering controls such as dust collection systems, fume hoods, and vacuums;
- Avoiding cleanup techniques for workplace surfaces in facilities using engineered nanoscale materials that are likely to disperse materials such as dry wiping or cleaning with blasts of compressed air;
- Using high efficiency particulate air (HEPA) certified respiratory devices;
- Preventing the consumption of food and beverages in the nano-workplace;
- Providing clothes changing and showering facilities; and
- Considering undertaking baseline worker health surveillance efforts.

NIOSH has also published a formal research plan to close the information gaps it has identified regarding possible workplace exposure, as well as general safety guidelines for employers and employees working with engineered nanoscale materials (Centers for Disease Control and Prevention, 2008). NIOSH is also conducting its own primary workplace exposure and material toxicity research and sponsors a valuable program through which it conducts field studies of nanomanufacturing facilities in order to gather exposure data and to help employers make their work areas as safe as possible for workers using engineered nanoscale materials (National Institute for Occupational Safety and Health, 2009).

In the EU, concerns are of course similar to those of the US, albeit the regulatory structure is quite different. The most relevant law is Framework Directive 89/391/EEC "on the introduction of measures to encourage improvements in the safety and health of workers,"[18] which has a variety

[18] Official Journal [1989] L183.

of so-called daughter Directives some of which may be relevant for nanoparticles. However, neither in the framework Directive nor in the daughter Directives, are there as yet any specific provisions on nanotechnologies, instead contenting itself with generic provisions such as that employers need to ensure the safety of their workers and organize relevant data gathering and consultation to that effect. Moreover, the European Agency for Safety and Health at Work, commonly known as "OSHA," does not have the kind of regulatory powers which NIOSH has in the US. In the EU, this role is fulfilled by agencies at the national level in conjuncture with the European Commission (EC). As a result of restrictions under European law, agencies cannot be tasked with duties which are truly executive, making them, like OSHA, more of a data clearing house and advisory organization. Moreover, under the aforementioned framework directive, Member States may take measures that go beyond what the EU itself has ruled—although in the case of nanotechnology, none of them have done so.

4.2.3 Worker's compensation

Under traditional US workplace and occupational liability laws, an employer is required to provide worker compensation insurance to cover possible injuries to employees resulting from their employment. These laws are applicable in the event of any workplace injury resulting from exposure to engineered nanoscale materials. Thus, rather than sue an employer for a workplace injury, the worker is compensated out of an insurance-type fund.

Workers' compensation laws vary from state to state. Every nanotechnology company should make itself knowledgeable concerning the specific state laws governing the operation of its facilities. Typically, an injured worker submits a claim to his or her employer which is substantiated by a treating doctor's medical records. The insurer then investigates the claim to determine whether the employment and injury are legitimate, the injury was work-related, and that the work in question was a substantial factor leading to the injury. Usually, a worker's compensation claim must be filed within a specified time of the alleged injury—6 months to 3 years depending upon the state—and the employer must be notified of the injury during the employee's period of employment.

Workers' compensation payments typically cover lost wages and medical treatment. Additionally, if a worker suffers a permanent injury, he or she can receive a lump sum payment for the disability under some States workers' compensation statutes. The system is "no fault" in that an employee does not have to show or allege that the employer acted negligently or did something wrong.[19] A simple "on the job injury" is enough. On the other hand, the worker himself may have done something inadvertently to cause his or her own injury. Compensation is still allowed under workers' compensation laws under such circumstances because negligence is not an issue.[20]

Many workers' compensation statutes provide the exclusive remedy for workers injured on the job and do not allow workers to sue employers or co-workers.[21] Thus, in many states an injured worker can receive worker's compensation benefits, but then cannot turn around and sue the employer for his or her injuries.[22] There are, naturally, exceptions to this rule including intentional torts.

Much like in the US, the European system for worker's compensation and healthcare cover is organized at the national (compared with state) level, the EU not having much of a formal role to play in this policy area. Cover is typically more generous than in the US, although it is impossible to generalize on this issue.

With studies reporting toxicity in high doses and under specific circumstances, and for specified nanoscale materials, it is clear that employers must no longer assume that nanoparticles are always going to be able to be handled in the same way as their larger cousins. While lack of specific data prevents employers from rolling out exact measures to deal with nanotechnologies, there would seem to be an increasing relevance in making sure that a number of basic precautions are taken. This would include measurement and detection of nanoparticles in the workplace.

4.2.4 Intentional workplace torts

In some narrow cases workers' compensation statutes may allow an injured employee to sue an employer even if he or she first collects worker's compensation when the law deems the injury to be "intentionally" caused by the employer. In these limited instances, "intentional" means: (1) knowledge by the employer of the existence of a dangerous employment condition that rises above the general hazards of standard employment; (2) knowledge by the employer that an injury is substantially certain to occur if the employee is subjected to the condition; and (3) the employer requires the employee to

[19] *See, e.g., Alaska Packers Ass'n v. Industrial Acc. Com'n*, 294 US 532 (1935).

[20] *See, e.g., New York Cent. R. Co. v. White*, 243 US 188 (1917).

[21] *See, e.g., US v. Demko*, 385 US 149 (1966).

[22] *See, e.g., Blankenship v. Cincinnati Milacrom Chem., Inc.*, 433 N.E.2d 572 (Oh. 1982).

continue to perform the task despite such knowledge. "Requires" can often be inferred from policies and procedures and need not be a direct command or instruction.[23] "Mere knowledge and appreciation of a risk—something short of substantial certainty—is not intent."[24] Mere recklessness is also insufficient. This is a very difficult legal standard to meet, but because of potential punitive damages based on intentional conduct, such lawsuits are not infrequent, especially when the alleged injury is severe or other employees have suffered the same or similar injury.

To reduce exposure to this type of liability, nanotechnology companies must ensure that they consistently monitor the most up-to-date scientific literature regarding the potential exposure risks posed by any engineered nanoscale material used in the workplace. Eventually, enough scientific literature may accumulate to allow a creative plaintiff's attorney to argue that an employer "knew" the potential EHS risks (or even consciously avoided such knowledge). Once such knowledge is established, a plaintiff's attorney will typically be able to locate some alleged defect in the company's occupational hygiene process and then attempt to link the defect to his client's purported inhalation or dermal exposure injury.

4.2.5 Commercial and contractual liability

Commercial and contractual liability is most prevalent in the transitions from the supplier stage to the manufacturing stage and from the manufacturing stage to the intermediate use or consumer stage. Of all the potential legal risks confronted by a nanotechnology company, it is the easiest to manage (Figure 4.4).

A contract is an agreement, obligation, or legal tie by which a party binds itself or becomes bound, expressly or implicitly, to pay a sum of money or to perform or omit to do some certain act or thing.[25] It has also been defined as a set of promises for the breach of which the law gives a remedy, or the performance of which the law in some way recognizes a duty.[26] Exact definitions differ in the EU, however, the basic idea remains the same.

---

[23] *See, e.g., Kerg v. Atlantic Food and Die Co.*, 892 N.E.2d 481, 485 (Oh. 8th Dist. 2008); *Russell v. Lexis-Nexis*, 2007 WL 949520 (Ohio App. 2 Dist. 2007).

[24] *See, e.g., Kerg v. Atlantic Food and Die Co.*, 892 N.E.2d 481, 485 (Oh. 8th Dist. 2008); *Russell v. Lexis-Nexis*, 2007 WL 949520 (Ohio App. 2 Dist. 2007).

[25] 17A Am Jur 2d §1 (2004); *Norfolk and Western Ry. Co. v. American Train Dispatchers Ass'n*, 499 US 117 (1991).

[26] Restatement Second, Contracts §1.

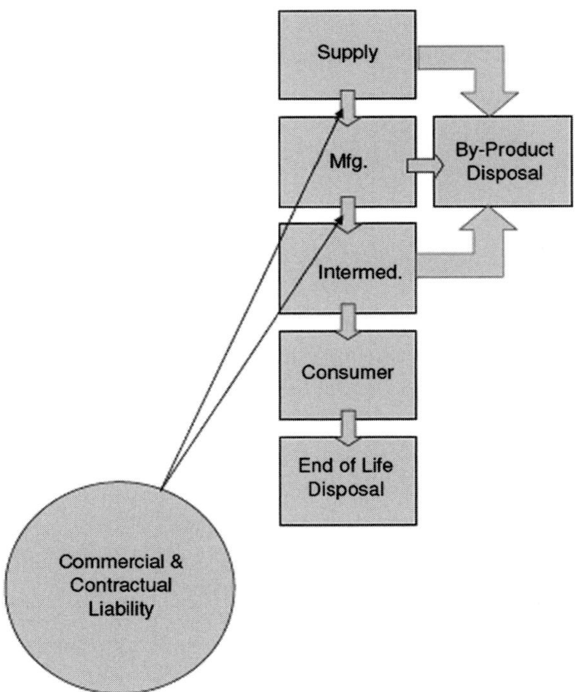

FIGURE 4.4 *Commercial and Contractual Liability.*

Despite this legal mumbo jumbo, most nanotechnology business people already intuitively know what they want out of their business contracts and which areas are most important to them. There are, of course, an almost infinite different type of contracts used for different purposes: employment agreements, confidentiality agreements, supply agreements, service agreements, leases, purchase and sale agreements, financing, stock purchase agreements, government contracts, construction agreements, surety agreements, insurance contracts, guarantees, agency agreements, franchise, distribution, and joint development agreements, manufacturing agreements, master services contracts, and technology licensing agreements...you get the idea. Any or all of these contracts may involve nanotechnology businesses.

Some general considerations all nanotechnology businesses should keep in mind are that certain contracts must be in writing to be enforceable; contracts are generally construed against their drafter (thus it is important for a business to make sure the contract says exactly what it wants)[27]; courts

[27] *See, e.g., Mastrobuono v. Shearson Lehman Hutton, Inc.*, 514 US 52 (1995).

endeavor to give contracts a reasonable, fair, and practical construction[28]; and while the language of contract is normally given its ordinary meaning, ambiguity and vagueness often require judicial interpretation.[29] Additionally, businesses should be aware of the effect of prior negotiations and oral agreements on entering into a formal written contact.[30] Further, because laws vary from state to state, a nanotechnology business must make sure it avails itself of the most favorable applicable law and consider including an alternative dispute resolution clause to limit potential legal costs in the event of a future dispute. Attorney's fees provisions and legal forum selection clauses[31] should also be considered to make sure a company ends up in the most favorable court in the event of a dispute.

4.2.6 Government regulation

Nanotechnology-specific regulation must be carefully and thoroughly considered by every nanotechnology business. There is very little nano-specific regulation as of the date of this text. However, as nanotechnology progresses and matures, businesses will find that potential regulation may be prevalent in all stages of the nanotechnology legal product life cycle, especially in the supply, manufacturing, and disposal stages. In the US, federal regulation of engineered nanoscale materials is most likely to take place through the Environmental Protection Agency (EPA), the Food and Drug Administration (FDA), and the Consumer Product Safety Commission (CPSC). Workplace issues involving NIOSH and OSHA are discussed above. In the EU, regulatory authority is much more centralized. While there are a wide variety of agencies and committees which play an important preparatory role, it is always the European Commission, together with the European Parliament and the Council of Ministers, which prepares the actual regulation (Figure 4.5).

4.2.6.1 Consumer product safety

In the US, the CPSC is tasked with protecting the public against unreasonable risk of injury associated with consumer products.[32] A consumer product is an

---

[28] *See, e.g., Giove v. Department of Trans.*, 230 F. 3d 1333 (Fed. Cir. 2000).

[29] *See, e.g., Republican Nat. Committee v. Taylor*, 299 F.3d 887 (D.C. Cir. 2002).

[30] *See, e.g., Lanier Professional Services, Inc. v. Ricci*, 192 F.3d 1 (1st Cir. 1999).

[31] *See, e.g., Stephen A. Goldberg Co. v. Remsen Partners Ltd.*, 170 F.3d 191 (D.C. Cir. 1999).

[32] Consumer Product Safety Act, 15 U.S.C. §2051(b)(1) (2007), *available at* http://www.herc.org/library/cpsa.pdf.

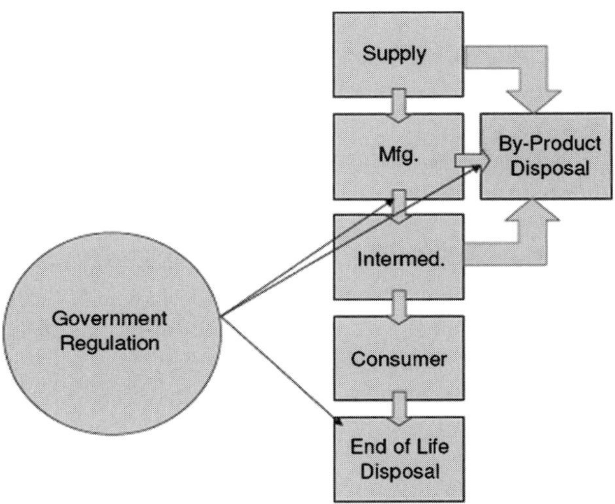

FIGURE 4.5 *Government Regulation.*

"article or component thereof used for the personal use, consumption or enjoyment of consumers."[33] It does not include tobacco, motor vehicles, pesticides, firearms, aircraft, boats, drugs, medical devices, cosmetics, or food, which are all regulated by other federal entities. The CPSC has broad powers to issue new safety standards, require product labels and warnings, require detailed written instructions, or even completely ban a product if it finds that it poses an unreasonable risk of injury to consumers.[34] Under the CPSC's statutory authority, a new consumer product rule, however, cannot be promulgated unless it is first determined to be "reasonably necessary to eliminate or reduce an unreasonable risk of injury associated with such product."[35] Additionally, the first step in any CPSC restriction is the application of existing voluntary standards, then mandatory standards if voluntary standards are inadequate, and finally resort to a product ban or labeling or other remedial measure which used if certain legal and factual findings are met.

The key to the process is that the CPSC must select the least burdensome requirement to prevent or adequately reduce the specific, targeted risk of injury. Beyond rule making power, the CPSC also has the legal authority

[33] Consumer Product Safety Act, 15 U.S.C. §2052(a)(1) (2007), *available at* http://www.herc.org/library/cpsa.pdf.

[34] Consumer Product Safety Act, 15 U.S.C. §2056(a)(1)–(2) and 2057 (2007), *available at* http://www.herc.org/library/cpsa.pdf.

[35] Consumer Product Safety Act, 15 U.S.C. §2058(f)(3)(A)–(F) (2007), *available at* http://www.herc.org/library/cpsa.pdf.

to bring a lawsuit to seize dangerous products or prevent their manufacturer or distribution if they present an imminently hazardous consumer risk. An "imminent risk" means a product that presents an "imminent and unreasonable risk of death, serious illness, or severe personal injury."[36] The CPSC also has complete legal authority to require manufacturers to recall or repair defective products and has access to civil and criminal penalties for noncompliance.

All existing consumer products containing engineered nanoscale materials are subject to existing consumer product safety laws. The jurisdiction and legal authority of the CPSC is more than broad enough to cover any potential risk posed by the use of nanoscale materials in consumer products (Innovation Society, 2007). Currently, there is no substantial evidence supporting the theory that the use of engineered nanoscale materials in existing consumer products poses any EHS dangers. This may change in the future.

While legal authority is not a major obstacle for the CPSC in dealing with potential nano-related EHS risks, funding and staff are. As of March 2007, the CPSC had only spent $US 20 000 on nanotechnology EHS research which primarily consisted of a literature review.[37] Appropriations for the CPSC for fiscal years 2009 and 2010 for nanotechnology EHS issues, however, total approximately $US 1 million each year.[38] In 2007 the Commissioner of the CPSC made a telling statement:

> *other agencies are asking for, and getting, millions of dollars for research in this area. Given the many products already on the market using nanotechnology, from computer chips to Docker pants, I do not think it will be too long before the agency is asked to assess the risks of nanotechnology used in some consumer products under our jurisdiction. At this point in time we would be hard pressed to make such an assessment. We simply do not have the resources to get up to speed in this area.*[39]

---

[36] Consumer Product Safety Act, 15 U.S.C. §2061(a)(3) (2007), *available at* http://www.herc.org/library/cpsa.pdf.

[37] Statement of Commissioner Thomas H. Moore submitted to the Subcommittee on Consumer Affairs, Insurance, and Automotive Safety, Senate Committee on Commerce, Science, and Transportation, 7 (2007), *available at* www.cpsc.gov/pr/moore2007.pdf.

[38] CPSC Reform Act, §2663, http://thomas.loc.gov/cgi-bin/query/z?c110:S.2663 (last visited 4 March 2009).

[39] Statement of Commissioner Thomas H. Moore submitted to the Subcommittee on Consumer Affairs, Insurance, and Automotive Safety, Senate Committee on Commerce, Science, and Transportation, 7 (2007), *available at* www.cpsc.gov/pr/moore2007.pdf.

The EU does not have an agency along the lines of the CPSC. As in the US, many of the products which are exempt from the CPSC are regulated under specific approval processes with relevant agencies acting in various advisory capacities. This includes food, drugs, and medical appliances (see below). Where no specific agency with attached regulatory framework exists, European Union law falls back on either general product safety laws which are a power of the Member States or on sector-specific Directives without a specific agency that has authority over it. Toys and the toys safety Directives are a case in point. With respect to general product liability, while the European product liability Directive[40] has been found to go further than merely minimum harmonization,[41] the regime in practice leaves so much to the Member States than one wonders whether the extent of harmonization truly deserves anything else but the qualification "minimum." Indeed a large number of issues which one cannot but consider the core of liability considerations, such as causation, remoteness of damage, standard of proof, contributory acts, assessment of damages, and discovery, are all left to the discretion of domestic law (Faigrieve, 2005). Hence to truly have an insight into how product liability law impacts on the development of new technologies, one would have to review all case-law of the various Member States—or at least the key States. The danger of having 27 different liability regimes often is a strong incentive for the Commission to act on the basis of its powers for the preservation of the Internal Market: with manufacturers having to produce in accordance with agreed health, safety, and environment standards, the Internal Market may be safeguarded.

4.2.6.2 Environmental regulation

In the US, federal environmental regulation of engineered nanoscale materials is most likely to occur under the Toxic Substances Control Act, the Federal Insecticide, Fungicide, and Rodenticide Act, the Resource Conservation and Recovery Act, the Comprehensive Environmental Response Compensation and Liability Act, and other "traditional" environmental statutes which focus on "end of pipe" or "end of stack" emissions. Additionally, there is a slow but growing trend of local and state regulation. Government regulation is most likely to affect the manufacturing and disposal stages of the nanotechnology product legal life cycle. For most if

[40] Directive 85/374 on the approximation of the laws, regulations, and administrative provisions of the Member States concerning liability for defective products (1985) OJ L210.

[41] See the case-law of the European Court of Justice: Case C-183/00, *Gonzalez Sanchez v. Medicina Asturiana SA* (2002) ECR I-3901.

not all of these various sectors, there are equivalent legal instruments in the European Union, albeit with differing contents as we shall see below.

4.2.6.2.1 Toxic substances control act

The Toxic Substances Control Act (TSCA) is a comprehensive federal environmental regulatory scheme covering the manufacturing, distribution, sale, and use of all chemical substances. TSCA provides the US EPA with full legal authority to gather EHS information and to require research regarding chemical substances of potential concern.[42] The manufacture of existing chemical substances is strictly controlled and regulated. The manufacture of new chemical substances can only occur after proper application and safety documentation.[43] There are strict civil and criminal penalties for TSCA violations, including injunctive relief and large financial penalties.

4.2.6.2.1.1 New chemical substances

One of the key questions regarding engineered nanoscale materials under TSCA is whether they constitute new chemical substances and/or significant new uses of existing chemical substances for regulatory purposes. If an engineered nanoscale material falls into either of these categories, a manufacturer must submit a pre-manufacturing notice and application to EPA substantiating the safety of the product given the proposed use.

In 2007, EPA published an issue paper explaining its treatment of engineered nanoscale materials under TSCA and whether it considered any or all of them new or existing chemical substances for regulatory purposes (Environmental Protection Agency, 2007). The EPA indicated that it does not consider *all* nanoscale materials to be new chemical substances just because of their diminutive size. Rather, a particular engineered nanoscale material must have a new and distinct molecular identity not shared with any other existing chemical substance on the TSCA inventory before it is considered a "new" chemical substance. EPA indicated that it was going to examine each nanoscale material in question on a case-by-case basis to determine whether it was in fact a new or existing chemical substance for purposes of TSCA and would make no blanket statements in this regard.

In October 2008, EPA issued a federal register notice reiterating its position that it would not treat all nanoscale materials as new chemical substances under TSCA (Environmental Protection Agency, 2008a). However, EPA also classified carbon nanotubes as new and distinct chemical

---

[42] *Chemical Manufacturers Association v. EPA*, 259 F.2d 977, 979 (D.C. Cir. 1988).

[43] Toxic Substances Control Act, 15 U.S.C. §2604(a) (2007), *available at* http://epw.senate.gov/tsca.pdf.

substances from graphite or other carbon allotropes previously listed on TSCA inventory and stated that they are subject to pre-manufacturing notice and application requirements. EPA encouraged all carbon nanotube manufacturers to submit pre-manufacturing notice applications under TSCA as quickly as possible and indicated that it would start enforcing its ruling regarding carbon nanotubes in March of 2009 (Environmental Protection Agency, 2008a). The EPA also recommended that companies in doubt as to whether their specific engineered nanoscale material constitutes a "new" chemical substance for TSCA purposes should submit a request for an inventory search to clarify the issue.

Beyond its TSCA guidance documents, thus far, EPA has entered into two consent orders under TSCA requiring the manufacturer to conduct 90-day inhalation studies to analyze the acute toxicity of the products in question (Office of Pollution Prevention and Toxics, 2008). The agency's impetus for these consent orders was its lack of knowledge concerning their possible health effects on humans coupled with purported tests on analogous substances which showed potential toxicity concerns. Specifically, while EPA predicted poor human absorption of carbon nanotubes through all exposure routes, it expressed concern regarding possible lung irritation and exposure from analogous respirable, poorly soluble particles. Accordingly, EPA stated that there might be a potential risk to workers exposed to carbon nanotubes through inhalation and/or dermal exposure. The agency further noted a potential risk to the public from water and landfill disposal or the incineration of carbon nanotubes.

4.2.6.2.1.2 Significant new uses of existing chemical substances

Beyond "new" chemical substances, if EPA determines that a specified use of an existing chemical substance constitutes a "significant new use" of that substance, pre-manufacturing notice and approval requirements are also triggered. The relevant factors in determining whether a proposed use constitutes a significant new use are the projected volume of manufacturing and processing of the substance; the extent to which there are changes in the type or form of exposure resulting from the specified use; whether there is an increase in the magnitude or duration of exposure from the proposed use; and the methods of manufacturing, processing, distributing, and disposing of the chemical substance.[44] No factor is conclusive by itself. Some EHS advocates have lobbied EPA to issue a blanket rule stating that the use of all nanoscale

---

[44] Toxic Substances Control Act, 15 U.S.C. §2604(a)(2) (2007), *available at* http://epw.senate.gov/tsca.pdf.

materials constitutes "significant new use" of an existing substance under TSCA (Section of Environment, Energy, and Resources, American Bar Association, 2006). The agency, however, has indicated that it has no intent to issue a categorical significant new use rule for all nanoscale materials, rather it intends to examine them on a case-by-case basis considering the four above-reference factors (Monica, 2007).

Applying these factors, EPA has issued significant new use rules for two engineered nanoscale materials used as additives in other chemical products as of the date of this text.[45] The engineered nanoscale materials in question were siloxane-modified silica nanoparticles and siloxane-modified alumina nanoparticles. Each chemical substance was the subject of a pre-manufacturing notice submission under TSCA which triggered EPA's review. The agency made it clear that possible dermal and inhalation exposure to the substances was not anticipated under the uses set forth in the applications. The agency further declined to determine whether the substances actually posed unreasonable risks, but expressed concern that based on analogous materials, the engineered nanoscale materials in question might present inhalation and/or dermal penetration concerns. Accordingly, EPA's significant new use rules required the manufacturers to ensure that the materials were not used in occupational settings without the use of impervious gloves and NIOSH approved respirators. Additionally, the significant new use rules prohibited the use of the substances in powder form.

4.2.6.2.2 Nanoscale materials stewardship program

Most of EPA's efforts under TSCA thus far address the potential EHS concerns accompanying the use of certain engineered nanoscale materials are focused on its Nanoscale Materials Stewardship Program (NMSP) which was created and implemented under TSCA (Environmental Protection Agency, 2008a). The NMSP was first implemented in February 2008 and is designed to collect existing data from manufacturers of engineered nanoscale materials for later use in possible regulation. While EPA has publicly stated that regulation is not the inevitable outcome of the NMSP, few nanotechnology companies believe otherwise.

The NMSP asks participants to submit information and data regarding their engineered nanoscale materials to EPA under two plan levels.

The first, "basic" plan level seeks data regarding existing material characterization, hazard, use, potential exposure, and risk management practices.

[45] Significant New Use Rule on Certain Chemical Substances, 40 CFR §721.10119 (2008), *available at* http://edocket.access.gpo.gov/2008/E8-26409.htm.

EPA believes this information should be readily available to most nanoscale material manufacturers. As of December 2008, 29 companies had submitted basic information covering 123 nanoscale materials under the "basic" plan level. The second, "in depth" level of the NMSP asks companies to partner with each other and EPA to generate new data on specific nanoscale materials of interest. This portion of the NMSP will take several years to complete. As of December 2008, four companies had committed to working with EPA under the "in depth" program.

In January 2009, EPA published an interim report on the successes and failures of its NMSP to date (Office of Pollution Prevention and Toxics, 2009). The agency admitted mixed results. On the one hand, EPA stated that "the program has sufficiently advanced EPA's knowledge and understanding to enable the agency to take further steps towards evaluating and, where appropriate, mitigating potential risks to health and the environment." On the other hand, the agency noted that at least 90% of the existing nanoscale chemical substances which are commercially available were not reported under the program thus far. The report also found that "the low rate of engagement in the in-depth program suggests that most companies are not inclined to voluntarily test their nanoscale materials" (Office of Pollution Prevention and Toxics, 2009, p. 27).

EPA will issue a final report on the NMSP in 2010. Unless something surprising develops, it is difficult to imagine that it will be possible to genuinely characterize the NMSP as successful.

4.2.6.2.3 Reach

As for the European counterpart for TSCA, the Regulation on the Registration, Evaluation, Authorization, and Restriction of Chemicals (REACH) (Regulation 1907/2006) (European Commission, 2006), signaled a fundamental shift in the way in which manufactured and imported chemical substances are regulated within the EU (Bowman and van Calster, 2007a, 2007b). REACH prohibits the manufacture or sale of any chemical substance in the EU that has not been registered with the agency. Unlike the previous EU chemical regulatory regime, which somewhat arbitrarily differentiated between chemical substances on the basis of being "existing" or "new," REACH creates a uniform regime for the registration of all substances. Registration is volume-based, with registration and risk assessment requirements dependent upon the mass of the chemical substance manufactured, imported, or produced by each manufacturer, importer, or producer (the registrant) each calendar year. As with the previous regime, REACH does not differentiate substances on the basis of their size, but rather on the basis of the substance's Chemical Abstract Service (CAS) number. However, in

light of the ultimately unsuccessful last minute attempt by Members of the Committee on the Environmental, Public Health, and Food Safety of the European Parliament to include specific provisions on engineered nanoparticles (Committee on the Environment, Public Health and Food Safety of the European Parliament, 2006), uncertainty remains as to how nanoscale substances may be treated by the regulator, the newly established European Chemicals Agency, as REACH is rolled-out. Review has already led to a removal of nanoparticles from the exemption of "naturally occurring substances" such as carbon, and the Head of the agency announced as recently as June 2009 that the agency is likely to adapt specific rules as to how nanoparticles will be treated under REACH.

4.2.6.2.4 Federal insecticide, fungicide, and rodenticide act

EPA has also levied a fine against one US nanotechnology company under the Federal Insecticide, Fungicide, and Rodenticide Act for marketing a product containing engineered nanoscale materials using claims that the product killed germs and microbes (Environmental Protection Agency, 2008b). The company was based in California and was selling computer mice and keyboards coated with nanoscale silver claiming that the coatings killed germs and pathogens. Once such claims are made, the product is treated as a pesticide under the Federal Insecticide, Fungicide, and Rodenticide Act.[46] At that point, any antimicrobial or germ killing claims must be substantiated through formal data submissions.[47] Because the company made the claims without first registering the product as a pesticide and/or submitting substantiating data, EPA fined the company $208,000.

There are numerous examples of products claiming to contain engineered nanoscale materials that are used to kill germs. Undoubtedly, EPA will similarly pursue these companies in the coming years.

4.2.6.2.5 Resource conservation and recovery act

The disposal stage in the nanotechnology product legal life cycle also presents specific issues regarding engineered nanoscale materials. The primary statutes in the US used to regulate the disposal of chemical substances are the

---

[46] Federal Insecticide, Fungicide, and Rodenticide Act, 7 U.S.C. 136(mm)(1) (2008), *available at* http://www.law.cornell.edu/uscode/html/uscode07/usc_sup_01_7_10_6_20_II.html.

[47] Federal Insecticide, Fungicide, and Rodenticide Act, 7 U.S.C. 136a(c) (2008), *available at* http://www.law.cornell.edu/uscode/html/uscode07/usc_sup_01_7_10_6_20_II.html.

Resource Conservation and Recovery Act (RCRA) and the Comprehensive Environmental Response Compensation and Liability Act.

Under RCRA, the federal government regulates the disposal of both solid wastes and hazardous wastes. A substance can only be a hazardous waste if it is first determined to be a "solid waste" under RCRA's analysis. The disposal of "hazardous wastes" is regulated much more strictly than the disposal of simple solid wastes. A solid waste is broadly defined as "any garbage, refuse, sludge from a waste treatment plant, water supply treatment plant, or air pollution control facility and any other discarded material, including solid, liquid, semi solid, or contained gaseous material resulting from industrial, commercial, mining, and agricultural operations, and from community activities."[48] Although no engineered nanoscale materials are currently specifically denominated solid wastes under RCRA, the definition is broad enough to capture almost any such material. Solid wastes must be disposed of in strict conformance with state or regional waste plans and may only be disposed of at sanitary landfills. These same requirements also apply to waste streams from manufacturing processes using engineered nanoscale materials.

Beyond solid wastes, a chemical substance may be labeled as a "hazardous waste" under RCRA if it is listed as a hazardous waste by EPA or if it is determined to be a characteristic "hazardous waste" that exhibits high ignitability, corrosivity, reactivity, or toxicity. Once a material is labeled as a hazardous waste, the material is tracked and permitted at all stages of the manufacturing, use, and disposal process.[49] Generators of hazardous wastes are required to keep detailed records from cradle to grave of the substance to ensure unintended releases and environmental contamination do not occur.[50]

In the EC, attention to the waste side of nanotechnologies has been slow in uptake, to say the least. The European Commission's line on waste and nanotechnologies is that in light of the generic nature of the provisions of the relevant Directives, the issues are at least covered in principle (European Commission, 2008). As we shall see below, the European Parliament in particular is ever less likely to buy this line.

---

[48] Resource Conservation and Recovery Act, 42 U.S.C. §6903(27) (2002), *available at* http://www4.law.cornell.edu/uscode/42/ch82.html.

[49] Resource Conservation and Recovery Act, 42 U.S.C. §6941 (2002), *available at* http://www4.law.cornell.edu/uscode/42/ch82.html.

[50] Resource Conservation and Recovery Act, 42 U.S.C. §6922 (2000), *available at* http://www4.law.cornell.edu/uscode/42/ch82.html.

4.2.6.2.6 Comprehensive environmental response compensation and liability act

The Comprehensive Environmental Response Compensation and Liability Act was first enacted in 1980 with the purpose of cleaning up abandoned hazardous waste sites and assigning financial responsibility. CERCLA applies very broadly to all "hazardous substances." These include many substances on specific lists created by EPA under the act, as well as other substances designated as hazardous under other federal statutes.[51] Because it is so broad, the definition of "hazardous substance" under CERCLA covers virtually any engineered nanoscale material which might present EHS risks. Thus far, no engineered nanoscale materials have been treated as a hazardous substance under CERCLA simply because it is a nanoscale material. The biggest hurdle for applying CERCLA to a specific engineered nanoscale material is determining whether it is deemed a hazardous substance under the statute. Once this scientific determination is complete, CERCLA's broad cleanup and cost apportionment provisions would apply (Section of Environment, Energy, and Resources, American Bar Association, 2006).

Perhaps the points nanotechnology companies should remember most about CERCLA are (1) it can be applied retroactively and (2) liability can be joint, individual, and several (Section of Environment, Energy, and Resources, American Bar Association, 2006). The first point is important because even if engineered nanoscale materials are not considered a hazardous substance today, they may be considered as such tomorrow after the fact. The second point is important because a company with deep pockets may find itself liable for the entire cleanup costs of a contaminated site even if it only contributed a relatively small amount of material to the site. This may be especially important years down the road when other companies which may have been primary contributors have been long dissolved.

The EU's *environmental liability* regime[52] imposes inter alia a strict liability regime for operators carrying out "hazardous" activities. They will be held strictly liable (i.e., there will be no need to show fault or negligence) for preventing or restoring any damage caused by those activities to land, water, and protected habitats and species. It is noteworthy that the liability Directive does not cover "traditional damage," i.e., personal injury and damage to personal goods and property—for such damage, the various liability regimes of the Member States apply.

---

[51] Comprehensive Environmental Response Compensation and Liability Act, 42 U.S.C. §9601(14), *available at* http://www4.law.cornell.edu/uscode/42/ch103.html.

[52] Directive 2004/35, OJ (2004) L143/56.

"Hazardous activities" include manufacture, use, storage, processing, filling, release into the environment, and onsite transport of those substances which are classified as dangerous substances under the EU's chemical legislation, referred to above. Hence there is a direct link between the classification under the EU's chemical policy and the ensuing liability.

Again, though, no specific proviso has been made in the liability Directive for nanotechnology per se. Interestingly, at the time of negotiation of the Directive, the need was discussed for a specific liability regime for genetically modified organisms (GMOs), so as to address the uncertainty associated with the technology. Eventually, a consensus was found to leave GMOs within the standard remit of the Directive, pending further evaluation of the need to review this, by the Commission. Hence the Directive fully applies to GM technology, including the Directive's defenses: if the release of the GMO was specifically authorized or if it was not possible to anticipate the damaging effect on the basis of the state of scientific and technical knowledge at the time, and if the operator was not negligent, all of which the operator has to prove, the competent authorities can exempt him/her from liability. For example, an operator would be negligent and thus liable if it does not follow the instructions provided by the GMO manufacturer or the competent authority authorizing the release (European Commission, 2004).

Similar considerations obviously apply to nanotechnology. In the current regulatory state, nanotechnological applications are not likely to have been specifically authorized, hence the defense one would have to raise relates to it not having been possible to anticipate the damaging effect on the basis of the scientific knowledge at the time.

4.2.6.2.7 Traditional end of pipe environmental regulation

Finally, the applicability of "traditional" end of pipe and end of stack environmental regulations such as the Clean Air Act,[53] Clean Water Act,[54] Safe Drinking Water Act,[55] and similar instruments in the EC to engineered nanoscale materials has been questioned because these regulations typically rely on mass determinants which may be inappropriate for engineered nanoscale materials. Simply put, number of particles and surface area may be

[53] Environmental Protection Agency, Clean Air Act, History of the Clean Air Act, http://www.epa.gov/air/caa/caa_history.html (last visited April 3, 2009).

[54] Clean Water Act, 33 U.S.C. §§1251(a), *available at* http://www.law.cornell.edu/uscode/html/uscode33/usc_sup_01_33_10_26.html.

[55] Safe Drinking Water Act, 42 U.S.C. §300g (1996), *available at* http://www.law.cornell.edu/uscode/42/usc_sup_01_42_10_6A_20_XII_30_B.html.

more appropriate measures for the potential toxicity and hazards presented by certain engineered nanoscale materials rather than mass. Thus, traditional statutory triggers may be inappropriate. Whether these regulations need to be amended to encompass nanoscale materials is a subject of much debate. Of course, these statutes in their current form already apply to the bulk versions of certain nanoscale substances and there is no current substantial scientific evidence that they should be treated otherwise.

4.2.6.2.7.1 Food and drug regulation

The US FDA formed a Nanotechnology Task Force in August 2006 to assess the state of scientific knowledge concerning nano-related EHS concerns and evaluate the effectiveness of existing food and drug regulations to deal with any unique issues raised by nanotechnology (Food and Drug Administration, 2006). The Nanotechnology Task Force issued its first written report in July 2007 which did not call for any new FDA regulatory authority to cover engineered nanoscale materials and concluded that the use of nanomaterials in FDA-regulated products presents completely manageable challenges similar to those posed by other existing FDA-regulated products (Food and Drug Administration, 2007). However, FDA admitted that some of the unique properties exhibited by certain engineered nanoscale materials could at some point create regulatory challenges and recommended developing guidance documents to clarify what information manufacturers should provide to FDA about nanotechnology products and the circumstances under which the regulatory status of certain products might change. As of May 2009, there is no intent to update, modify, or change the FDA's report.

The European Parliament on 24 April 2009 adopted a resolution[56] on regulatory aspects of nanomaterials and also voted to include nano-specific provisions in cosmetics and food legislation. The Resolution includes some important regulatory constraints for the nanotechnologies sector, in particular for those incorporating nanomaterials in products. Most importantly, the text testifies to the increased readiness within the regulatory community to adopt targeted, nano-specific regulation. Parliament has employed its regulatory powers by proposing a much more proactive approach to nanoregulation in two areas: the review of cosmetics law in Europe (Bowman and van Calster, 2008) and a similar update for so-called novel foods (van Calster et al., in press), where it proposes special treatment of nanoparticles and nanomaterials.[57]

[56] European Parliament, Resolution of 24 April 2009 on regulatory aspects of nanomaterials, P6_TA(2009)0328.

[57] European Parliament legislative resolution of 24 March 2009 on the proposal for a regulation on novel foods, A6-0512/2008.

According to the proposal, nano-specific test methods should be developed as a matter of urgency and nanomaterials present in food should be entered on a list of approved nanomaterials, for food contact materials accompanied by a limit on migration into or onto the food products contained in such packaging. This means that until such methods have been developed in practice, no such materials will be allowed in the market—in other words, a moratorium.

The European Parliament also proposes to amend the definition of a "novel food" to include food containing or consisting of "engineered nanomaterials," however, Members of the European Parliament did not support the inclusion of terminology referring to "produced with the aid of nanotechnology." All ingredients present in the form of nanomaterials will have to be clearly indicated in the list of ingredients. It is not clear at the moment whether Parliament will have enough support from Council for it to push through its proposals. "Engineered nanomaterials" is defined by Parliament as:

> *any intentionally produced material that has one or more dimensions of the order of 100 nm or less or is composed of discrete functional parts, either internally or at the surface, many of which have one or more dimensions of the order of 100 nm or less, including structures, agglomerates or aggregates, which may have a size above the order of 100 nm but retain properties that are characteristic to the nanoscale. Properties that are characteristic to the nanoscale include: (i) those related to the large specific surface area of the materials considered and/or (ii) specific physico-chemical properties that are different from those of the non-nanoform of the same material.*

Parliament advocates in other words a freeze on market authorization for products with nanoparticles that are not readily soluble or biodegradable. In its view this would be an implied consequence of the precautionary principle.

The move is highly significant, as it would be the first time a major jurisdiction adopts specific regulations to deal with the risks perceived from nanotechnologies.

4.2.6.3 Local and State regulation in the United States

4.2.6.3.1 Berkeley, California

In December 2006, Berkeley, California indicated that it was tired of waiting for EPA to specifically regulate nanotechnology and amended its own hazardous material ordinance to encompass engineered nanoscale materials. The City's amended ordinance now states that "all facilities that manufacture or use manufactured nanoparticles shall submit a separate written disclosure of the current toxicology of the materials reported, to the extent known, and how the facility will safely handle, monitor, contain, dispose, track inventories, prevent release and mitigate such material."[58] Nanoscale materials covered by the ordinance include "all manufactured nanoparticles defined as a particle with one axis less than 100 nanometers in length."[59]

The City further issued disclosure guidelines in the Spring of 2007 for companies seeking more information on exactly how to comply with the amended ordinance (City of Berkeley, 2007). The guidelines indicated that the City was seeking five types of toxicity data: inhalation, dermal, oral, genotoxic, and reproductive. Recognizing that this extensive toxicity data may not be available for most engineered nanoscale materials, the City's guidelines stated that "if an exposure potential is present but insufficient toxicological information is available, a precautionary approach should be taken which assumes that the material is toxic." Additionally, the guidelines mandate that companies reporting under the ordinance prioritize their activities involving engineered nanoscale materials into four control bands depending upon the uncertainty of the toxicity and the possibility of exposure.

4.2.6.3.2 Cambridge, Massachusetts

In January 2007, Cambridge, Massachusetts considered whether it needed its own nanomaterials ordinance patterned after Berkeley, California. The City Manager asked Cambridge's Director of Environmental Health to create a committee of experts to recommend a subsequent course of action (Cambridge Nanomaterials Advisory Committee, Cambridge Public Health Department, 2008). The Director put together a nanotechnology advisory committee which met for 6 months to consider various options. The committee was made up of public citizens, academic experts, private consultants, lawyers, industry representatives, and representatives from non-governmental organizations. Rather than jumping to conclusions, the committee heard detailed presentations on nanotoxicology issues, the oversight of nanomaterials in an academic setting, an overview of existing federal laws and regulations pertaining to nanoscale materials, and an overview of existing nanoscale material risk management frameworks. In May 2008, the committee reported back to the City Manager with a written report primarily

[58] Berkeley, Cal. Ordinance ch. 15.12, §15.12.040(I) (2006).

[59] Berkeley, Cal. Ordinance ch. 15.12, §15.12.050(C)(7) (2006).

focused on potential workplace exposure risks and those possibly posed to the general public through manufacturing processes (Cambridge Nanomaterials Advisory Committee, Cambridge Public Health Department, 2008). The report concluded that while the City should continue to monitor scientific and legal developments, the existing science was too inconclusive to recommend creating any new city ordinance specifically aimed at engineered nanoscale materials.

4.2.6.3.3 State of California

In January 2009, California's Department of Toxic Substances Control issued a formal chemical information call in letter to 26 entities involved in the manufacturing of carbon nanotubes. The manufacturers have 1 year to respond to the letter under California Health and Safety Code Chapter 699.[60] The data requested by the State include information regarding the specific products in which the carbon nanotubes are used; quantities used; major customers; sampling detection and monitoring methods; quality assurance and quality control protocols; potential environmental risks; knowledge of the safety of carbon nanotubes in terms of occupational safety, public health, and the environment; worker protection methods; and environmental protection methods. The letter also poses three questions recipients should carefully consider before answering: "When released, does your material constitute a hazardous waste under California Health and Safety Code provisions? Are discarded off spec materials a hazardous waste? Once discarded are the carbon nanotubes you produce a hazardous waste?"

California has indicated that its data call in efforts for engineered nanoscale materials will not end with carbon nanotubes. Rather, it intends to issue a series of letters over the coming months, focusing on various types of engineered nanoscale materials of potential concern.

4.2.7 Product and tort liability in the United States

As noted, in the EU, product and tort liability are organized exclusively along national lines, and a review within the context of this article is meaningless. Product and tort liability may be prevalent in all stages of the nanotechnology product legal life cycle, especially in the supply, manufacturing, and disposal stages. In the US, key tort liability theories are negligence, strict product

[60] Cal. Health & Safety Code, ch. 699, §57019 (2008) *available at* http://www.leginfo.ca.gov/cgi-bin/waisgate?WAISdocID=21332418341+0+0+0&WAISaction=retrieve.

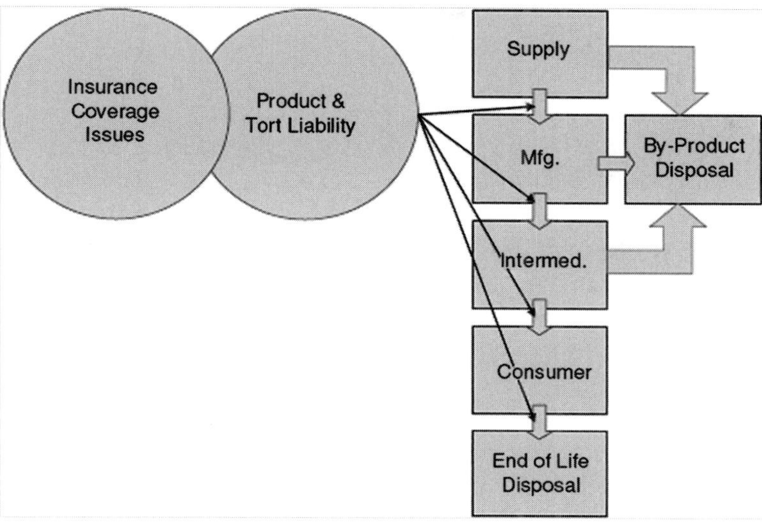

FIGURE 4.6 *Product and Tort Liability.*

liability, and intentional or reckless torts which may generate punitive damages. One of the biggest issues accompanying such potential tort liability is insurance coverage (Figure 4.6).

4.2.7.1 Negligence

If a manufacturer or supplier negligently makes a product which is then sold and injures a third party, that company may face lawsuits regarding the most basic form of tort liability—negligence. Simply put, a company may be found liable for the tort of negligence if the company failed to act reasonably in light of the circumstances presented in the case and that failure was a cause of a person's actual injury.[61] The factual focus under this theory is whether the manufacturer acted reasonably in the particular situation at hand and owed the injured party that duty.[62] The tort theory of negligence became most prominent in the 1940s and 1950s. Injured plaintiffs had to prove that a manufacturer acted outside the standard of normal care. This was sometimes difficult to prove, and courts ultimately

[61] *See, e.g., Briggs v. Washington Metropolitan Area Transit Authority*, 481 F.3d 839 (2007); *Japan Airlines co., Lt. v. Port Authority of New York and New Jersey*, 178 F.3d 103 (2d Cir. 1999).

[62] *Alexander v. Pathfinder, Inc.*, 189 F.3d 735 (8th Cir. 1999).

started pushing strict liability toward manufacturers for public policy reasons. In the 1960s, California led the way toward modern strict liability for product defects without regard to fault or negligence by the manufacturer.

4.2.7.2 Product liability

Rather than focusing on a manufacturer's conduct, the legal theory of strict product liability focuses on the product itself. If the product is defective in any demonstrable way, liability attaches and the manufacturer may be held liable for the injuries of anyone hurt by the product. This type of tort liability is most prevalent in the manufacturing stage of our nanotechnology product legal life cycle.

According to Black's Law Dictionary (1979, p. 1275), strict liability means liability "without fault, when neither care nor negligence, neither good faith nor bad faith, neither knowledge nor ignorance will save the defendant." Product liability is strict liability. A manufacturer can be liable for injuries related to its product even if it did not act negligently, in bad faith, or in ignorance. Damages may include compensation for economic pain and suffering, as well as punitive damages in certain circumstances. There are three primary types of product liability claims: design defect, manufacturing defect, and failure to adequately warn or instruct users.

4.2.7.2.1 Design defects

"Design defect" claims are those that are brought against a manufacturer or supplier when reasonably foreseeable risks of injury from the product could have been reduced or avoided through the implementation of a reasonable alternative design. A design defect occurs when there is something fundamental to a product's design that causes unreasonable risk of injury. Under the Restatement of Torts, a product is defectively designed when it is sold if "the foreseeable risks of harm posed by the product could have been reduced or avoided by the adoption of a reasonable alternative design, and the omission of the alternative design renders the product not reasonably safe."[63] When determining whether a design was defective in any given case, courts often balance the likelihood and gravity of potential injury against the utility of the product, the availability of other safer products to meet the same need, the obviousness of the use and potential injury, and the ability to eliminate or minimize the danger without seriously impairing the product or making it

[63] Restatement (Third) of Torts §2 (1998).

unduly expensive.[64] Thus, determining whether a product has a design defect is often a complicated task. Design defect claims are the most likely type to be asserted against manufacturers using engineered nanoscale materials in their products. A consumer who is exposed to nanoscale materials from a product he or she purchases and is subsequently injured will most likely claim that the very design of the product was defective. The consumer's attorney will allege that existing scientific studies at the time of manufacture highlighted the potential exposure risks to the particular nanoscale material in question and that the use of this material in the product was unreasonable given these risks. The scientific literature has not yet reached the point to make these types of claims attractive to plaintiffs' attorneys. Thus far, there have been no design defect product liability claims filed against a manufacturer of engineered nanoscale materials.

4.2.7.2.2 Manufacturing defect

"Manufacturing defect" claims are those that are asserted against a manufacturer or supplier when a product is safely designed, but the product in question departed from its intended design and injured someone.[65] A manufacturing defect occurs when a "product departs from its intended design even though all possible care was exercised in the preparation or marketing of the product."[66] An example would be if the design of a product is completely safe and called for the use of one specific engineered nanoscale material, but the manufacturer substituted a cheaper alternative and the substitution somehow ended up hurting a consumer. If the use of the substituted material causes a consumer injury and the consumer's lawyer learns of the deviation, he may allege that because the design was not followed to the letter the product was defectively manufactured and the manufacturer is strictly liable for his client's injuries. Again, a manufacturing defect product liability claim is a strict liability tort. Liability may be imposed regardless of the amount of effort a manufacturer puts into the manufacturing and quality control processes. The theory is that strict

---

[64] Restatement (Third) of Torts §2 cmt. d, ¶ II(B) (1998) (quoting *Radiation Technology, Inc. v. Ware Constr. Co.*, 445 So.2d 329 (Fla. 1983)) (emphasis added). For other examples of courts applying this basic reasoning *see also, Brooks c. Beech Aircraft Corp.*, 902 P.2d 54 (N.M. 1995); *Claytor v. General Motors Corp.*, 286 S.E.2d 129 (S.C. 1982) (describing South Carolina's risk balancing test).

[65] Restatement (Third) of Torts §2(a) (1998). *See, also, Caterpillar Tractor Co. V. Beck*, 593 P.2d 871, 881 (Alaska 1979); *Barker v. Lull Engineering Co.*, 573 P.2d 443, 454 (Cal. 1978) (defining a manufacturing defect as one that "differs from manufacturer's intended result or other ostensible identical units of the same product line").

[66] Restatement (Third) of Torts §2 cmt. a. (1998).

liability makes a good deterrent and increases safety.[67] Thus far, there have been no manufacturing defect claims against a manufacturer of an engineered nanoscale product based on the "nano-ness" of that product.

4.2.7.2.3 Failure to adequately warn or instruct

Product liability claims for failure to adequately warn or instruct a consumer about the dangers presented by a product arise when the foreseeable risk of injury could have been avoided through use of reasonable instructions or warnings provided by the manufacturer. As a legal matter, inadequate instructions or warnings result "when the foreseeable risks of harm posed by the product could have been reduced or avoided by the provision of a reasonable instructions where warnings, and the omission of the instructions or warnings renders the product not reasonably safe."[68] Generally, warnings and instructions accompanying a product must "alert users and consumers to the existence and nature of product risks so that they can prevent harm either by appropriate conduct during use or consumption or by choosing not to use or consume."[69] Additionally manufacturers are required to warn users about nonobvious and not generally known risks that are inherent in using the product. The issue of how much warning is sufficient is generally driven by the facts and circumstances in a particular case. Generally under the Restatement of Torts, "warnings must be provided for inherent risks that reasonably foreseeable product users and consumers would reasonably deem material were significant in deciding whether to use or consume the product."[70] On the other hand, warnings are not generally required for open and obvious risks. Currently, the science is still out regarding whether engineered nanoscale materials may present EHS risks in realistic exposure settings. Manufacturers, however, should be aware of this developing body of scientific literature, determine whether their products are sufficiently safe in light of these studies, and carefully consider what nano-specific safety warnings and instructions (if any) should accompany products under these standards.

4.2.7.2.4 Punitive damages

Punitive damages are awarded in civil tort actions in excess of actual compensatory damages due to a defendant's conduct which the judicial system finds particularly egregious or malicious. There is no independent

[67] *Hoven v. Kelble*, 256 N.W.2d 379, 391 (Wis. 1977).

[68] Restatement (Third) of Torts §2(c) (1998).

[69] Restatement (Third) of Torts §2(c) cmt. i (1998).

[70] Restatement (Third) of Torts §2(c) cmt. i (1998).

cause of action for punitive damages, and simply committing a "standard" tort will not warrant punitive damages by itself. The conduct in question must be reckless, egregious, "ruthless," outrageous, "evil," and/or with malice.[71] Punitive damages are awarded to punish and make an example out of the defendant to deter similar future behavior.[72]

Although it is sometimes hard to determine from awards in modern tort cases, punitive damages are (or used to be) generally disfavored by the law and only awarded in very limited circumstances. Because of complaints about monetary "windfalls" to successful plaintiffs and their attorneys, some states have capped punitive damage awards and the US Supreme Court has determined that punitive damages must bear some reasonable relationship and size to the underlying conduct which generated the tort claim.[73] For purposes of our nanotechnology product legal life cycle, punitive damages for intentional torts may occur at any juncture a tort may occur. "Intentionally" setting out to hurt someone is never part of a business plan, however, nanotechnology businesses must be aware that if they conceal potential EHS risks posed by their products—or turn a blind eye toward them—they may be open to intentional tort claims supporting punitive damages.

4.2.7.3 Commercial insurance coverage

One of the largest issues accompanying potential product and tort liability claims is whether commercial insurance will cover any such occurrences. Without insurance, it is almost impossible to successfully operate in the modern commercial world. From the insurers' perspective, it is difficult to determine exactly how to insure a potential new risk with unknown health effects and exposure rates.

One insurer theorizes that nanotechnology insurance coverage issues will appear in three stages (Blaunstein, 2006). First will be the Early Study Period during which nanotechnology risks may already be covered by existing commercial insurance policies, but are not separately delineated. It is during this stage that the insurance industry will strive to assess potential risks and exposures. The second stage is the Apprehensive Phase during which the insurance industry may attempt to reduce coverage exposure by using sublimits and claims made coverage. The third and final phase is the Mature

---

[71] *See, e.g., Choctaw Maid Farms, Inc. v. Hailey*, 822 So.2d 911 (Miss. 2002); *Wearer v. Stafford*, 8 P.3d 1234 (Id. 2000); *Doe v. Isaacs*, 579 S.E.2d 174 (Va. 2003); *Horner v. Byrnett*, 511 S.E.2d 342 (N.C. 1999).

[72] *See, e.g., PPG Industries, Inc. v. Transamerica Inc. Co.*, 975 P.2d 652 (Ca. 1999).

[73] *See, e.g., Pacifico Mut. Life Ins. Co. v. Haslip*, 499 US 1 (1991).

Phase during which insurance companies offer specialized and customized insurance, solutions for their nanotechnology insureds. As of 2006, this insurer believed that we are in the Early Study Period.

In 2008, Lloyd's of London identified several options for insurers seeking to deal with the potential risks posed by issuing commercial insurance coverage for products and operations involving engineered nanoscale materials (Baxter, 2008). Lloyd's noted that insurers could choose to completely exclude coverage for nanotechnology, exclude nanotechnology from full coverage and then provide separate limited coverage for those risks, and/or only accept claims within a fixed period of time after a policy is written which would limit latent exposure. In the interim, Lloyd's noted that it will continue to monitor and research emerging risks potentially related to engineered nanoscale materials. Most other major commercial insurers are taking this same "wait and see" approach (Germano, 2008).

In the fall of 2008, however, one US insurance company—Continental Western Insurance Group—issued the first nano-specific commercial insurance exclusion in the US. The company explained that "the intent of this exclusion is to remove coverage for the, as of yet, unknown and unknowable risks created by-products and processes that involve nanotubes. The exclusion is being added to make you and your customers explicitly aware of our intent not to cover injury and/or damage arising from nanotubes, as used in products and processes" (Monica, 2008). Continental compared the possible risks insurers face by covering applications involving carbon nanotubes to those created by insuring asbestos in its early days. The specific exclusion issued by Continental covers "bodily injury, property damage, and personal and advertising injury related to the exposure of nanotubes and nanotechnology in any form. This includes the use of, contact with, existence of, presence of, proliferation of, discharge of, dispersal of, seepage of, migration of, release of, escape of, or exposure to nanotubes or nanotechnology" (Monica, 2008).

It remains to be seen whether Continental actually implemented its nano-specific exclusion. Shortly after posting these documents on its website, BNA published an article about the exclusion which created a stir. The documents were then quickly removed from Continental's website.

4.3 CONCLUSION

The regulatory debate on nanotechnologies is heating up. Were the European Parliament's amendments on nanotechnology in foodstuffs and cosmetics to be accepted—which they probably will be, industry will be faced with a much more urgent risks assessment and risk management exercise than previously

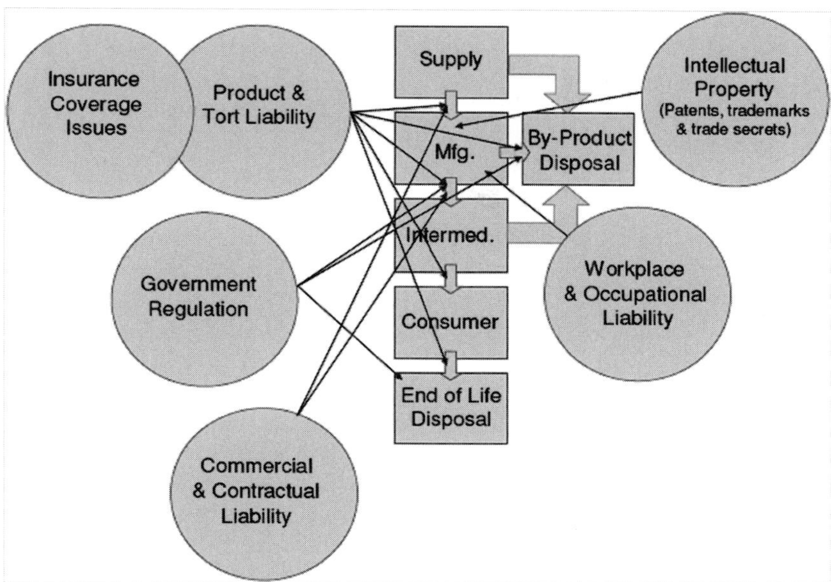

FIGURE 4.7 *Summary—A Complex Legal View.*

envisaged. Under the new US administration, too, various agencies have been tasked to review the regulatory oversight of nanotechnologies more urgently. In such a regulatory environment, monitoring manufacturer compliance and potential liability over the full product life cycle becomes even more important. The legal framework set forth above provides a good starting point for this analysis when overlaid by the various regulatory and/or liability pressure points. As Figure 4.7 depicts, taken all at once a complex legal web develops which can appear daunting. However, breaking down the issues piece-by-piece as outlined above should prove useful to attorneys, businesses, regulators, and non-governmental organizations examining these issues. By recognizing how the various stages of a nano-product's life cycle interact with legal and regulatory issues, a flexible nanotechnology legal framework results, which should be valuable to those examining nano-related EHS legal issues.

REFERENCES

Baxter, D., 2008. Nanotechnology: An Insurer's Perspective. Lloyd's of London, London.

Bawa, R., 2004. Nanotechnology patenting in the US. Nanotechnology Law and Business 1 (1), 31–51.

Black's Law Dictionary, 1979. West Publishing St. Paul.

Blaunstein, R., 2006. Unfamiliar exposure, insurance networking news. Available at: <http://www.insurancenetworking.com/issues/20061101/4372-1.html>.

Bowman, D.M., van Calster, G., 2007a. Reflecting on REACH: global implications of the European Union's chemicals regulation. Nanotechnology Law and Business 4 (3), 375–384.

Bowman, D.M., van Calster, G., 2007b. Does REACH go too far? Nature Nanotechnology 1, 525–526.

Bowman, D.M., van Calster, G., 2008. Flawless or fallible? A review of the applicability of the European Union's cosmetics directive in relation to nanocosmetics. Studies in Ethics, Law, and Technology 2 (3), 1–35.

Burge, D.A., 1984. Patent and Trademark Tactics and Practice. John Wiley & Son, New York.

Cambridge Nanomaterials Advisory Committee, Cambridge Public Health Department, July 2008. Recommendations for a Municipal Health & Safety Policy for Nanomaterials. A Report to the City Manager. Cambridge, Mass. Available at: <http://www.nanolawreport.com/Cambridge(1).pdf>.

Centers for Disease Control and Prevention, Department of Health and Human Services, 2006. Approaches to Safe Nanotechnology: An Information Exchange with NIOSH. National Institute for Occupational Safety and Health, Washington, DC. Available at. <http://www.cdc.gov/niosh/topics/nanotech/pdfs/Approaches_to_Safe_Nanotechnology.pdf>.

Centers for Disease Control and Prevention, Department of Health and Human Services, 2008. Draft Strategic Plan for NIOSH Nanotechnology Research and Guidance: Filling the Knowledge Gaps. National Institute for Occupational Safety and Health, Washington, DC. Available at. <http://www.cdc.gov/niosh/nas/RDRP/appendices/chapter7/a7-1.pdf>.

City of Berkeley, August 2007. Manufactured Nanoscale Materials Health & Safety Disclosure. City of Berkeley, California. Available at: <http://www.ci.berkeley.ca.us/uploadedFiles/Planning_(new_site_map_walk-through/Level_3_-_General/Manuffactured%20Nanoscale%20Materials.pdf>.

Committee on the Environment, Public Health and Food Safety of the European Parliament, 2006. Draft Recommendation on Second Reading. European Parliament, Brussels.

Cummings, S., 2008. The role of trade secrets in today's nanotechnology patent environment. Nanotechnology Law and Business 5 (1), 41–52.

Du Mont, J., 2008. Trademarking nanotechnology: nano-lies and federal trademark registration. American Intellectual Property Law Association Quarterly Journal 36 (2), 148.

Dunens, O., Mackenzie, K.J., Chee, H., Harris, A.T., 2008. Inconsistencies in the carbon nanotube patent space: a scientific perspective. Nanotechnology Law and Business 5 (1), 24–40.

Environmental Protection Agency, 2007. TSCA Inventory Status of Nanoscale Substances—General Approach. EPA, Washington, DC. Available at. <http://www.epa.gov/oppt/nano/nmsp-inventorypaper.pdf>.

Environmental Protection Agency, 2008a. Toxic substances control act inventory of carbon nanotubes. Federal Register 73 (212), 64946–64947.

Environmental Protection Agency, 5 March 2008b. News releases from region 9: U.S. EPA fines Southern California technology company $208,000 for "nano coating" pesticide claims on computer peripherals. Available at: <http://yosemite.epa.gov/opa/admpress.nsf/2dd7f669225439b78525735900400c31/16a190492f2f25d585257403005c2851!OpenDocument> (last visited April 3, 2009).

European Commission, 2004. Memo 04/78 of 1 April 2004. EC, Brussels. Available at: <http://europa.eu/old-address.htm>.

European Commission, 2006. REACH: Commission Welcomes European Parliament Vote on New EU Chemicals Legislation, 13 December (IP/06/1799). EC, Brussels.

European Commission, 2008. Regulatory Aspects of Nanomaterials: Summary of Legislation in Relation to Health, Safety and Environment Aspects of Nanomaterials, Regulatory Research Needs and Related Measures. EC, Brussels.

Faigrieve, D., 2005. Product Liability in Comparative Perspective. Cambridge University Press, Cambridge.

Food and Drug Administration, 10 October 2006. Transcript: Nanotechnology Task Force Public meeting on nanotechnology materials in FDA regulation products. Available at: <http://www.fda.gov/ScienceResearch/SpecialTopics/Nanotechnology/NanotechnologyTaskForce/ucm111425.htm> (last visited February 17, 2009).

Food and Drug Administration, 2007. Nanotechnology—A Report of the U.S. Food and Drug Administration Nanotechnology Task Force. Washington, DC, FDA. FDA, Washington, DC.

Germano, C., 2008. Managing the emerging risks of nanotechnology, ACE casualty risk. Available at: <http://www.aceusa.com/News/Pages/Articles Speeches.aspx> (last visited 6 March 2009).

Gwinn, M., Vallyathan, V., 2006. Nanoparticles: health effects—pros and cons. Environmental Health Perspectives 114 (12), 1818–1825.

Innovation Society, 2007. Regulation of Nanotechnology in Consumer Products. Innovation Society, St. Gallen.

Matsuura, J., 2006. Nanotechnology Regulation and Policy Worldwide. Artech House, Norwood.

Maynard, A.D., Aitken, R., Butz, T., et al., 2006. Safe handling of nanotechnology. Nature 444 (16 November), 267–269.

Maysinger, D., Behrendt, M., Przybytkowski, E., 2006. Death by nanoparticles. NanoPharmaceuticals Online Journal 1 (October), 1–21. Available at: <http://nanopharmaceuticals.org/files/Death_by_Nanoparticles_nanopharmaceuticals2.org_OCT_2006.pdf>.

Miller, J., Serrato, R., Represas-Cardenas, J.M., Kundahl, G. (Eds.), 2005. The Handbook of Nanotechnology: Business, Policy, and Intellectual Property Law. John Wiley & Sons, New York.

Monica, J.C., 2 August 2007. EPA has no immediate plans to issue comprehensive SNUR under TSCA covering all nanoscale materials. Nanotechnology Law Report Available at: <http://www.nanolawreport.com/2007/08/articles/epa-has-no-immediate-plans-to-issue-comprehensive-snur-under-tsca-covering-all-nanoscale-materials> (last visited April 3, 2009).

Monica, J.C., 24 September 2008. First commercial insurance exclusion for nanotechnology. Nanotechnology Law Report Available at: <http://www.nanolawreport.com/2008/09/articles/first-commercial-insurance-exclusion-for-nanotechnology/> (last visited March 6, 2009).

Mouttet, B., 2005. Nanotech and the U.S. Patent & Trademark Office: the birth of a patent class. Nanotechnology Law and Business 2 (3), 260–264.

National Institute for Occupational Safety and Health, 2009. Nanoparticle Information Library (NIL). NIOSH, Washington, DC. Available at: <http://www2a.cdc.gov/niosh-nil/index.asp> (last visited February 25, 2009).

Oberdörster, G., Maynard, A.D., Donaldson, K., et al., 2005. Review: principles for characterizing the potential human health effects from exposure to nanomaterials: elements of a screening strategy. Particle and Fibre Toxicology 2 (8), 1–35.

Office of Pollution Prevention And Toxics, 2008. Regulation of a New Chemical Substance Pending Development of Information. Re: Premanufacture Notice Number P-08-0177, Consent Order and Determinations Supporting Consent Order. Environmental Protection Agency, Washington, DC. Available at: <http://www.nanolawreport.com/EPA%20Premanufacture%20Notice%20Number%20P-08-0177.pdf>.

Office of Pollution Prevention and Toxics, 2009. Nanoscale Materials Stewardship Program, Interim Report. Environmental Protection Agency, Washington, DC. Available at: <http://www.epa.gov/oppt/nano/nmsp-interim-report-final.pdf>.

O'Neill, S., 2007. Broad claiming in nanotechnology patents: is litigation inevitable? Nanotechnology Law and Business 4 (1), 29–40.

Project on Emerging Nanotechnologies, 2008. Nano-product inventory—analysis of on-line inventory. Available at: <http://www.nanotechproject.org/inventories/consumer/>.

Section of Environment, Energy, and Resources, American Bar Association, 2006. CERCLA Nanotechnology Issues. American Bar Association, Washington, DC. Available at. <http://www.abanet.org/environ/nanotech/pdf/CERCLA.pdf>.

Smith, G., Parr, R.L., 2005. Intellectual Property: Valuation, Exploitation, and Infringement Damages, third ed. John Wiley & Sons, Inc., New York.

Troilo, L., 2005. Patentability and enforcement issues related to nanotechnology inventions. Nanotechnology Law and Business 2 (1), 36–44.

United States Patent and Trademark Office, 2008. Patents Inventors Resources and Information. USPTO, Washington, DC. Available at: <http://www.uspto.gov/web/offices/com/iip/patents.htm> (last visited February 25, 2009).

van Calster, G., Bowman, D.M., D'Silva, J., 2008. Sufficient or Deficient? A Review of the Adequacy of Current European Legislative Instruments for Regulating Nanotechnologies across Three Industry Sectors, paper presented at the Tilting perspectives on regulating technologies, 10–11 December, Tilburg.

SECTION 3

Management

CHAPTER 5

Nanotechnology Risk Management: An Insurance Industry Perspective

Robert Blaunstein and Igor Linkov

CONTENTS

5.1 INTRODUCTION

The expectation that nanotechnologies will greatly enhance our lives in ways that push the limits of our imagination has long been the technological topic of the day. Research momentum is in full gear, and hundreds of products containing nanomaterials have already found their way to the commercial marketplace. Given the rapid pace with which nanotechnology is developing, it is likely that by the time this book reaches the public, an even greater number of products containing nanomaterials will have moved farther along the development pipeline and into the commercial realm.

As definitions and technical aspects of nanomaterials and nanotechnologies are discussed elsewhere in this book, this chapter will focus on risk management considerations in general and, specifically, how insurance companies perceive emerging nanotechnologies and the companies responsible for developing and commercializing them. Also presented in this chapter will be specific tools and strategies that emerging companies might adopt in order to reduce their risks and liability as well as successfully present themselves to insurers to obtain appropriate insurance coverage. Likewise, in consideration of the tools available to assist insurers with quantitative assessments of risk, we will review the application of Multi-Criteria Decision Analysis (MCDA) in context.

Of particular importance in this chapter is that, in terms of "Risk Governance," there is an implicit understanding that the nature of managing risk requires the collaboration and coordination between several different stakeholders: specifically regulators, insurance companies, and potential insureds.

Nanotechnology Environmental Health and Safety

5.2 RISK MANAGEMENT STRATEGIES

First, principles of corporate management require that any company, nanotechnology-focused or otherwise, newly emerging or mature, must identify its risks; that is, identify those events that, when triggered, may cause significant problems for the organization. Once identified, the risks must be assessed by their probability of occurrence and potential severity of loss. The fundamental difficulty in making such an assessment is that, unless quantifiable statistical data are readily available, both probability and severity are difficult to calculate.

Once risks have been identified and assessed, however, managing each of the risks falls into one or more of the following categories:

- Avoidance;
- Mitigation (reduction);
- Retention (self-insure);
- Transfer to another party.

5.2.1 Risk avoidance

Risk avoidance includes performing only those activities that carry no significant risk. An example would be choosing not to purchase a piece of property because of potential liability or choosing not to use certain chemicals in a manufacturing process because they are hazardous. Although this may appear to be a simple answer to risk avoidance, it could also mean neglecting the gains that could be made by accepting the risk. Clearly, choosing not to enter into a business investment to avoid risk also eliminates potential advances and profits.

5.2.2 Mitigation

Mitigation involves using methods that could reduce the severity of loss. Examples include employing fire sprinklers to reduce the risk of loss by fire, placing hazardous chemicals in special containers to avoid risk of spills or corrosion, or using detection devices to signal unwanted dispersion of hazardous materials into the air, water, or onto the land.

5.2.3 Retention (self-insurance)

In this scenario, the company accepts the loss when it occurs. This is true "self-insurance," a viable strategy for small losses, where the cost of insuring against the loss is greater than the cost of the loss. Losses that are not insured or avoided are retained by default. This is also applicable when insurance is not available, such as in times of war, or the cost of transferring the risk is so great that doing so would hinder organizational goals.

5.2.4 Transfer the risk (insurance)

In this scenario, the company transfers the risk, for a premium, to another party, usually an insurance company. The insurance company issues a policy (a contract), stating under what conditions it will be liable to pay for any unexpected occurrence. This scenario provides the policyholder a large resource for an unexpected occurrence, a viable alternative when the company can obtain the resource for an acceptable premium.

5.3 WHICH STRATEGY TO CHOOSE?

Most often, emerging technology companies take a proactive approach by employing both mitigation and risk transfer. This combination provides for risk control and for substantial financial protection at an affordable premium, allowing the company to retain funds for activities focused on its business objectives.

The following section discusses risk transfer and insurance in further depth.

5.3.1 The role of insurance

The role of insurance as a risk management strategy has not changed significantly in concept over several hundred years. Its aim is to reduce financial uncertainty and make accidental loss manageable by providing a transfer of risk. This is accomplished by an insurance company agreeing to provide compensation for specific future losses in exchange for a periodic payment. This means, for a given amount of money (premium), the insurance company (the insurer) will accept a defined risk transferred from the insured. The definition of the risk, the amount of premium, the conditions and amount of insurance payments, limits of the policy (the policy is a contractual agreement), term of the policy, exclusions, are all defined in the insurance policy.

Insurance is exceedingly important in attracting investors or lenders for new businesses, innovative product development or research. Without the safety net of insurance, investors may be unwilling to risk funds without this measure of guarantee against unexpected loss. In an emerging field like nanotechnology, the nanotechnology company has many potential risks, including property damage, general liability, worker's compensation, product liability, environmental liability, professional liability, and employment liability. The company benefits by reducing its risk, while at the same time coveting monies that need to be expended for development and production. The insurance company benefits as nanotechnology represents new business opportunities for accepting risk and gaining premium. The challenge for the two parties is to develop a contract agreement that is acceptable to both, stimulating this symbiotic relationship.

5.3.2 Relationship between insurance and innovation

Risk is generally a major barrier to innovation, yet taking a risk is the first step to making progress. The productivity of the global economy depends on companies that are willing and able to find new and better ways of doing things despite potential pitfalls. If they start to be ruled by fear of impending liability, our global economy can stagnate. By helping businesses manage the risks associated with product development, production, and distribution, insurers play an important role in stimulating innovation and helping in the growth of the global economy. From the early days of marine exploration, to the first satellite launch, to the development of cutting-edge technologies, to today's proclaimed nanotechnology revolution, insurers have provided a critical safety net that has supported and encouraged the creative process. This is a particularly difficult challenge when a new industry is operating in a time of technical, social, and commercial uncertainty.

From the insurance company's perspective, innovations from an emerging technology may provide substantial benefits in unexpected ways. New materials may provide for increased structural strength, reduction of damage from natural disasters, or replacement of hazardous materials with fire-retardant, environmentally friendly ones. Or, new materials may comprise entirely of new products that could help in cleansing contamination. Additionally, medical innovations can improve diagnostic procedures that provide early warning before health problems become unmanageable and costly, while curative procedures could reduce sick time and cost.

Given the revolutionary potential of nanotechnology and its anticipated use in virtually every industrial segment imaginable, insurers can be expected to be supportive and to develop a thorough understanding of the risks involved.

5.4 INSURANCE EXPOSURE AND TOOLS FOR RISK MANAGEMENT

As this chapter focuses on issues that relate to risk tolerance, the salient question is "What are an insurance company's concerns regarding exposure and risk?"

In the 1970s, the early days of environmental insurance, and for some years thereafter, insurance underwriters were extremely cautious about environmental, health, and safety (EH&S) coverage. There were multiple reasons for their caution, some of which include:

1. The environmental impacts of new chemicals were projected to be very large. There were insufficient data to enable characterization of the exact extent and nature of contamination, making clean-up projections very difficult to quantify;
2. Transport models were not in place to describe the movement of contaminants through the ecosystems;
3. Instrumentation did not have the ability or the sensitivity to detect all types of contaminants;
4. There was disagreement on which materials were to be considered contaminants so that they could be defined appropriately in an insurance contract;
5. Reliable and proven clean-up technologies did not exist;
6. If contamination was discovered in soil, it was difficult, if not impossible, to determine if it was a new release or a prior release; and
7. Environmental regulations were in the nascent stages.

Insurance underwriters, therefore, often sought copious amounts of information from their prospective insureds, so that they could get a "handle" on the facilities or services to be covered. This requirement for information has persisted over the years; however, policy premiums have seen a dramatic reduction, as more environmental data became available and underwriters gained experience.

5.4.1 Exhibit 1—A template for informing insurer concerns about EH&S risks

An environmental insurance policy provides coverage for an incurred liability resulting from the release of a contaminant into the atmosphere, into water, or onto land. Coverage is for property damage, bodily injury to a third party, and clean-up. Exhibit 1 is an outline for information often requested by environmental insurance companies providing such coverage. More often than not, a potential insured can expect an insurance company site inspector to visit his facility seeking detailed information included in this exhibit. As such, this exhibit provides companies with a valuable risk management tool for assessing and controlling their environmental exposures.

5.4.1.1 EXHIBIT 1. Outline for environmental site management and risk control

This outline is not alleged to be complete, or meeting any regulatory or other legal guidelines. Its purpose is to provide general guidance for site management and risk control.

1.0 NAME AND LOCATION OF CORPORATION AND LOCATION OF FACILITIES

2.0 CORPORATE GOVERNANCE

- 2.1 Identify individuals with specific responsibility for Environmental Management
- 2.2 Does the board follow governing principles such as "Responsible Nano Code"?

3.0 DESCRIPTION OF FACILITY

- 3.1 Provide location and site history of facility(s)

4.0 ENVIRONMENTAL SETTING

- 4.1 Describe surrounding land use and population
- 4.2 Describe the geology, groundwater, surface waters and surface drainage routes
- 4.3 Are there special or sensitive environmental conditions near the site?

5.0 OPERATIONS

- 5.1 a. Describe the major products and by-products used
  - b. What are the end uses of the products and who are the users of products?
- 5.2 Raw materials
  - ■ Quantities and hazard classes. Are MSDS' on file and easily accessible?
- 5.3 Description of operations at the site
  - ■ Describe the operational components including:
    - ■ Hazardous materials handled
    - ■ Emergency systems

6.0 ENVIRONMENTAL HAZARDS AND CONTROLS

6.1 Loading/unloading

- Identify each loading/unloading area
- Describe the containment or drainage collection system used
- Operational considerations

Develop written procedures for loading/unloading

6.2 Waste management procedures for hazardous and non-hazardous materials

- Identify wastes generated or received
- Describe general waste management procedures

6.3 Wastewater management:

- Identify wastewater streams
- Identify wastewater treatment facilities:
  a. Biological treatment components
  b. Physical/chemical treatment facilities
- Permitting elements:
  a. Identify discharges to surface waters
  b. Identify discharges to POTW
- Describe effluent treatment facility
- Effluent testing
  a. Identify frequency and test conducted

6.4 Storage tanks:

Above ground tanks

- Materials stored in each tank:
  a. By type (i.e. products, raw materials, wastes, fuels)
  b. By hazard classes or hazardous properties
- Description of containment system
- Inspection procedures and fire protection specifications

Underground tanks

- Identify each underground tank unit and specifications
- Materials stored in each tank
  a. By type (i.e. products, raw materials, wastes)
  b. By hazardous classes or hazardous properties
  c. Determine if product(s) is a CERCLA regulated substance
- Containment system
  a. Concrete vault, synthetic liner, compacted clay
- Leak testing
  a. Frequency of leak testing
  b. Date and results of most recent leak test
  c. Leak test method (does method meet NFPA criteria)
- Inventory monitoring procedures

6.5 Drum and container storage areas:

- Materials stored
- Description of drums
  a. Describe construction materials and condition of containers and labeling
- Describe secondary containment

6.6 Monitoring of air emissions:

- Identify all stationary and fugitive sources of air emissions
- Permit/regulatory requirements:
  a. Identify all existing operational permits for stationary and fugitive sources.
  b. Identify emission permit(s) or regulatory limitations for sources.
- Monitoring data:
  a. Review emissions data from facility, compared to permit or regulatory limits

b. Is there any ambient monitoring conducted at site?

c. Is there any personnel monitoring in effect for specific chemical exposures?

6.7 Groundwater monitoring

- Describe existing groundwater monitoring systems
- Water level and groundwater gradient:

a. Determine the upgradient/downgradient directions

- Evaluation and assessment:

a. Evaluate water quality compared to federal drinking water standards, RCRA groundwater protection standards, State standards or Alternate Concentrations Limits (ACL's)

b. Review the extent of any contaminant plume, if existing

c. Is there potential for offsite migration or contamination to underlying aquifers?

6.8 PCB equipment:

- Identify PCB equipment at site
- Evaluate containment systems for PCB-containing equipment

7.0 ENVIRONMENTAL MANAGEMENT

7.1 Procedures to prevent and control hazards:

- Are there preparedness, prevention, and response documents in place, including:

a. Site emergency response plan

b. Hazardous waste contingency plan

c. SPCC plan?

7.2 Describe internal inspection programs for:

a. Bulk storage tanks

b. Drum storage areas

c. Air emission control equipment

d. Wastewater treatment facilities

e. Waste management units

f. PCB equipment

- Describe personnel training programs
- Describe management of environmental information and data
- Environmental auditing programs
- SARA Title III Notification and Compliance reporting procedures

7.3 Security:

- Are there barriers to areas of unauthorized entry?

7.4 Fire protection systems:

- Are fire protection systems for individual components or units in place?

8.0 REGULATORY AND LIABILITY ISSUES

8.1 Is there a history of spills, releases, or pollution events?

- Identify all past spills, accidental releases, or events (i.e. fires explosions, uncontrolled reactions)
- Identify third party actions and complaints
- Are there regulatory issues pending?

Exhibit 1 provides an extensive list of environmental and safety risk management considerations that a company can use to manage and control its EH&S exposures. The answers to these questions also provide a database for underwriting an environmental policy. The information feeds into an analytical model which provides a premium as a function of policy limits, retention, policy period, and first and third party coverages.

Today, a myriad of human and environmental health and safety regulations (see Linkov and Satterstrom, in press, for review) as well as analyses of past spill and clean-up data, coupled with analytical models, provide an underwriter with a reasonable degree of comfort in addressing the task of underwriting risk with much more understanding and knowledge. The result has been that over the past 20 years, environmental insurance premiums have decreased by as much as 10-fold as compared to those in the 1970s. Concomitantly, policies now have broader coverage and clearer policy language; as more knowledge developed, an increasing number of insurance companies entered the environmental insurance market, creating competition.

It is likely that underwriting of emerging nanotechnologies will follow a similar trend, where initial premiums may be increased to reflect preliminary uncertainty, but will decrease considerably as more information emerges about nanotechnology risks and associated underwriting strategies.

5.4.2 A nanotechnology risk management framework

Although the items in Exhibit 1 address hazardous materials, *they do not specifically address nanomaterials*. What additional precautions, therefore, should a company handling nanomaterials establish to address its risk controls?

A *proactive* approach to nanotechnology EH&S risk control has recently been published by the Partnership of the Environmental Defense and DuPont (June 2007) called "Nano Risk Framework." The authors state, "This is our proposal for a comprehensive, practical, and flexible Nano Risk Framework—a systematic and disciplined process—to evaluate and address the potential environmental, health and safety risks of nanoscale materials." While addressed by Ostraat elsewhere in this book and in more detail, the Nano Risk Framework is a disciplined approach, structured in six steps and is described by the framework authors in the following manner.

Step 1. Describe the Material and Application

For this step, a general description of the nanomaterial and its intended uses is developed.

Step 2. Profile Lifecycle(s)

This step defines a process for developing the following three sets of profiles:

1. A profile of the nanomaterial's properties, which identifies and characterizes the material's physical and chemical properties;

2. A profile of the nanomaterial's inherent hazards, which identifies and characterizes the material's potential environmental, health, and safety hazards;

3. A profile identifying the associated exposures throughout the material's lifecycle, which identifies and characterizes the opportunities for human and/or environmental exposure to the nanomaterial. Potential exposure includes both intended use and accidental release.

The nanomaterial's full lifecycle is addressed, from material sourcing, through production and use, to the end-of-life disposal or recycling.

This last aspect is of particular importance in the United States, wherein compliance with the regulatory requirements of the Comprehensive, Environmental Response, Compensation and Liability Act (CERCLA) must be ensured.

Step 3. Evaluate Risks

Using the information generated in Step 2, identify and characterize the nature, magnitude, and probability of risks presented by the particular nanomaterial and its anticipated application. Data used are that which are known, or newly generated, or by using "reasonable worst case" assumptions or values.

Step 4. Assess Risk Management

This step evaluates the available options for managing risks identified in Step 3 and recommends a course of action. Options include engineering controls, protective equipment, risk communication, and product or process modification(s). This step is essentially a mitigation strategy, described in Section 5.2.2 of this chapter.

Step 5. Decide, Document, and Act

In this step, an appropriate review team decides in what capacity, if at all, to continue development and production.

Step 6. Review and Adapt

This step provides for regularly scheduled reviews, at which time updates and risk evaluations are again conducted. This ensures that the risk management systems are working as expected and tests them against new information regarding hazard data and/or new or altered exposure patterns.

5.4.3 Exhibit 2—An insurer's translation of the Nano Risk Framework

Exhibit 2 is a worksheet adapted directly from the Nano Risk Framework. This worksheet details the six steps described in the previous section, providing a descriptive and analytical basis for nanomaterial risk control. It can be viewed as a template to organize and evaluate the information in the Framework and outline subsequent decisions.

5.4.3.1 EXHIBIT 2. Output worksheet

Nanomaterial Risk Assessment Document — [nanomaterial]

Section 1: Describe Material and Its Applications

Develop basic descriptions — general overviews — of the nanoscale material and its intended uses. In filling out this section, users may wish to consider the longer list of key questions included in the framework.

A. General overview[1]

B. Material description

  a. Material source or producer

  b. Manufacturing process

  c. Appearance

  d. Chemical composition

  e. Physical form/shape

  f. Concentration

  g. Size distribution

  h. State of aggregation or agglomeration

  i. Solubility

  j. Material CAS number (if applicable)

C. Main applications (current or expected)

D. Stage of development

E. General physical and mechanical properties of this material

F. Past experience with this material or a similar material

G. Potential benefits/positives of the material

H. Potential risks/negatives of the material

Section 2: Profile Lifecycles

Define and catalog the known and anticipated activities in a material's lifecycle in the following table, detailing both the product form and the operations and activities that occur at that stage of the product lifecycle. Include activities within the user's control as well as those activities upstream or downstream of the user.

---

[1] The general overview should contain descriptions sufficient to guide development of more detailed profiles of the material's properties related to hazard and exposure potential at various lifecycle stages (such as manufacture, use, and end-of-life). This overview should be developed from information in the possession of the user or available in the literature.

Lifecycle Profile		
Material Lifecycle Stage	**Material Form(s)**	**Operations and Activities**
Material sourcing (e.g., producer, supplier)		
Manufacturing level I (e.g., processor)		
Manufacturing level II (e.g., product fabrication)		
Manufacturing level III (e.g., filling/packaging)		
Distribution (e.g., retailer)		
Use/Reuse/Maintenance (e.g., consumer)		
End of life (e.g., recycling, disposal)		

Section 2A: Develop Lifecycle Properties Profile
Identify and characterize the nanoscale material's physical and chemical properties, including property changes throughout the full product lifecycle.
Summary:
Data needs and actions:

Lifecycles Properties — Summary Table			
Lifecycle Stage*			
Technical or Commercial Name			
Common Form			
	Result	**Method**	**Remarks*****
Chemical Composition (including surface coatings)			
Component 1:			
Component 2:			
Component n:			
Crystal phase/molecular structure			
Physical form/shape			
Particle size and size distribution			

Continued

Surface area
Particle density
Solubility
Bulk density
Agglomeration/aggregation state
Porosity
Surface charge

User may create rows for data on additional properties, if available.
* *Repeat table entries for each lifecycle stage if properties change.*
*** *E.g., reference, source of data, degree of certainty.*

Additional Notes:

Section 2B: Develop Lifecycle Hazard Profile

Gather information and characterize the material's potential health, environmental, and safety hazards over the entire lifecycle.

Summary:

Data needs and actions:

Nanomaterial Lifecycle Hazard Profile — Base Set

Route	Hazard (characterization [e.g., low, moderate, high] and quantification if available [e.g., LOAEL = x mg/kg])	Source of Information (e.g., report number)
Health hazard data		
1. Short-term toxicity a. Pulmonary toxicity b. Oral toxicity		
2. Skin sensitization/irritation		
3. Skin penetration*		

Continued

4. Genotoxicity
a. Gene mutation in prokaryotic cells b. Chromosomal aberration
Environmental hazard data
Aquatic Toxicity
1. Fish (fathead minnow or trout)
2. Invertebrate (Daphnia)
3. Aquatic Plant (algae)
Terrestrial toxicity (if significant release to terrestrial environments)
1. Earthworms
2. Plants
Environmental fate data
Water solubility
Octanol-water partition coefficient
Vapor pressure
Aggregation or disaggregation (in applicable exposure media)
Adsorption/desorption coefficients in release medium (soil/sludge)
Persistence potential screen
Bioaccumulation potential screen
Base set of safety hazard data
Flammability
Explosivity
Incompatibility
Reactivity
Corrosivity

Additional tests on an "as needed" basis

Nanomaterial Lifecycle Hazard Profile — Additional Tests		
Route	**Hazard (e.g., low, moderate, high)**	**Source of Information (e.g., report number)**
Health hazard data — additional tests as needed		
Biological fate and behavior		
Chronic inhalation studies		
Chronic ingestion studies		
Chronic dermal irritation/sensitization studies		
Reproductive and developmental toxicity		
Neurotoxicity studies		
More extensive genotoxicity studies		
Focused toxicity studies		
Environmental hazard data — additional tests as needed		
ADME studies on aquatic organisms		
Chronic toxicity to soil microorganisms and sediment- and soil-dwelling organisms		
Further testing for terrestrial toxicity		
Avian toxicity		
Population/ecosystem-level studies		
Environmental fate data — additional tests as needed		
Activated sludge respiration inhibition		
Microorganism toxicity		
Persistence potential in relevant media		
Potential for transformations via oxidation–reduction reactions		

Section 2C: Develop Lifecycle Exposure Profile

Assess potential for exposure from direct human contact or release to the environment at each stage of the lifecycle. The key deliverable from Step 3 is the *Exposure Characterization* — a summary and synthesis of the gathered exposure information.

Summary:

Data needs and actions:

Potential for Direct Human Context — Summary Table			
Lifecycle Stage*			
Material Form			
Material			
Step (e.g., process step, transfer step, cleanup/disposal procedures)	Engineering Controls	Personnal Protection Equipment (PPE)	Exponent Potential

* Repeat table entries for each lifecycle stage.

Elaboration

a. Lifecycle stage

b. Step name

c. Material form

d. Number of people potentially exposed

e. Potential routes for exposure (e.g., inhalation, ingestion, eye, dermal)

f. Personal protective equipment

g. Engineering controls

h. Procedures

i. Exposure potential

j. Estimated exposure and dose

k. Unknowns and uncertainties

Potential for Environmental Release — Summary Table			
Lifecycle Stage*			
Material			
Step (e.g. process step, transfer step)	**Potential Release Medium (e.g., water soil)**	**Engineering Controls**	**Release Potential**

* *Repeat table entries for each lifecycle stage.*

Elaboration

a. Lifecycle stage

b. Step name

c. Potential release medium (i.e., routes of entry)

d. Engineering controls

e. Procedures

f. Release potential

g. Map fates of the material (e.g., degradation, transformations, or transfers to other media)

h. Estimated exposure and dose

i. Unknowns and uncertainties

Questions

a. What is the ultimate environmental fate of the material?

b. Does it accumulate in a particular environmental sink?

c. What are the populations that may be exposed?

d. What is the bioaccumulation potential?

Exposure Data — Summary Table

Nanomaterial Manufacture		
		Information
Stage of development		
Number and Location of manufacturing sites		
Annual production volumes (current and expected)		
Manufacturing site's NAICS code		
Manufacturing method		
Number of workers handling nanomaterials at the manufacturing site		
Industrial functions (e.g., adhesive, coloring agent)	Percent of production	Physical form & concentration
Function 1:		
Function 2:		
Function 3:		
Function n:		
Material processing		
Type of downstream industrial processing or use		
Number of processing or commercial use sites		
NAICS code of processors		

Continued

Industrial functions	Percent of production	Number of sites	Numbers of workers at site	Number of workers exposed	
Function 1:					
Function 2:					
Function 3:					
Function n:					
Material use					
Commercial or consumer product types	Percent of production	Setting for use (homes, outdoors)	Concentration in product	Released during use	Est. Number of Exposed Users
product Type 1:					
product Type 2:					
product Type 3:					
product Type n:					

Distribution/storage		
Methods of delivery and storage		
Manufacturer		
Processors		
Distributors		
Retailers		
Consumers		
Post-use management		
	Expected disposal methods	Expected recovery/reuse/recycle methods
Manufacturer		
Processors		
End-users		

Elaboration

a. Types of employees

b. Handling practices

c. Environmental containment and control equipment

d. Exposure potential at the manufacturing site(s)

e. Exposure potential at downstream processing site(s)

f. Use of the material in commerce

g. Exposure potential in commerce

h. Recommended controls

i. Product recovery or recall techniques

j. Potential for use by children or other sensitive groups

k. Post-use management of the material across the lifecycle

Section 3: Evaluate Risks

Using a synthesis of information collected in Step 2, produce a *Risk Evaluation*: estimates of the nature, likelihood, and magnitude of adverse effects on human health and the environment.

Summary:

Data needs and actions:

Section 4: Assess Risk Management

Risk Evaluation—Summary Table*

Risk Type	Nature, Magnitude, and Probability	Source(s) of Risk Assessment
Human		
Respiratory	Nature: Magnitude: Probability:	
Dermal	Nature: Magnitude: Probability:	

Continued

Ingestion	Nature: Magnitude: Probability:
Other health (e.g., reproductive, developmental, neural)	
Environmental	
Aquatic	
Avian	
Mammalian	
Terrestrial	
Other (e.g., sludge)	

* *Information contained in this table is based on existing studies. Where no information is available, a reasonable worst-case assumption may be made.*

Determine how to minimize or eliminate any potential adverse impacts throughout the product's lifecycle. The key deliverable from Step 4 is the *Plan for Risk Management, Monitoring, Compliance, and Reporting*, based on the gathered exposure information.

Summary:

Data needs and actions:

Review cycle and conditions:

Plan and timeline for risk management, monitoring, compliance, and reporting:

Material Safety and Handling (manufacturer of nanomaterial)		
Material Hazard Event	**Recommended Precaution/Action**	**Expected effectiveness of recommended action (e.g., what level of exposure will be achieved)**
Receipt		
Processing		
Storage		
Handling		

Continued

Spills		
Transport		
Packaging		
Use		
Recycling		
Disposal (including packaging materials)		
Other:		
	Material Safety and Handling (nanomaterial user)	
Material Hazard Event	Recommended Precaution/ Action	Expected effectiveness of recommended action (e.g., what level of exposure will be achieved)
Receipt		
Processing		
Storage		
Handling		
Spills		
Transport		
Packaging		
Use		
Recycling		
Disposal (including packaging materials)		
Other:		
	Material Safety and Handling (end-product user)	
Material Hazard Event	Recommended Precaution/ Action	Expected effectiveness of recommended action (e.g., what level of exposure will be achieved)
Receipt		
Storage		
Handling		
Spills		
Transport		

Continued

Packaging		
Use		
Recycling		
Disposal (including packaging materials)		
Other:		
	Material Safety and Handling (end-of-life)	
Material Hazard Event	Recommended Precaution/Action	Expected effectiveness of recommended action (e.g., what level of exposure will be achieved)
Receipt		
Processing		
Storage		
Handling		
Spills		
Transport		
Packaging		
Use		
Recycling		
Disposal (including packaging materials)		
Other:		

User may add tables for additional steps in the value chain as appropriate.

Section 5: Decide, Document, and Act

Cross-functional review team critically examines compiled information, analyzes the options, documents the resulting analysis, makes decisions, and takes appropriate actions.

- Go/no-go/redirect decision and rationale:
- Additional data needs:
- Additional data-collection assignments:
- Product steward:
- Review team:

- Product review cycle:
- Needed actions and responsible persons:

Step 6. Review and Adapt
User implements a series of periodic and as-needed reviews to ensure that the information, evaluations, decisions, and actions of the previous steps are kept up-to-date.

- List of reviews held (dates):
- Conditions that triggered review(s):
- Changes made in report and rationale (e.g., changes to lifecycle profiles):
- Actions taken and rationale (e.g., revised risk management practices):

Additional References:
User may add additional references as appropriate.

Thus, when used in concert, Exhibits 1 and 2 provide a roadmap for responsible risk management. Nanotechnology risks are eligible for a wide variety of insurance policies including product liability, worker compensation, professional liability, environmental liability, and general liability. Therefore, seeking and documenting the information outlined in these exhibits, being as transparent as possible and consistent with protection of confidential business information and using a conservative approach when data are not available, can establish a sound risk management strategy.

While some may argue that such risk management approaches are imperfect for an assortment of reasons, insurance carriers can look to this information in evaluating nanomaterial users and would be expected to be more positively inclined to offer coverage if information is presented in this manner. Even though the Environmental Defense/DuPont Nano Risk Framework is gaining increased attention, there are other risk management frameworks proposed by different agencies and organizations (see Linkov et al., 2009 for review). MCDA approaches discussed below provide an approach that the insurance industry could implement in concert with Nano Risk Framework or another regulatory or risk assessment framework.

5.4.4 Selecting the "Best" nanotechnology risk management option: MCDA as a tool

Given data on EH&S risks and an informed risk management framework, a range of specific risk management options can be derived both from the perspectives of organizational EH&S managers to those of insurers. However, the task of selecting which of those options is most appropriate for a particular scenario can be daunting. Elsewhere in this book—in chapters by Ostraat and Hull—the development and selection of risk management frameworks for large and small organizations are described. But how does one determine specifically which risk management framework is most appropriate for a particular situation? This section illustrates one example of how decision analysis tools, specifically Multi-Criteria Decision Analysis (MCDA) methods, can aid nanotechnology risk-management decision-making with a particular focus on insurers.

MCDA refers to a group of methods used to impart structure to the decision-making process. MCDA methods consist of four steps:

1. Creating a set of criteria relevant to the decision at hand;
2. Defining the preference parameters of the model (criteria weights, thresholds, etc.);
3. Measuring the performance of each alternative with respect to each criterion on possibly heterogeneous scales; and
4. Aggregating the information defined in Steps 1–3 to solve the question at hand: to choose the best alternative, to rank the alternatives, or to sort them into pre-defined categories.

Most MCDA methodologies, including Multi-Attribute Utility Theory (MAUT), Analytical Hierarchy Process (AHP), and outranking, share similar steps (Steps 1 and 3), but diverge on their approach to Steps 2 and 4. A detailed analysis of the theoretical foundations of different MCDA methods and their comparative strengths and weaknesses is presented in Belton and Steward (2002).

Over the past several decades, decision-making strategies for EH&S risks have become increasingly more sophisticated and now include expert judgment, cost–benefit analysis, toxicological risk assessment, comparative risk assessment, and a number of methods for incorporating public and stakeholder values. This evolution has led to an improved array of decision-making aides, including the development of MCDA tools that offer a scientifically defensible decision analytical framework. Several MCDA methods have been automated in commercially available software programs, each of which can vary with respect to their practicality, mathematical rigor, assumptions and simplifications, and requirements of decision-makers or other participants. Linkov et al. (2007, in press) and Tervonen et al. (2009) include additional discussion on MCDA use for nanotechnology risk assessment and management.

Considering the insurance industry's decision-making problem in particular, insurers must decide on a particular level of risk that they are willing to accept, as well as establish a premium that prospective clients will pay in exchange for that risk burden. Such decisions are not made without due consideration; those affected by and involved in the decision-making process must also decide what specific risk concerns will be involved in the decision, how they will prioritize those concerns, and how premiums should be structured to ensure that business objectives are met. Typically, a range of possible management strategies will emerge and the insurer must then select the option that best suits their business interests. MCDA methods may be employed to address this decision problem in several ways:

- *Sorting* alternative clients/policies into classes/categories (e.g., "unacceptable," "possibly acceptable," and "definitely acceptable,");
- *Screening* alternative policies—a process of eliminating those alternative policies that do not appear to warrant further attention, i.e., selecting a smaller set of alternatives that (very likely) contains the "best" alternative;
- *Ranking* alternative policies (from "best" to "worst" according to a chosen algorithm);
- *Selecting* the "best alternative" from a given set of alternatives;
- *Designing* (searching, identifying, creating) a new action/alternative to meet goals; and
- *Exploring* the interaction between alternatives and decision-makers to learn more about the feasibility, acceptability, or potential conflicts and opportunities for compromise.

In this discussion, we will consider the use of MCDA for insurer portfolio selection decisions. Diversification is an important strategy for mitigating risks while maximizing benefits; high risks in one area can be offset by comparatively lower risks in another. MCDA methods can be applied to assist insurers with achieving a tolerable balance of risk in their portfolios of nanotechnology clients. Diversification of an insurance portfolio can be achieved through a variety of ways based on, for example, the type of company (business process, business dynamic), the nature of the product (technology, materials, value), or the details of the insurance agreement (extent of coverage and premium cost). These elements can be represented using multiple criteria (Figure 5.1) and prioritized using MCDA methods.

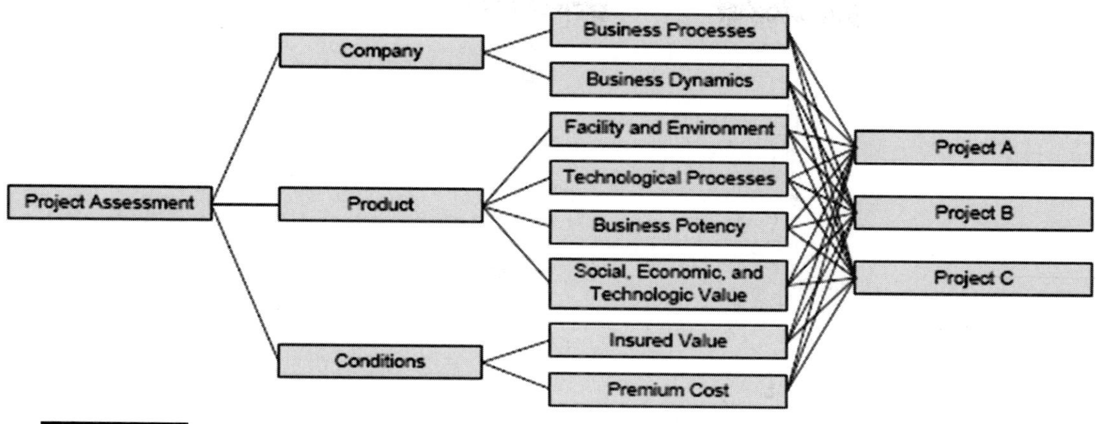

FIGURE 5.1 *Prioritization of Potential Clients/Projects Using MCDA Methods: Criteria and Metrics*

In addition to the multi-criteria representation of the problem, relationships between projects, companies, and products should be taken into account. In such assessments, premium cost and maximal insured value can be found using Multi-Objective Decision-Making (MODM) methods and solving as a multi-criteria optimization problem (Figure 5.2); the same criteria can be reused for insurance portfolio optimization, and in the case of discrete alternatives (premium cost or insured value), the Multi-Attribute Decision-Making (MADM) approach can be used. Different risk assessment approaches can be adapted for MCDM; for example, product lifecycle can be presented in detail and/or insured accidents can be presented implicitly along with business opportunities and other benefits.

In summary, the availability of information on nanotechnology EH&S risks and comprehensive organizational frameworks are critical first tiers in the risk management process. But ultimately, this information must be translated into informed decisions that help accomplish important business objectives. In the context of the insurance industry, this means that such decisions should establish risk management options that allow insurers to provide insureds with reasonable levels of protection from nanotechnology EH&S risks in exchange for commensurate premiums. As described here, tools such as MCDA can provide insurers, and other stakeholders, with a systematic and open method for selecting nanotechnology EH&S risk management options that are best suited for organizational needs.

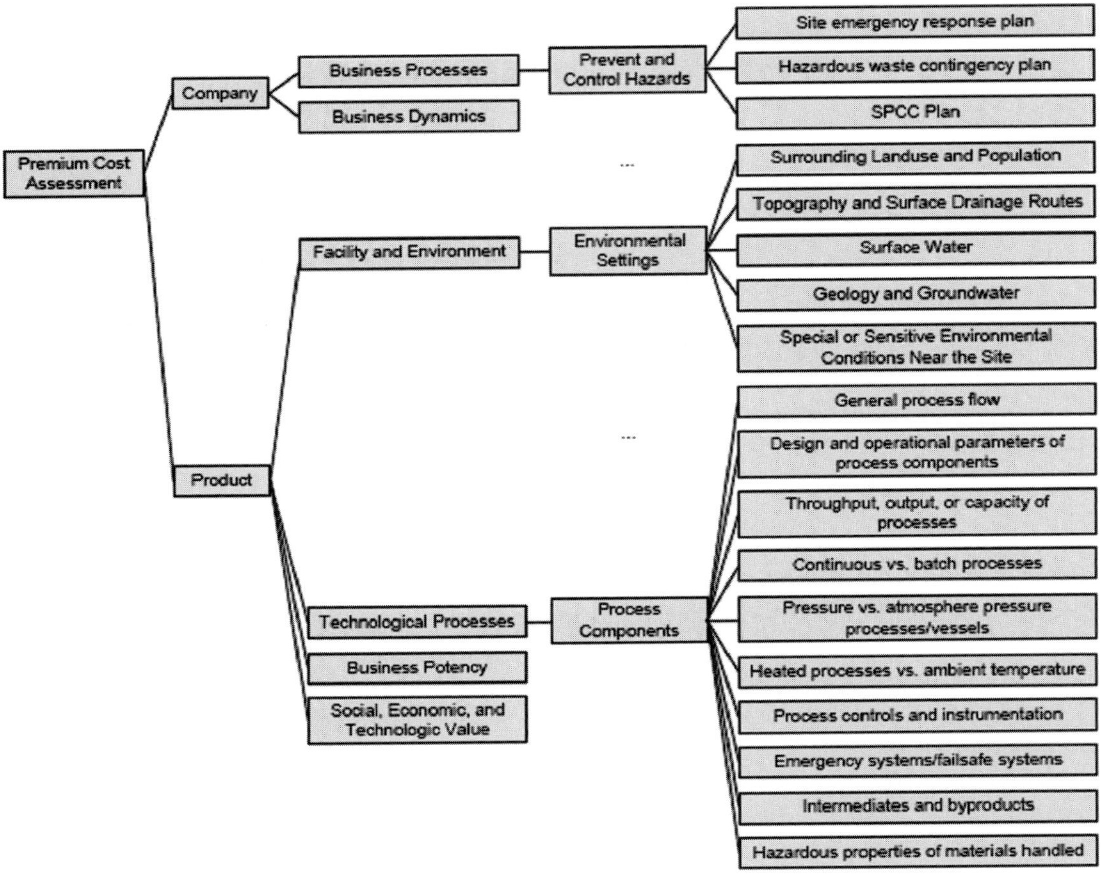

FIGURE 5.2 *Example of how MODM Methods can be Applied to Determine Premium Cost from the Relationships Between Projects, Companies, and Products*

5.5 RISK MANAGEMENT AND REGULATORY ISSUES FOR NANOMATERIALS

Currently, the most adverse issues associated with nanotechnologies are those dealing with environmental, health, and safety (EH&S) exposures. As a result, risk management issues relating to EH&S are at the forefront of regulatory considerations. Companies involved with nanomaterials are cognizant of the special controls that are often needed to address their unique properties. Likewise, these new properties and their potential for creating new health and environmental risks are causing governmental agencies to scramble to provide responsible regulatory guidance in a timely manner. The problem each faces is the paucity of data relating to the environmental, health, and safety exposures of nano-sized materials and whether nanomaterials can be appropriately regulated in the same manner as other materials. The availability of information regarding chronic, long-term health effects is altogether absent from the literature, which poses unique downstream challenges for nanotechnology companies and insurers alike.

EPA, for example, in its White Paper on Nanotechnology, has openly expressed concern over this lack of data and has questioned the use of the very models it employs to predict movement of substances through the environment because these models are based on macro-scale substances. The reactivity and mobility associated with nanoscale materials could dramatically alter the models currently used.

Under pressure to provide interim guidance, particularly under the Toxic Substance Control Act (TSCA), EPA in July 2007 issued guidance on determining whether a new nanoscale material is considered an existing chemical covered by inventory listing or a new chemical subject to Premanufacture Notification (PMN) reporting requirements. Specifically, are nanomaterials automatically considered New Chemicals under the TSCA or may they be considered as Existing Chemicals?

The answer currently lies in TSCA's definition of "chemical substance." EPA has decided that until there are changes in the regulations, any nanomaterial that has the same molecular identity as a non-nanoscale substance already listed on the inventory may be considered as "existing," even though they differ in particle size and certain physical and/or chemical properties resulting from this difference in particle size. This opens the door for manufactured nanomaterials to reach the marketplace much quicker. However, in determining whether a specific substance does not require a Premanufacture Notice (PMN), the agency encourages the manufacturer or importer of the nanoscale substance to contact the New Chemicals Program to arrange a prenotice consultation.

Although insurers have not as yet responded to EPA's guidance, it is expected that they will take a conservative approach to reporting.

5.6 LIKELY INSURANCE SCENARIOS

Although the future evolution of insurance coverage is difficult to predict, one could expect nanotechnology coverage to evolve in a similar fashion as did other emerging technologies, including computerization, e-commerce, and, more recently, security.

The evolution of insurance coverage often develops in three stages:

- The Early Study Period
- The Fear Phase
- The Mature Phase

5.6.1 Stage 1: The early study phase

This stage, which typifies the current state of nanotechnology, is characterized by continuance of existing policy coverages and efforts by insurers and reinsurers to become more familiar with those special exposures and risks posed by nanotechnology. This phase is well underway.

Several of these special EH&S risks include dispersal and movement of nanoparticles through the environment (air, water, and land), potential for nanomaterials to enter the body with easier movement, and uncertain results if they enter human cells or penetrate the blood–brain barrier.

Underwriters' response to applications may be positive initially, as the technologies represent increased premium, and there are no early definitive studies that validate potential risk. Therefore, there have been no broad decisions to exclude nanotechnologies from policy coverage. The reasons for this include:

- Exposure to the general public is still low;
- The various nanotechnologies encompass a wide array of activities and products without a uniform description and with different risk characteristics; and
- Within most insurance portfolios, there is significant diversification between the various nanotechnologies, mitigating generalization of adverse effects of single technologies.

However, this scarcity of data may be short-lived as governments worldwide are funding research and insurers are gathering information about the impact of environmental, health, and safety of nanotechnologies. Additionally, companies that produce nanomaterial-containing products are coalescing to study these issues and develop appropriate stewardship and governance. The National Industries Association (NIA), UK, is a prime example, having developed programs in governance, health, and environment to attempt to develop a roadmap for Responsible Technology Development.

The United States under its National Nanotechnology Initiative included fiscal 2008 expenditure of $1.445 billion, which included $59 million to study the EH&S impacts of nanotechnologies. The results of these studies will eventually generate a more stable regulatory landscape, which in turn, will provide an improved opportunity for insurers to analyze their risk.

The three objectives of the National Nanotechnology Initiative, as well as its international counterparts are as follows:

- To expand the scope of information on the behavior of nanomaterials;
- To develop instruments capable of measuring and testing nanomaterials and monitoring exposure; and
- To assess the environmental, health, and safety of nanomaterials across all areas of usage.

Concurrent with government and industry research, insurers are gathering their own information about businesses that produce, store, or dispose of nanomaterials and/or products containing nanomaterials. As can be deduced from Exhibit 1, the insurance industry is assessing potential property damage, bodily injury to workers and the public, and the environmental liabilities associated with businesses handling and using nanomaterials.

5.6.2 Stage II: The fear phase

This phase is characterized by growing anxiety about impending liability. In fact, recent discoveries suggesting that carbon nanotubes have asbestos-like behavior (Poland et al., 2008) or suggestions to halt nanoscale research altogether (ETC Group, 2003) indicate that with respect to nanotechnology, the Fear Phase may have already arrived. Along with these reports and unless data show otherwise, insurance companies and reinsurers begin to harbor fear that the risks associated with these technologies may be higher than anticipated. Media hype has increased, raising doubts among insurance company CEO's and inspiring them to consider reducing limits and policy coverage. Risk transfer becomes more limited through the use of sub-limits and claims-made coverage.

At this time it is too early to predict the impact of the Fear Phase or how long it will last. Environmental health and safety research results are published on a daily basis and often appear to be conflicting due to differences in nanomaterial structure, purity, temperature, cell type (if studied in vivo), residence time in the body, soil conditions, inter-laboratory variability, and various other parameters. These differences often go undetected by the media and, until results of further studies are reported, may produce unwarranted public concern or, conversely, unwarranted positive acceptance.

Some consequences of the Fear Phase might include alternative actions taken by insurers and governments. Fearing the worst, insurers may begin to pull out of the market, leaving insureds "bare," that is, with no available risk transfer products. Without a risk transfer resource, companies may be forced to self-insure. However, considering the international importance of nanotechnology in areas such as healthcare, energy, and defense, we are likely to see governments proposing alternative solutions in the absence of other commercially available forms of insurance. The following summaries provide two examples of how government intervention can create alternative insurance solutions in support of potentially high-risk activities of national interest.

5.6.2.1 States create pool solutions

States may initialize pools of insurance companies to ensure availability of insurance. Under this arrangement, pools assume the most volatile aspects of the technology by mutualizing and balancing the funding exposures across all nanotechnology insureds, thus enabling insurers to provide a lower premium cost to their clients.

5.6.2.2 Governments provide direct support

Lacking quantified risks, national governments may step in as a back-stop to limit the liability of nanotechnology industries.

There is precedent for this action in the US Congress' enactment of the 1957 Price-Anderson Act. This act limited the liability of the nuclear industry in the event of a nuclear accident in the United States.

Under the Act, each nuclear energy utility is required to maintain the maximum amount of coverage available from the private insurance industry, which today is $200 million per reactor. For coverage above that amount, the Act establishes two insurance tiers. The first tier requires every nuclear operator to pay $88 million for each reactor it operates and is triggered if claims following a nuclear accident exceed the coverage provided by private insurers. If the first tier is depleted, any additional claims are paid by the government.

In a similar fashion, in order to accept the unknown risks of nanotechnology, it may be necessary for insurers to establish a no-fault system in which the nanotechnology industry funds the first layer of insurance according to a predetermined scheme and any claims above that amount would be covered by the national government.

5.6.3 Stage III: The mature phase

At this stage, insurers will know more precisely the type, frequency, and severity of losses that are likely to occur as a result of emerging nanotechnologies. When these risk factors are better understood and more data are available to characterize them, insurers can predict with more precision the types of losses that may be expected. As a result, customized solutions should become available at reasonable rates, both in the insurance and reinsurance markets. At this point, standard forms applicable to the new exposures can be developed.

Three separate forms of coverage in this phase can be envisaged:

- Coverage based on legislation, similar to that of Environmental Impairment Liability (EIL) policies;
- Stand-alone policies, similar to the EIL and Employee Practices Liability (EPLI);
- Coverage integrated into standard policies.

5.7 CONCLUSIONS

As with most emerging technologies, nanotechnologies present uniquely challenging risks with many unknown variables. These challenges are complicated by the fact that there are few risk-related forecasts that have been scientifically confirmed. Further complications derive from the uniquely complex physical and chemical nature of nanomaterials. A new materials science is emerging and reliable risk information is critically needed to codify it.

The approach described in this chapter is developed from extant practice and can provide the nanomaterial user an initial framework from which to develop responsible risk management strategies. Likewise, insurance carriers can use the framework as an informational tool for developing policy analyses and for assessing potential clients. The combination of the framework with decision analysis tools such as MCDA can provide quantitative assessments of risk amidst significant uncertainty.

It is imperative that manufacturers, governments, scientists, the legal community, and the insurance industry work together in taking a proactive approach in identifying and quantifying the risks of nanotechnology. Public response and the legal climate are critical to the health of the industry, both of which will depend upon the availability and accuracy of risk-related information.

REFERENCES

Belton, V., Steward, T., 2002. Multiple Criteria Decision Analysis: An Integrated Approach. Kluwer Academic Publishers, Boston.

Carpenter, G., 2006. Nanotechnology: The Plastics of the 21st Century. Available at: <http://gcportal.guycorp.com>.

Department of Energy, 2008. Nanoscale Science Research Centers: approach to nanomaterial ES&H, revision 3a. Available at: <http://orise.orau.gov/ihos/Nanotechnology/files/NSRCMay12.pdf>.

Environmental Defense and DuPont, 2007. Nano Risk Framework. EDF, New York.

Environmental Protection Agency, 2007a. TSCA Inventory Status of Nanoscale Substances—General Approach.

Environmental Protection Agency, 2007b. Nanotechnology white paper. Available at: <http://es.epa.gov/ncer/nano/publications/whitepaper12022005.pdf>.

ETC Group, 2003. The big down: Atomtech—technologies converging at the nano-scale. Available at: <www.etcgroup.org/upload/publication/171/01/thebigdown.pdf>.

Harville, D.A., 2003. The selection or seeding of college basketball or football teams for postseason competition. Journal of the American Statistical Association 98 (461), 17–27.

International Risk Governance Council, 2006. White paper on nanotechnology risk governance. Available at <www.irgc.org/IMG/pdf/PB_nanoFINAL2_2_.pdf>.

Linkov, I., Satterstrom, K., Steevens, J., Ferguson, E., Pleus, R., 2007. Multi-criteria decision analysis and environmental risk assessment for nanomaterials. Journal of Nanoparticle Research 9, 543–554.

Linkov, I., Satterstrom, K., in press. Nanomaterial risk assessment and risk management: review of regulatory frameworks. In: Linkov, I., Ferguson, E., Magar, V. (Eds.), Real Time and Deliberative Decision Making. Springer, Amsterdam.

Linkov, I., Steevens, J., Adlakha-Hutcheon, G., Bennett, E., Chappell, M., Colvin, V., Davis, M., Davis, T., Elder, A., Foss Hansen, S., Hakkinen, P., Hussain, S., Karkan, D., Korenstein, R., Lynch, I., Metcalfe, C., Ramadan, A., Satterstrom, F.K., 2009. Emerging methods and tools for environmental risk assessment, decision-making, and policy for nanomaterials: summary of NATO advanced research workshop. Journal of Nanoparticle Research 11, 513–527.

Linkov, I., Satterstrom, F.K., Monica, J.C., Jr., Foss Hansen, S., Davis, T.A., 2009. Nano risk governance: current developments and future perspectives. Nanotechnology Law and Business 6 (2), 203.

Poland, C.A., Duffin, R., Kinloch, I., Maynard, A., Wallace, W.A.H., Seaton, A., Stone, V., Brown, S., MacNeel, W., Donaldson, K., 2008. Carbon nanotubes introduced into the abdominal cavity of mice show asbestos-like pathogenicity in a pilot study. Nature Nanotechnology 3, 423–428.

Royal Society, Insight Investment, Nanotechnology Industries Association, Nanotechnology Knowledge Transfer Network, 2007. Responsible Nanotechnologies Code: Consultation Draft—17 September 2007 (Version 5). Responsible NanoCode Working Group, London.

Swiss Re, 2004. Nanotechnology: Small Matters, Many Unknowns. Swiss Reinsurance Company, Zurich.

Tervonen, T., Linkov, I., Figueira, J., Steevens, J., Chappell, M., Merad, M., 2009. Risk-based classification system of nanomaterials. Journal of Nanoparticle Research 11 (4), 757–766.

von Winterfeldt, D., Edwards, W., 1986. Decision Analysis and Behavioral Research. Cambridge University Press, Cambridge.

CHAPTER 6

Industry-Led Initiative for Occupational Health and Safety

Michele L. Ostraat

CONTENTS

The commercialization of nanotechnology-enabled products is expected to reach US $2.6 trillion worldwide by 2014, representing 15% of global manufacturing output. To achieve these numbers, it is estimated that 11% of all manufacturing jobs will involve building or handling products that contain nanomaterials (Lux Research, 2004). In 2006, industrial investment in nanotechnology and commercialization is estimated to be US $5.3 billion, representing a 19% growth from 2005, while worldwide government funding for nanotechnology-related science and technology is estimated to be US $6.4 billion, representing a 10% growth from 2005 (Holman, 2007). The U.S. Federal Government budget request is in excess of US $1.4 billion for 2008, a 13% increase from 2007, and triple the US $464 million in 2001 (National Nanotechnology Initiative, 2008). With this funding increase, nanotechnology patent filings in the US, Europe, and Japan have also increased, gaining approximately 25% for a number of years (Li et al., 2007). Within the increased US Federal Government spending, approximately US $48 million in 2007 and US $59 million requested for 2008 is dedicated to programs supporting nanotechnology safety, health, and environmental issues. Additionally, industry contributes funding and resources toward initiatives focused on safety, health, and environment objectives, either internally or through national and international collaborations, such as NANOSAFE2 (Nanosafe2, 2007).

In 2007 alone, there have been a number of conferences dedicated either exclusively or partially to topics related to nanotechnology and safety, health, and the environment, including the 3rd International Symposium on Nanotechnology, Occupational and Environmental Health in Taipei, Taiwan, EuroNanOSH 2007 in Helsinki, Finland, as well as topical sessions within the annual conferences of the American Institute of Chemical Engineers (AIChE) in Salt Lake City, UT and the American Association of Aerosol Research (AAAR) in Reno, NV.

Throughout these collaborations and conference discussions, an overriding theme is that the potential societal benefits and issues associated with commercial-scale deployment of nanotechnology have raised many safety, health, and environmental questions about nanotechnology that must be addressed, including potential inhalation exposure of nanoparticles and potential risks associated with this exposure (Aitken et al., 2004; Royal Society and Academy of Engineers, 2004; Warheit, 2004; Pritchard, 2004). Engineered nanoparticles, as defined currently by the National Nanotechnology Initiative (National Nanotechnology Initiative, 2007), have at least one dimension in the range of 1-100 nm and possess unique properties and functions because of their nanometer-scale dimensions. Although there are several potential exposure routes, including ocular, dermal, and inhalation, within the scientific community, the route considered to have a greater risk of occupational exposure is inhalation. Employees with the highest exposure potential are those who are exposed to aerosolized nanoparticles that are either released or become airborne during the course of their materials handling activities. In order to protect workers from potential occupational exposure, academic and government safety and industrial hygiene groups are actively developing protocols and equipment to assess the effectiveness of workplace controls and to monitor workplace conditions for protecting their employees from exposure to aerosolized nanoparticles (Maynard and Kuempel, 2005; Liu et al., 1993). With current practices largely designed to protect in the >100-nm size range, the effectiveness of current containment and control procedures must either be verified for nanoparticles <100 nm or new methods for reducing inhalation exposure risk to nanoparticles must be developed (NIOSH, 1996, 2004, 2005). Specifically, the health, safety, and environmental community is actively involved in addressing several critical questions, including the following:

- Are new or different health or environmental concerns observed from a material with nanoscale dimensions versus the same material with greater than nanoscale dimensions?
- Will traditional air cleaning systems currently used to clean ambient workplace air operate correctly in the presence of nanoparticles?
- Will existing engineering controls designed to control dust or emissions function properly when nanoparticles are present?

- Will present personal protective equipment provide an effective barrier to nanoparticles? and
- Does the presence of nanoparticles change the fire or explosion hazard of a process?

Areas considered to be of greatest potential for nanoparticle inhalation exposure (and, thus, areas critical for initial investigation) focus on process steps in which (1) the nanoparticle exists as an aerosol with inhalation potential or (2) forces within the process are sufficient to reaerosolize potentially agglomerated particles back into their aerosol primary particle size. Once the nanoparticle is placed into a liquid or bound into a final product, inhalation exposure risk should be minimized, though this is highly product dependent and must be verified. For this reason, safety and occupational health professionals are presently focusing upon identifying and implementing safety containment and control procedures during aerosol nanoparticle synthesis and during process steps involving potential nanoparticle handling. Current safety practice guidance to reduce the potential for inhalation of airborne nanoparticles recommends employees to utilize the full range of containment and control measures, e.g., inherently safer design of engineering control technologies, work practice protocols, and personal protective equipment (NIOSH, 2005).

This chapter details a journey starting in 2004 to the present with the early discussion of safety, health, and environment issues related to nanotechnology that have helped in part to raise the attention to and awareness of these activities worldwide, the formation of an international consortium of industry, government, and non-government organizations, outlines of the technical program, highlights of the technical achievements and their significance, and recommendations for future work. This chapter is a small snap shot of that journey that is still under way. The chapter concludes with a brief discussion of general lessons learned throughout this process and insights for other companies considering similar initiatives.

6.1 INCEPTION AND FORMATION OF THE CONSORTIUM

6.1.1 Assessing the opportunity and understanding the needs

In early 2004, four visionary people from four different companies convened to discuss the emerging area of nanotechnology from an industrial hygiene perspective that they had been observing from within their own companies and the implications of this emerging technology on occupational safety and health issues. Although the company applications, products, and markets were varied among these four participants, their companies had several common goals, including to:

- Be proactive in assessing and understanding potential occupational safety and health issues related to the synthesis, handling, and fabrication of products that fell under the emerging field of nanotechnology;
- Share this knowledge broadly with their co-workers and collaborators; and
- Develop professional networks upon which further discussions and collaborations could be built.

All the company representatives were sensing the strong and pronounced technology trends within their companies that were moving toward nanotechnology-enabled programs and products. As representatives of companies with a history of robust management systems and strong work practices with safety and as company stewards charged with the occupational safety and health issues, particularly in emerging technologies, these visionaries recognized the necessity for collaborative efforts.

The culmination of this meeting resulted in an open assessment of the state-of-the-art knowledge of nanoparticle occupational safety and health within these four companies. Condensed into four basic questions outlined in Table 6.1, it became apparent that there was much to learn about nanotechnology as it pertained to occupational safety and health. The questions were broad, but the message was clear. The occupational safety and health community needed science-derived information on nanoparticle occupational safety and health issues, with particular emphasis on linking scientific data to real-world applications and to workplaces where nanoscale materials are produced, handled, and processed.

The first three questions were immediately identified as being common issues among many companies and organizations and the answers to these

Table 6.1 Questions Identified that Indicate Focus Areas for Occupational Safety and Health of Nanotechnology

- What is known about engineered nanoparticles in the work environment?
- What do we need to know in order to manage safely and effectively the technology within our businesses?
- What engineering controls, work practice, and management systems are appropriate?
- What is known about the toxicology of nanoparticles?

questions could potentially be addressed with a common set of objectives. The fourth question was not perceived to share the commonality with the other three since toxicology is often believed to be materials- or chemistry-specific. The focus of these three general questions was on providing knowledge and developing tools, and their answers would enable individual practitioners to make better judgments on risk and controls for their specific and often proprietary business situations. The next challenge was to determine if any of those three questions could be answered, and if so, then when and how?

6.1.2 The technology offering

With the list of three basic questions in hand, the first draft of the technical proposal that would form the foundation of the consortium was created in July 2004.

From the onset, this proposal was broken into three separate but interrelated activities called Deliverables. These are outlined in Table 6.2.

The broad intent of Deliverable 1 was to develop and build multiple reactors that could easily and reproducibly generate robust and stable aerosol nanoparticles so that the technical team could have a readily available supply of aerosol nanoparticles of various chemistries with controlled particle size distributions and number concentrations in order to conduct the different programs within each deliverable. If successful, these aerosol reactors would enable the technical team to attach various aerosol generators upstream of

Table 6.2 Deliverables and Activities for Consortium Articulated in Early Proposal to Address Focus Questions

- Deliverable 1
  - Generate well-characterized aerosols of various particle chemistries
  - Evaluate commercial instrumentation to measure aerosol nanoparticles
  - Characterize aerosol behavior as a function of time
- Deliverable 2
  - Develop a portable air sampling method for daily monitoring of R&D and manufacturing settings
- Deliverable 3
  - Develop a test method capable of measuring filtration efficiency of filter media to aerosol nanoparticles
  - Measure barrier efficiency of materials to aerosol nanoparticles

test systems, including the commercial instrumentation for evaluation and the aerosol chambers for time studies. Furthermore, these aerosol generators would be critical to generate the aerosols required to develop concepts for the portable monitor in Deliverable 2 and to synthesize the challenge aerosols for the test method development and measurement of filtration efficiency in Deliverable 3. A second goal of the aerosol nanoparticle synthesis was to design and develop robust nanoparticle synthesis systems to facilitate additional testing of nanomaterials outside of the consortium for occupational safety and health experiments, as well as for environmental and toxicological testing. Additional goals of Deliverable 1 included the evaluation of several commercial aerosol instruments to enable scientists with diverse backgrounds, expertise, and instruments to ascertain how data from their particular aerosol equipment would compare to data obtained from equipment referenced in the literature or utilized either by other sites within their own company or by collaborators at different companies or organizations. The ability to measure aerosol nanoparticle behavior as a function of time was identified as a need to assess how aerosol nanoparticles behave and change over time in open environments or in gas handling equipment, including ventilation systems, or to understand how they may be transported or transformed throughout an occupational setting. This deliverable has important ramifications in providing knowledge on how to implement appropriate work practice controls to contain and to handle nanoparticles with either conventional or new gas handling equipment and containment practices.

The purpose of Deliverable 2 was to either internally develop a prototype concept or instrument or facilitate the external development of a portable aerosol monitor that could be used in a variety of occupational settings as a monitoring or detecting instrument. To be useful to industrial hygienists, this instrument would have to be capable of measuring an aerosol nanoparticle number concentration with limited size classification capability for broad aerosol particle chemistries. This instrument was envisioned to be similar to other industrial hygiene tools that probe indoor air quality, but it would be specifically designed to detect aerosol nanoparticles. In addition to assessing indoor air quality, this instrument would have additional value in verifying the effectiveness of work practice controls to contain nanoparticles and of gas handling and ventilation systems to remove or contain nanoparticles, and in detecting whether specific processes were responsible for the generation of aerosol nanoparticles.

The goal of Deliverable 3 was to measure the filtration efficiency of commercially available filter media to aerosol nanoparticles with a practical goal, namely, to inform members on how filter media being used in their companies performed toward filtration of aerosol nanoparticles under various process conditions. Upon review of the state of the art in the literature and after assessing certification standard test methods, this deliverable acquired an additional feature: to develop a test method that was capable of measuring filtration efficiency of filter media to aerosol nanoparticles, particularly in regard to industrially relevant particles and conditions.

6.1.3 Collecting early feedback on industry interest in a consortium

In October 2004, a letter was broadly circulated to all interested parties (1) to assess the level of interest in pursuing a collaborative consortium related to occupational safety and health of nanotechnology and (2) to determine the extent to which the proposed technical solution would meet the needs of a broad audience. The full text of the letter appears in the Appendix. Briefly, this letter included a description of the background and objectives of a consortium and the early draft of the technology proposal that included three deliverables, namely:

(1) Development of a method to generate a well-characterized aerosol of solid nanoparticles in air and evaluate instrumentation to measure solid nanoparticles in air in the aerosol generation equipment;

(2) Develop an air sampling method that can be used on a day-to-day basis in R&D or manufacturing settings; and

(3) Measure filtration or penetration/permeation and protection of protective clothing and materials with respect to specific engineered nanoparticles or nanomaterials. Provide measurement capability as a service.

As for the concept of a consortium to tackle these issues, the decision was a natural progression from the 2004 discussion between the four companies that resulted in the generation of the four questions from Table 6.1, especially considering the commonality of the needs in occupational safety and health issues involving nanotechnology.

6.1.4 Technical and uncertainty assessment—the peer review process

Since committed to the concept of a funded consortium and from the feedback from the October 2004 interest solicitation, it was determined that the proposal needed to be technically validated by a panel of independent, expert individuals who were neither associated with the proposal nor with potential members of the future consortium to refine the proposal to increase opportunities for success and to increase the acceptance of the technical proposal across broad audiences. The goal of this peer review process was to collect an assessment of the technical merits from an expert and independent panel to determine whether or not this proposal had a technical right to succeed and to determine if additional or different technical approaches may improve opportunities for success. The panel convened in Dec 2004 and included four academic experts and four nanotechnology experts from US national laboratories and facilities. In this peer review process, each of the elements of the three deliverables were presented and discussed in detail, including the overall goal of each deliverable and how the deliverables were interrelated, the objectives of the experimental plan and potential deviations or additions from that proposed plan, and the proposed technical solution, including instrumentation needs, milestones, and budgets. For each of the three deliverables, the panelists were asked to answer the following four questions as shown in Table 6.3.

From the discussion and formal feedback from the eight-member technical panel, this proposal was unanimously technically validated and was determined to be based on sound science with a technical right to succeed. As with any research proposal, technical challenges were acknowledged from the beginning by the technical representatives, particularly in the Deliverable 2 goals, and the expert panel acknowledged those same technical challenges as being the most ambitious and riskiest in their comments. However, they reiterated that these were the right objectives to be focused on since they had the highest needs among broad audiences. The proposed technical program was not going to be trivial to accomplish, but the proposal offered a sound technical plan to address many of the most important questions on nanoparticle occupational safety and health. Furthermore, the technical panel stated that they could not suggest an easier technical approach to address these objectives and that they knew of no existing literature data that could immediately address these objectives. However, several panel members highlighted relevant work in the early stages,

Table 6.3 Expert Panel Member Questions and Discussion Topics for Peer Review of Technical Proposal

- Does the approach we propose have a technical right to succeed?
- What are the major barriers we will need to overcome? Do you have any advice?
- Can you suggest an alternative approach to meet the deliverable that is (a) more certain to succeed or (b) faster or (c) lower cost?
- Are you aware of any other work that either makes what we are doing redundant or is something we can build on?

particularly in areas of measuring filtration efficiency of commercial and early production filter media.

6.1.5 Forming the consortium

In March 2005, a meeting was held in which all interested companies were invited to participate. Attendance included participants across broad industries and among all portions of the nanotechnology value chain, from raw materials suppliers, to materials compounders and integrators, and to device companies. Although mid- and large-size companies were well represented, start-up companies and small businesses also participated. At this meeting, the proposed technical approach to address the issues around occupational safety and health of nanoparticles was communicated. The merits and objectives of the proposal as well as the technical challenges were presented and discussed. This meeting served several purposes: it introduced the potential members of the consortium to the why, how, where, and when of the technical proposal to address the main objectives; it sought reinforcement of those initial objectives; it established a technical foundation to build on the technical components included in the proposal; and most importantly, it brought diverse professionals with broad backgrounds and perspectives from many companies and organizations together to discuss diverse issues involving individual and collective concerns over occupational safety and health of nanotechnology. Fortunately, it also illustrated the commonality of many of these concerns as identified by a diverse audience. This meeting emphasized the benefit of and necessity for undertaking this work as a collective group of interested and collaborative parties.

The culmination of the two-day event was a request to individual companies to determine whether or not they wanted to participate in the consortium. A maximum financial commitment and minimum member commitment was proposed: a maximum contribution of $68,000 and a minimum member commitment of 10 members. In August 2005, the formation of the Consortium was finalized. The membership included the companies listed in Table 6.4. Although additional members are participating, they require that the NOSH Consortium keep their membership confidential. From Table 6.4, it is clear that mid- and large-size companies were well represented. Although start-up and small companies participated in these earliest discussions, they expressed interest in contributing to the consortium through non-cash contributions, including supplying nanomaterials. These offers, although appreciated, were seen to be complicating an already complicated initiative, and majority decision dictated that cash and not in-kind payments would be required for membership in the consortium.

Table 6.4 NOSH Consortium Membership

Air Products & Chemicals, Inc.	
Boeing	Health & Safety Executive (UK)
Degussa	Intel Corporation
Department of Energy Office of Science	Kimberly-Clark
Dow Chemical	NIOSH
DuPont	PPG
Environmental Defense	Procter & Gamble
GE	Rohm & Haas

6.2 AIMS AND OBJECTIVES OF NOSH CONSORTIUM

6.2.1 High level consortium charter

With the widespread recognition that engineered nanoparticles are becoming incorporated into an increasing number of products across a wide variety of applications (Project on Emerging Nanotechnologies, 2008), opportunities and mechanisms for exposure are just as varied. As stated earlier, these routes can include inhalation, ingestion, and ocular and transdermal exposure (NIOSH, 2005). Although all exposure routes are critical, the immediate scope for this work was focused on understanding inhalation exposure and assessing behavior of solid-engineered aerosol nanoparticles.

6.2.2 The introductory advisory board meeting

Prior to the August 24–25, 2005 meeting, the Consortium was established. The formal contracts were signed and the legal procedures and requirements were established. Additionally, the technical objectives were broadly defined by a proposed technical plan, and a series of potential experiments to arrive at those objectives and a high level of procedural guidance was established in the signed contracts. The technical and logistical details, however, remained to be formalized. At the August 24 and 25 meeting, the meeting attendees and member representatives were charged with the task of agreeing on the specific details of the technical plan and on how the consortium would operate logistically. To initiate the consortium within a firm foundation, the high-level objectives were reiterated and the proposed work and technical plan were discussed in detail.

Within the technical proposal presentation, the first opportunity for open discussion and debate involved the decision on what nanomaterials chemistries would be synthesized as part of Deliverable 1. Prior to this meeting, several materials had been identified from a variety of perspectives as being most suitable to try and were included in the initial discussion. These materials had diverse, yet common synthesis methods. In some cases, these synthesis methods were well known in the literature or were being actively investigated by other groups. In some cases, these methods included procedures also used commonly in scaled-up manufacturing or occupational environments, such as thermal evaporation, spray pyrolysis, or thermal decomposition. They also included broad classes of material chemistries that were either industrially relevant due to their large-scale production at larger particle sizes or they could be in large-scale production at the nanoscale due to their commercially relevant properties. There were also materials selected for the sole purpose of being different from each other, such that any differences in their behaviors (through filter media or aerosol behavior over time, for example) could offer insights for future work and directions. This first broad sweep of materials included the following classes: inorganic amorphous metal oxides, inorganic crystalline metal oxides, noble metals, water soluble organics, natural nanoscale clay materials, particles with organically modified surfaces, and a standard reference material.

Through discussions with members, it became quite apparent that there was considerable interest in including carbon-based materials, such as carbon black, nanotubes, or other fullerenes. Recognized as a material of interest for occupational safety and health, carbon-based material also appeared to be undergoing significant scale-up work at a variety of companies and academic groups due to its potentially important and commercially relevant properties. However, there were several logistical and legal issues related to pursuing carbon-based fullerene materials that made including them in the technical program challenging (despite the obvious value of including fullerenes in the consortium work), including the fact that most synthesis methods for carbon nanotubes and fullerenes were proprietary or patented. The consortium would then either have to focus on investing time and resources in licensing a synthesis method in order to be able to produce aerosolized material in situ, have a member agree to disclose thoroughly their synthesis methods to the consortium membership and technical team, or develop new methods to generate fullerene material. Furthermore, at the time, no aerosol instrumentation had been calibrated for high aspect ratio materials, so even if fullerene synthesis methods were straightforward, a significant effort to assess the aerosol instrument performance to large aspect ratio materials or calibrate existing aerosol instruments for non spherical, high aspect ratio materials (e.g., nanotubes) would also be required. Undeniably, the company representatives agreed that this important work should be done, but the decision came down to the realization that licensing or developing fullerene synthesis and characterization methods was not really within the scope, budget, and timing of this program and that there were higher priority tasks to accomplish. Additionally, other groups were expressing an interest in including fullerene materials in their studies.

After brainstorming possible nanomaterials for study, the members used a power voting technique to select materials for inclusion in the study. The materials with the most votes would be highest priority and the one with the fewest votes would be lowest priority. The power voting results broke down into the following ranking as seen in Table 6.5.

Upon further refinement of this list, two additional materials were added after voting: a 100-nm polystyrene latex National Institute of Standards and Technology (NIST) standard reference material to calibrate the aerosol instrumentation and citric acid, a water-soluble organic material to include a material that has distinct aerosol behaviors due to its water soluble property although it is not industrially or commercially relevant to any member companies. During this day, the initial technical experimental plans were discussed. A considerable amount of time was also invested in educating and providing a common language that would be used in all subsequent consortium communications.

On day two of the meeting, the members discussed operationally how the meetings, interactions, communications, and other logistics would proceed. During this discussion, the name for the consortium was formalized as the Nanoparticle Occupational Safety and Health Consortium, or NOSH

Table 6.5 Results from Voting on Material Chemistries for Deliverable 1

Nanoscale Material	Number of Votes
Silica	17
Clay	11
Titanium Dioxide	10
Silver	9
Organofunctional Material	8
Nanotubes	4
Buckminster Fullerenes	3
Silicon Carbide	3
Carbon Black	3
Nickel Oxide	1
Indium Tin Oxide	1

Table 6.6 Roles and Responsibility of Advisory Board Members

(1) Act as technical consultants for the Project Manager.

- Understand the work plan—content/status/next steps
- Help in problem solving ("how to" and also strategic direction when circumstances change)
- Keep an eye on the big picture to ensure that strategic directives are met
- Agree on the materials to study in Deliverable 1

(2) Inform the Project Manager and other members of relevant work being done by other groups.
(3) Recruit agreed upon new members (2/3 majority vote). New members must add value and we should do "sensing" within the Advisory Board before we actively invite others to join.
(4) Act as the voice of the customer (e.g. for Deliverable 2, what does "portable" mean?).
(5) Approve external communications (straightforward majority vote).

- Initial announcement
- Ongoing communication plan
- Decide what, if anything, is confidential and agree on timing of release of information
- Publications

While collectively,
(A) The Advisory Board will support the project team without "micro managing".
(B) We will respect the diverse nature of the group.
(C) We will communicate with other relevant groups active in the field, will take their advice/suggestions into account when problem solving our work, and will communicate our results within the framework of our communication strategy.

Consortium. The membership also discussed confidentiality issues and requirements for communication. Advisory Board Meetings via conference call were to occur every quarter with an annual face-to-face meeting that would also include a lab tour of the facilities. The NOSH Consortium Advisory Board included a representative from each company contributing funding to the consortium as well as from non-contributing strategic members. The other product of this meeting was the definition of the roles and responsibilities of the Advisory Board as detailed in Table 6.6 and its interaction with the technical team.

6.3 THE TECHNICAL PROGRAM

As seen by the roles of the Advisory Board members (highlighted in Table 6.6, section 1), the entire technical plan for the NOSH Consortium was

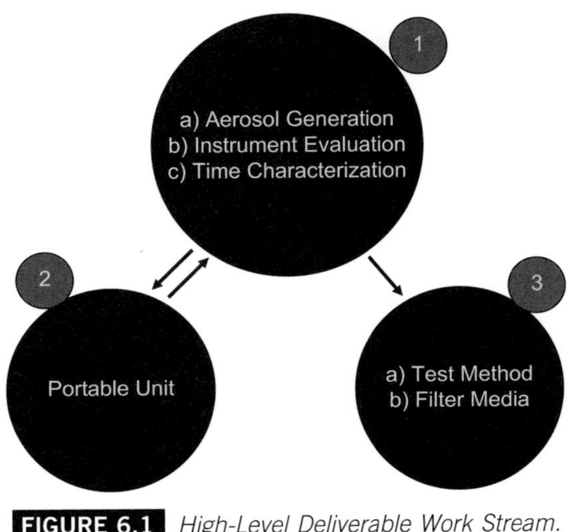

FIGURE 6.1 *High-Level Deliverable Work Stream.*

not rigidly fixed at the first meeting. Rather, there were some decisions that would be made as progress was completed and as information was generated to reflect the best state-of-the-art knowledge (inside and outside the NOSH Consortium) available at the time when the decisions were needed.

Rather than working on the deliverables consecutively and in series, work proceeded in order of practicality, need, and priority as illustrated in Figure 6.1. Efforts were initially started on Deliverable 1 SiO_2 aerosol nanoparticle synthesis in order to facilitate work on Deliverables 2 and 3. With the SiO_2 aerosol nanoparticle reactors up and running, work then progressed on each of the deliverables in parallel, with early emphasis on 1a, 1b, and 3 and followed by later emphasis on 1c and 2. Initial emphasis on 3 was high because members wanted to know as soon as possible the filtration efficiency behavior of commercially available filter media that they may be using in their individual companies based upon their specific business conditions and situations.

6.3.1 Deliverable 1

6.3.1.1 Aerosol nanoparticle synthesis

6.3.1.1.1 In situ aerosol nanoparticle synthesis

One objective of the NOSH Consortium was to develop robust synthesis methods to generate the broad particle chemistries using a variety of

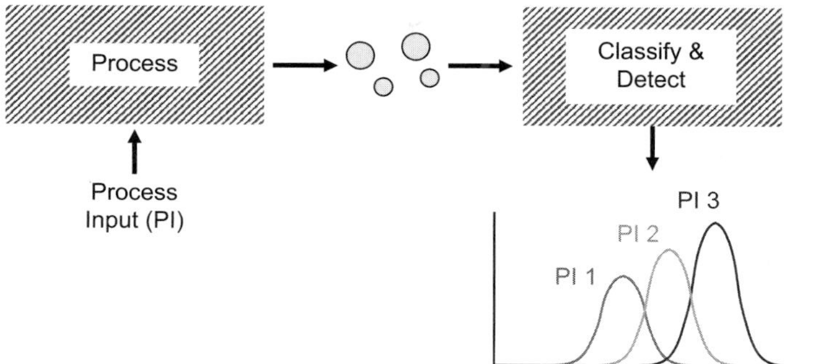

FIGURE 6.2 *Resulting Particle Size Distribution of In Situ Synthesized Aerosol Nanoparticles is a Function of Input Process Parameters.*

generation techniques. To address both priorities, SiO_2 and TiO_2 were selected for their industrial relevance and for their amorphous (SiO_2) and crystalline (TiO_2) metal oxide chemistries and were to be generated via thermal decomposition of liquid precursors. Citric acid was selected, not for its industrial relevance, but because it is an organic material and is water soluble and is, thus, very different from many of the other selected aerosol nanoparticles for this study. Citric acid was to be synthesized via spray atomization followed by drying. Silver was selected for its industrial relevance and for its crystalline metal chemistry and would be prepared via thermal evaporation of solid silver. Polystyrene latex was selected because it is a NIST Traceable standard material that is used frequently in aerosol research to calibrate and verify performance of aerosol instrumentation. Aerosols of polystyrene latex particles were to be generated using spray atomization of a polystyrene latex suspension. Because the SiO_2 aerosol nanoparticle system was developed first, most of the extensive characterization on aerosol instrumentation and filter media testing was done with this SiO_2 particle system.

As represented in Figure 6.2, the resulting particle size distribution of in situ synthesized aerosol nanoparticles depends upon the process and the process conditions used to synthesize the nanomaterials, such as precursor concentration, furnace temperature, vapor pressures, and precursor types.

6.3.1.1.2 Reaerosolization of bulk nanomaterials

Handling of nanoparticle powders may present a particle inhalation hazard (although this needs to be verified) but not necessarily in the nanometer size range. When nanoparticles are collected as powders, adhesion forces between adjacent particles are significantly large such that these materials may prove

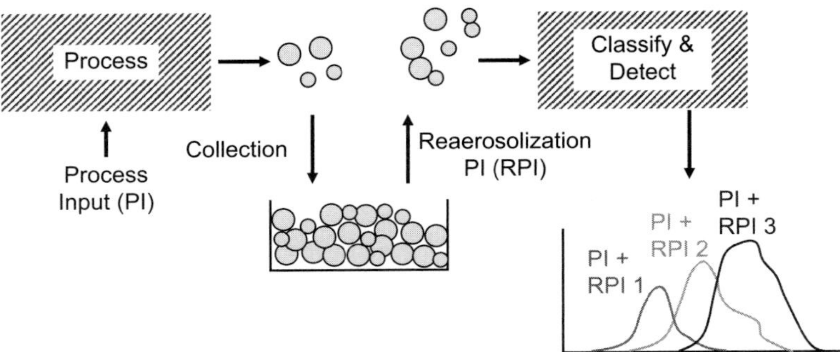

FIGURE 6.3 *Resulting Particle Size Distribution of Reaerosolized Nanoparticles from Bulk Nanopowders is a Function of Input Synthesis Process Parameters As Well As Input Process Parameters Used in the Reaerosolization Step.*

to be low-inhalation risk materials in the nanometer size range simply due to the extremely high energy required (1) to reaerosolize the materials and (2) to break them down into their primary nanoparticle size. To understand whether larger agglomerates of nanoparticles pose special risks requires additional investigation to determine whether, for example, these agglomerates break apart once in the body into their primary nanoparticle size. For these reasons, a natural nanomaterial of montmorillonite clay was selected for study. The notable difference between the montmorillonite clay and the other particle chemistries is that the montmorillonite clay would be aerosolized from bulk powder and not synthesized in situ.

As represented in Figure 6.3, the resulting particle size distribution of reaerosolized bulk nanomaterials depends not only upon the bulk nanopowder properties formed by controlling the process inputs, but also upon the parameters used in reaerosolization process, including reaerosolization method, pressures, and forces and not necessarily upon the original process conditions used to synthesize the nanomaterials prior to collection as bulk nanopowder.

6.3.1.1.3 Aerosol nanoparticle synthesis of various chemistries

6.3.1.1.3.1 Generation of stable SiO_2 aerosol nanoparticles

The initial technical requirement for the program was the ability to generate stable and reproducible aerosol nanoparticles of various chemistries in situ upstream of other aerosol instrumentation or experimental apparatus for the three deliverables. Once these aerosol nanoparticle reactors were developed, the objectives and goals of Deliverables 2 and 3 could be pursued.

Due to the behavior of aerosol nanoparticles and their instability as a function of time, aerosol nanoparticles currently cannot be collected and stored for future aerosol use while simultaneously preserving the original aerosol size distribution or properties. An aerosol of solid nanoparticles with a specific particle size, size distribution, and number concentration cannot be recreated simply by reaerosolizing that same solid material once it has been collected in bulk. For this reason, studies involving aerosol nanoparticles and their properties must maintain an aerosol nanoparticle reactor in situ within a process, upstream of characterization equipment, as well as upstream of any filter testing units or inhalation toxicology equipment. This tool must be easy to use and to operate and must demonstrate long-term, stable, reproducible generation of aerosol nanoparticles.

Aerosol particles have been synthesized in industrial quantities as aerosols for a number of years, including TiO_2, carbon black, and SiO_2. Numerous aerosol nanoparticle reactors are detailed in the literature that generate aerosols through various methods, including thermal evaporation to produce Ag particles (Kim et al., 2007), liquid spray to generate NaCl and DOP particles (Martin and Moyer, 2000), and thermal decomposition to produce Si particles (Camata et al., 1996). The variety of aerosol particle morphologies that can result may have important occupational health implications in that aerosol particles sintered into hard agglomerates may retain their structure after inhalation, whereas soft agglomerates may disperse in the lungs after inhalation. This issue poses additional opportunities for inhalation toxicology experiments that utilize aerosol reactors upstream of in vivo studies.

With the results from the power voting that indicated a high level of interest among the consortium members and the recognition that amorphous SiO_2 is an industrially relevant nanomaterial, the initial aerosol nanoparticle reactor was built to thermally decompose TEOS to generate SiO_2 aerosol nanoparticles. In the specific case of amorphous silica, various methods exist to synthesize SiO_2 aerosol nanoparticles, including spray pyrolysis, flame synthesis, thermal evaporation, and even spray drying of colloidal or precipitated particles (Biswas and Pratsinis, 1989; Xiong et al., 1993; Okuyama et al., 1991). Particularly in industrial scale reactors, the resulting aerosol is typically comprised of highly agglomerated nanometer-sized primary particles such that the final aerosol can be several hundred nanometers in mobility diameter. Extensive articles previously published in the literature have modeled and characterized many SiO_2 aerosol particle formation and growth mechanisms, including sintering of SiO_2 via viscous flow (Ulrich and Riehl, 1982) and high-temperature gas phase synthesis of SiO_2 to understand agglomerated particle formation by coagulation and sintering (Martin and Moyer, 2000). Ehrman (1999) also examined effects of SiO_2 particle size on coalescence rate. Tsantilis and Pratsinis (2004) further developed and improved a model to account for the effects of process parameters, including temperature, residence time, precursor concentration, and cooling rate on the degree of agglomeration of SiO_2 that accounts for simultaneous chemical reactions, coagulation, and sintering. For the purposes of the NOSH Consortium, the initial activities focused upon designing a high-temperature reactor to synthesize a stable source of SiO_2 aerosol nanoparticles with no halogen-containing reactants, products, or byproducts for occupational health and safety applications. As demonstrated by Ostraat et al. (2005), TEOS vapor can undergo homogeneous nucleation at sufficient rates to produce SiO_2 aerosol nanoparticles at reaction temperatures >800 °C. Although not suitable for large scale manufacturing of SiO_2 aerosol nanoparticles, it turns out that the TEOS reactor and corresponding classification and detection capabilities pictured in Figure 6.4 is ideal for studying aerosol behavior of nanoparticles, for measuring filter efficiency of media to nanoparticles, and for developing monitoring and sampling techniques and equipment for verifying workplace exposure assessments, protocols, procedures and containment methodologies.

The detailed schematic of this SiO_2 aerosol nanoparticle reactor is shown in Figure 6.5 with two differential mobility analyzers (DMAs) used for aerosol particle classification (nano-DMA and long-DMA) and two aerosol detectors, namely a condensation nucleus counter (CNC) and an aerosol electrometer (AE).

Data obtained from the SiO_2 aerosol nanoparticle reactor and classification and detection systems are tabulated in Table 6.7. As shown in Table 6.7, by changing two main process conditions, namely Q_{pr} and T_{furn}, the aerosol particle size distribution can be varied to produce particles from 7 nm $< d_{50}$ $<$ 45 nm at concentrations $\sim 10^5$–10^8 particles/cm^3, depending upon reactor configurations and tubing details.

These SiO_2 aerosol nanoparticles initially form by homogeneous nucleation and continue to grow by chemical vapor deposition and by particle

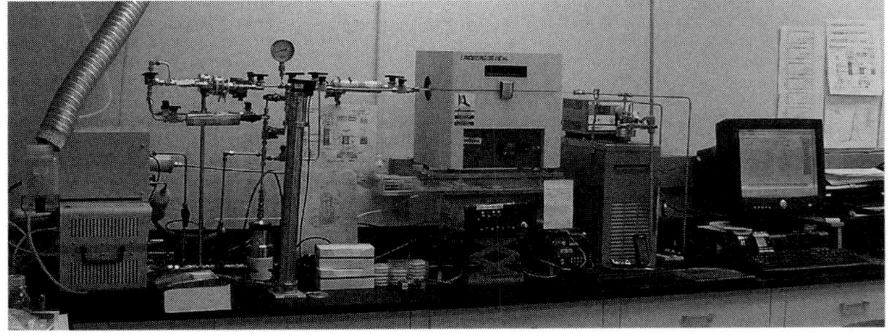

FIGURE 6.4 *Benchtop SiO_2 Aerosol Nanoparticle Reactor with Nanoparticle Synthesis on the Right Side and Classification and Detection Capabilities on the Left Side.*

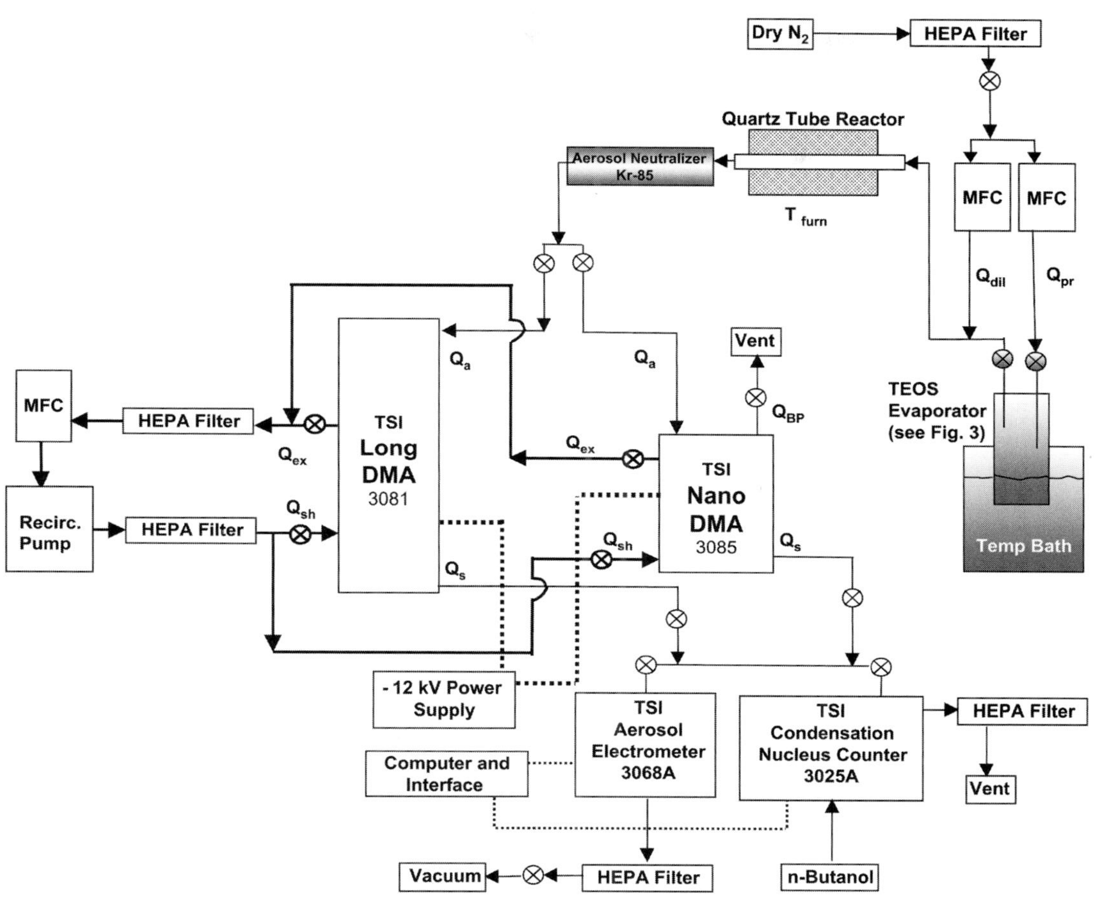

FIGURE 6.5 *Schematic of the SiO_2 Aerosol Nanoparticle Reactor with Classification and Detection Capabilities.*

coalescence as shown pictorially in Figure 6.6. Although the data are not shown, this reactor produces amorphous aerosol particles as measured by XRD and contains Si as measured by EDX.

Table 6.7 shows d_{50} in nm and σ_g as a function of Q_{pr} and T_{furn} for this reactor schematic as measured by the nano-DMA. By increasing Q_{pr} and maintaining a constant $T_{furn} = 750$ °C, the particle size distribution grows from $d_{50} \sim 7$ nm to $d_{50} \sim 20$ nm, whereas the σ_g does not clearly trend in one direction. However, due to the limitation of the nano-DMA at the specific flow values used, the particle distribution data becomes less reliable at particle sizes >60 nm. By increasing T_{furn} to 950 °C, a similar trend is observed. At increasing Q_{pr}, the d_{50} increases from $d_{50} \sim 15$ nm to $d_{50} \sim 42$ nm and the peak particle number concentration increases.

Table 6.7 SiO_2 Aerosol Nanoparticles with d_{50} in nm and σ_g as Classified by the Nano-DMA and Detected with the AE at Various Q_{pr} and T_{furn} Process Parameters

Q_{pr} (cm^3/min)	750 °C	850 °C	925 °C	950 °C
0.4		8.6 1.49		
1	6.7 1.45	10.7 1.64	12.7 1.61	15.1 1.51
3	6.7 2.04	18.4 1.64	21.0 1.60	24.7 1.56
5	9.6 1.87	23.7 1.63	25.6 1.58	31.3 1.51
10	15.0 1.75	32.5 1.56	39.5 1.53	41.7 1.48
15	19.3 1.91			

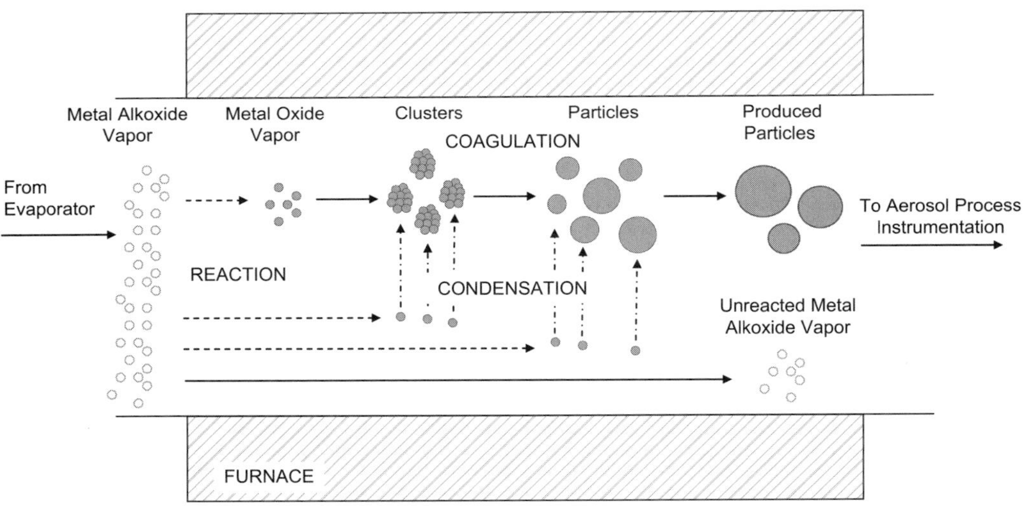

FIGURE 6.6 *Thermal Decomposition Process to Form Aerosol Nanoparticles. (Adapted from Okuyama et al., 1986.)*

In Figure 6.7, the particle size distributions as classified by the nano-DMA and detected by the AE show an increase in particle size and number concentration as Q_{pr} increases up to ~25 cm^3/min. After reaching the

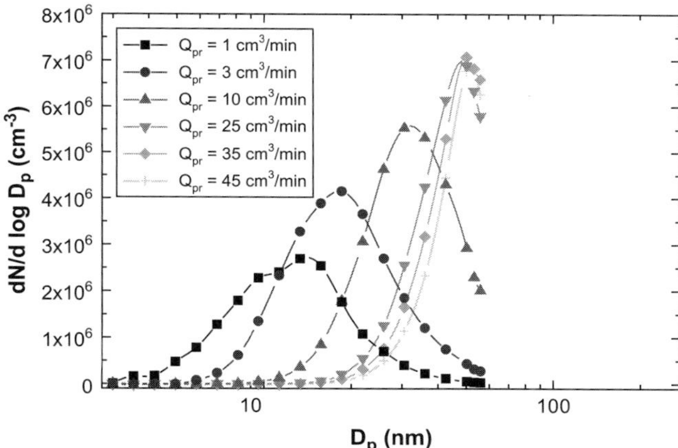

FIGURE 6.7 *Particle Size Distributions of SiO_2 Aerosol Nanoparticles Generated via Thermal Decomposition as Classified with a Nano-DMA.*

upper size classification of the nano-DMA, no significant changes in the particle size distribution are detected with the nano-DMA as Q_{pr} is further increased to 45 cm^3/min. At $Q_{pr} < 3$ cm^3/min, a size distribution with a double peak is recorded, indicating that particles are growing by nucleation and chemical vapor deposition (left peak) and growing by coalescence (right peak).

However, as seen in Figure 6.8, using a long-DMA increases the range of larger particle sizes that can be classified and resolved. Figure 6.8

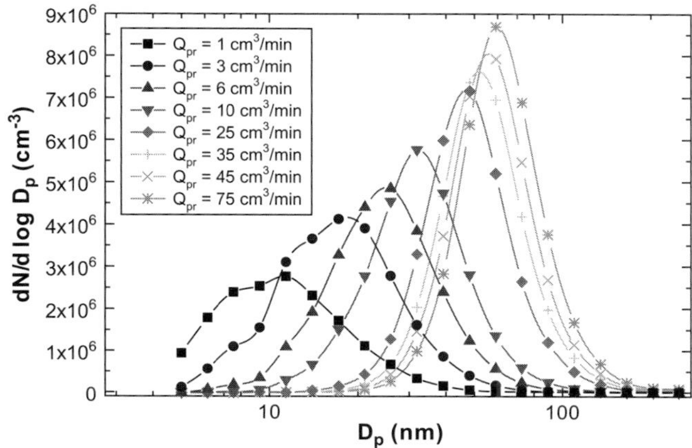

FIGURE 6.8 *Particle Size Distributions of SiO_2 Aerosol Nanoparticles Generated via Thermal Decomposition as Classified with a Long-DMA.*

demonstrates the increase in both the particle size and in the number concentration as Q_{pr} is increased beyond 45 cm^3/min to 75 cm^3/min. Above 75 cm^3/min, no further increase in size or number concentration is observed. This may be due to the limited rate of TEOS delivery available from the current TEOS evaporator design. As seen with the nano-DMA, the long-DMA is also able to resolve the double peak at $Q_{pr} < 3$ cm^3/min.

6.3.1.1.3.2 Long-term stability of SiO_2 aerosol nanoparticle generation

Long-term stability of the reactor has been verified for daily operation ~6 months for multiple process conditions for the variables $T_{furn} = 850$ °C and $Q_{pr} = 1$, 10, and 75 cm^3/min. As illustrated in Figure 6.9 by particle size distributions selected randomly from measurements taken during each of five successive months at $Q_{pr} = 10$ cm^3/min, the long-term stability of the generation system is very high. A minimum of two particle size distributions per day have been measured and documented to verify and to establish the daily and long-term stability of this reactor configuration, although only illustrative data for process conditions $Q_{pr} \sim 10$ cm^3/min and $T_{furn} = 850$ °C are shown in this chapter. In this five-month period, the stability of the reactor was such that the particle diameter differences were <10%, within the instrument resolution of the DMAs. The number concentration data did not show significant differences at the peak particle diameter. These data indicate that the system is stable and that the reactor

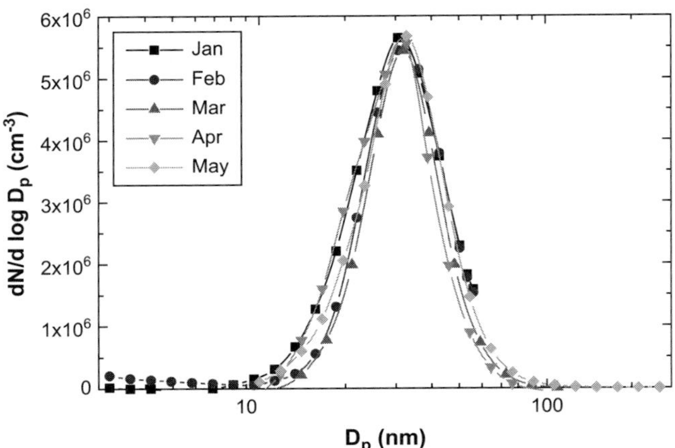

FIGURE 6.9 *Long-Term Stability of the SiO_2 Aerosol Nanoparticle Reactor with Five Randomly Selected Particle Size Distributions at $T_{furn} = 850$ °C and $Q_{pr} = 10$ cm^3/min Over 5 Months.*

system can be operated without constant aerosol monitoring. Thus, once the aerosol reactor is characterized and as long as the TEOS is kept dry, the reactor scheme described can produce a stable, reproducible source of SiO_2 aerosol nanoparticles for at least 6 months. The demonstrated daily and long-term stability of this reactor makes this reactor an accessible and acceptable source of SiO_2 aerosol nanoparticles to a broad audience, including to the non-aerosol community for occupational health and safety testing and to users who do not have dedicated aerosol classification and detection instrumentation for daily monitoring. The stability of the reactor could be further improved if the applications require more rigorous control over long-term particle size distributions and particle number concentrations.

6.3.1.1.3.3 Significance of the SiO_2 aerosol nanoparticle reactor

A useful and simple reactor was developed to produce stable, well-controlled amorphous SiO_2 aerosol nanoparticles in the <100-nm size range. By varying the partial pressure of TEOS introduced into a tube furnace and the TEOS reaction temperature, nanoparticles with peak particle diameter from 10 to 70 nm can be produced with stable results for at least 6 months. Additionally, the SiO_2 aerosol nanoparticles can be produced at number concentrations from $\sim 10^3$ to 10^8 particles/cm^3 depending upon dilution following synthesis, providing a useful tool to measure the effect of aerosol nanoparticle concentration on occupational safety and health studies. Although not scaleable to larger volumes as a manufacturing source of nanoparticles, this reactor design is ideal for the synthesis of a well-characterized, stable aerosol for applications in occupational health and safety studies. Long-term stability of this reactor scheme enables researchers to do periodic aerosol monitoring of the reactor, allowing access to in situ synthesized aerosol nanoparticles for groups that do not have dedicated aerosol classification and detection equipment available on a daily basis for their activities. The data indicates that this aerosol reactor and process can be used to deliver reproducible, stable particle diameters and known concentrations of amorphous SiO_2 aerosol nanoparticles for inhalation toxicology programs, explosion studies, filter efficiency studies, and industrial hygiene monitoring and sampling needs for workplace exposure methodologies.

6.3.1.1.3.4 Titanium dioxide nanoparticle synthesis

Schematically, the TiO_2 nanoparticle system is similar to the SiO_2 reactor system, except for the liquid precursor used in the evaporation. The silicon dioxide system uses TEOS, whereas the titanium dioxide system uses titanium isopropoxide. Because these two liquid precursors have different

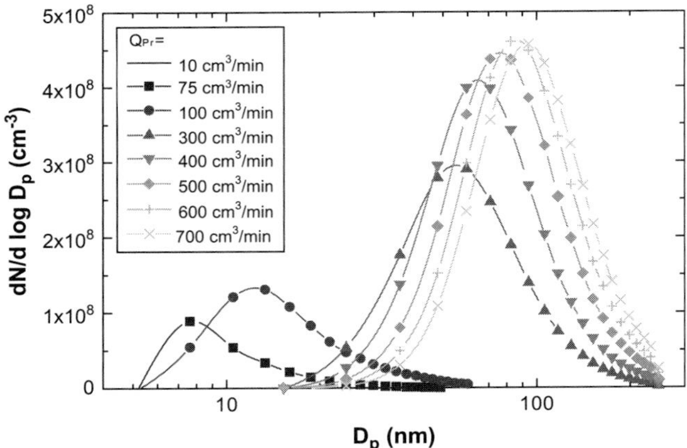

FIGURE 6.10 *TiO_2 Aerosol Nanoparticle Size Distributions Classified with a Nano-DMA for Q_{pr} = 10-75 cm^3/min and with a Long-DMA for $Q_{pr} > 75$ cm^3/min to Obtain The Full Size Range from 10 nm $< d_p <$ 200 nm.*

physical and chemical properties, different process conditions must be used to generate aerosol nanoparticles of similar particle diameters.

The following graph in Figure 6.10 details the particle size distribution of titanium dioxide particles that results from a reactor with the following process parameter fixed at $T_{pr} = 40\,°C$ and $T_{furn} = 900\,°C$. By varying the Q_{pr}, the particle size distribution and the number concentration can be controlled.

From the TEM in Figure 6.11 taken from the Q_{pr} = 700 cm^3/min, these particles do not appear to be single particles. These particles, however, are crystalline with an anatase phase (XRD data not shown).

6.3.1.1.3.5 Citric acid nanoparticle synthesis

Citric acid nanoparticles were produced using a common aerosol technique, known as spray atomization. In spray atomization, high-pressure gas is used to shear off liquid particles through an orifice to produce liquid droplets with a well-controlled diameter. In the setup used to support the NOSH Consortium effort, the as-generated liquid particle size distribution is centered at $d_{50} \sim 350$ nm with a σ_g that is preserved through the solid aerosol formation. By varying the concentration of citric acid dissolved in water as the liquid precursor, the constant output spray atomizer and diffusion dryer can be used to produce dry particles of different sizes within a certain range according to the following approximation in Equation 1 that correlates the wet to dry particle relationship.

$$d_{dry} \approx d_{wet}\left(\frac{C_{wet}}{\rho_{dry}}\right)^{\frac{1}{3}} \tag{1}$$

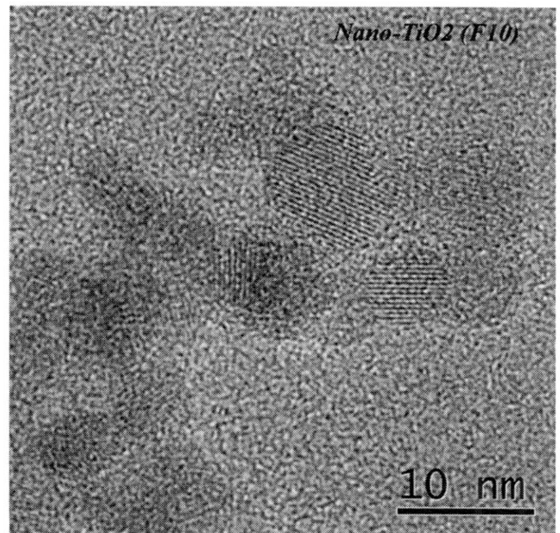

FIGURE 6.11 *Transmission Electron Micrograph of Crystalline TiO_2 Synthesized at $T_{furn} = 900\,°C$.*

where d_{dry} and d_{wet} are the dry and wet particle diameters, respectively, C_{wet} is the concentration of the liquid precursor, and ρ_{dry} is the density of the dry particle.

The following graph in Figure 6.12 illustrates the size distribution of dry citric acid nanoparticles generated with the constant output atomizer as a function of precursor concentration. By increasing the citric acid

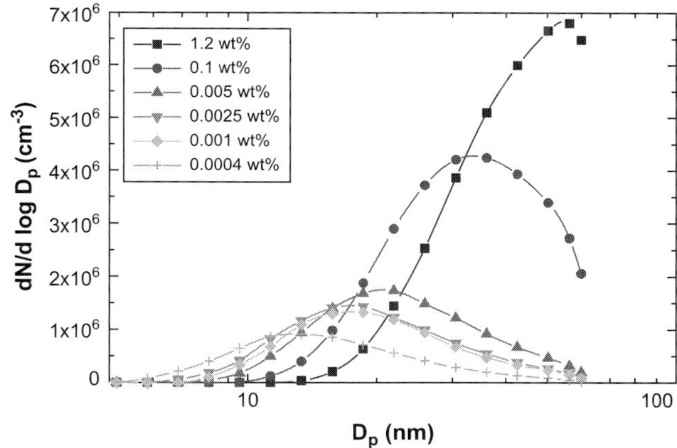

FIGURE 6.12 *Citric Acid Aerosol Nanoparticle Size Distributions Generated via Spray Atomization and Diffusion Drying.*

concentration in the liquid precursor, the dry particle diameter increases. These results can be readily transferred to other solvent and solute systems.

6.3.1.1.3.6 Silver nanoparticle synthesis

Silver nanoparticles were generated using a common technique known as thermal evaporation. The synthesis of aerosol particles of metal via thermal evaporation is shown schematically in Figure 6.13, in which a source of silver is placed into the hot zone of a furnace, heated to create vapor of the solid silver material, and cooling to nucleate and grow aerosol nanoparticles.

This technique to produce aerosols of silver nanoparticles has been discussed in the literature (Kim et al., 2007). Although several process parameters can be varied to change the resulting particle size distribution, such as gas flow rate and residence time, the process parameter selected for the NOSH Consortium effort was furnace temperature. By varying the temperature of the furnace, the particle size distribution can be changed as seen in the resulting size distributions for silver particles in Figure 6.14.

6.3.1.1.3.7 Polystyrene latex particle synthesis

Polystyrene latex (PSL) particle suspensions are common calibration materials for aerosol research and aerosol instrumentation and the National Institute of Standards and Technology (NIST) has several spherical nanoscale standard reference materials available, including SRM1963a (d_p = 100 nm) and SRM1964 (d_p = 60 nm) that are suitable for calibration of aerosol

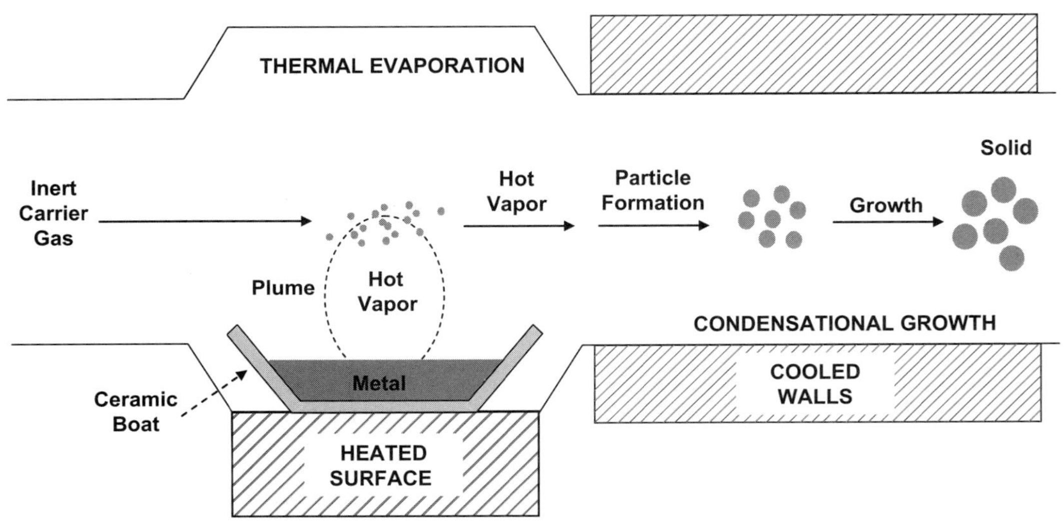

FIGURE 6.13 *Thermal Evaporation of Solid Material to Form Aerosol Nanoparticles. [Adapted from* Aerosol Processing of Materials *(Kodas and Hampden-Smith, 1999)].*

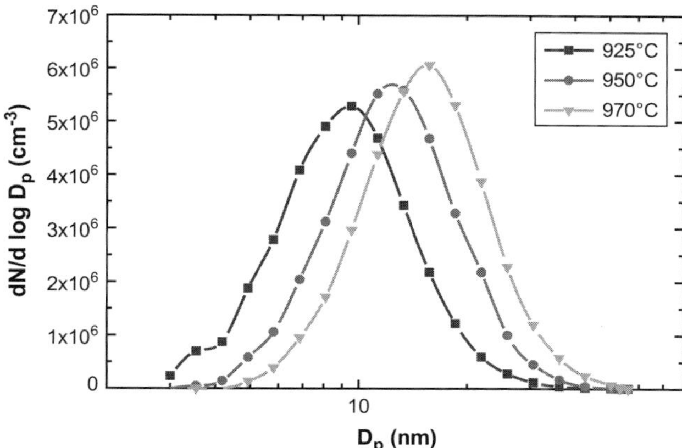

FIGURE 6.14 *Silver Aerosol Nanoparticle Size Distributions via Thermal Evaporation by Varying Furnace Temperature.*

instrumentation. For the NOSH Consortium effort, two types of PSL particles were selected, one a NIST SRM1963a and the other a commercial suspension of $d_p = 100$ nm PSL. Briefly, the PSL aerosol is generated using a constant output atomizer (similar to the citric acid aerosol nanoparticle generation) of liquid precursor, but unlike the soluble citric acid precursor, the liquid precursor for PSL generation already contains solid PSL particles present in the precursor as a suspension. The generated liquid aerosol is passed through a diffusion dryer to remove excess water, drying the aerosol such that only solid polystyrene latex particles remain in the gas. The resulting particle size distribution in Figure 6.15 indicates not only the presence of singly charged particles centered at 100 nm, but multiply charged single particles and single charged multiplets of particles as peaks on both sides of the 100-nm calibration peak. As a matter of note, the presence of surfactant can alter the presence and magnitude of these secondary peaks.

6.3.1.1.3.8 Summary of aerosol synthesis

Several aerosol nanoparticle reactors have been built and characterized in which one or more convenient process parameters can be used to control the particle size distribution, including particle diameter and number concentration. To address the diverse needs of the NOSH Consortium membership, various aerosol nanoparticle synthesis methods have been employed, including thermal decomposition of liquid precursor vapors, spray atomization of liquids of soluble materials or solid suspensions, and thermal vaporization of solid metals. These aerosol nanoparticle reactors are used in subsequent NOSH Consortium activities as detailed in the remaining

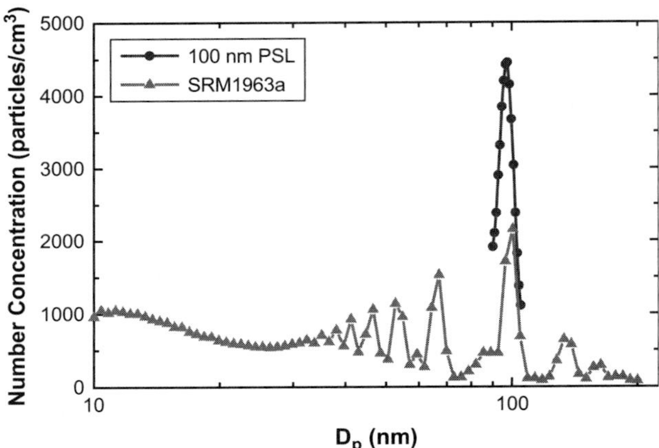

FIGURE 6.15 *Calibration Particle Size Distributions Using Spherical Polystyrene Latex Suspension via Spray Atomization and Diffusion Drying.*

chapter sections, with primary focus on the extremely stable SiO_2 aerosol nanoparticle reactors.

6.3.1.2 Aerosol instrumentation

One of the stated goals of the NOSH Consortium is to evaluate commercial aerosol instrumentation with the purpose to report on the instrument specifications, ease of use, applicability to different operating conditions, and types or form of data generated to the membership, and to discuss these results with particular emphasis in communicating issues or sensitivities that are relevant to occupational safety and health issues. Major focus areas were in comparing commercial classification and detection instrumentation: (1) nano-DMA and long-DMA, (2) ELPI and DMA, and (3) CNC and AE.

Although this chapter is not meant to provide a complete tutorial on aerosol instrumentation, there are a number of excellent resources on many aerosol concepts and instruments used in the NOSH Consortium. These references are included in Table 6.8.

6.3.1.2.1 Nano-DMA and long-DMA

The SiO_2 aerosol nanoparticle reactor previously discussed was built with flexibility to enable classification with either the nano-DMA or the long-DMA as well as to enable detection with either the CNC or the AE. Data obtained from the SiO_2 aerosol nanoparticle reactor scheme is tabulated in Table 6.9 with d_{50} in nm and σ_g values for $T_{furn} = 850$ °C as classified by the nano-DMA and the long-DMA.

Table 6.8 Selected Aerosol Concepts and Instruments with References

Aerosol Concept	Aerosol Instrument	Reference
Fuchs charging efficiency		Fuchs, 1963, Wiedensohler, 1988
	^{85}Kr aerosol neutralizer	Whitby, 1968
Rapid size classification		Wang, 1990
Step size classification		Fissan, 1983, Ehrman, 1999
Particle size distribution data inversions		Knutson, 1976, Hoppel, 1978, Hagen, 1983
	Differential mobility analyzer	Knutson, 1975
	Nano-differential mobility analyzer	Chen, 1998
	Condensation nucleus counter	Bricard, 1976, Sinclair, 1975
	Aerosol electrometer	Liu, 1975

From the data in Table 6.8, negligible differences are observed between the nano- and long-DMA. The performance of the nano- and long-DMA with the same processing conditions, namely $T_{\text{furn}} = 850$ °C and Q_{pr}, are directly compared in Figure 6.16 as particle size distributions with open symbol data referring to the nano-DMA and the solid symbol data referring to the long-DMA. These data verify that both instruments are required to resolve the entire particle size distribution in the range of 10 nm-100 nm. Based upon the design intent of the long- and nano-DMAs, the long-DMA is more ideally suited to resolve the particle size distribution at $d_p > 60$ nm, whereas the nano-DMA is designed to have improved resolution capability at $d_p < 20$ nm for the given flow conditions of the aerosol system being described. However, in the overlap region 20 nm $< d_p <$ 60 nm, agreement between the two classification instruments is quite good, both in terms of particle size and number concentration.

6.3.1.2.2 ELPI and DMA

Operationally, the ELPI and the DMA classification systems are quite different. The ELPI operates as an inertial classifier with particles being classified based upon the ratio of their inertial (particle) to viscous (gas) forces, whereas the DMA operates as an electrostatic classifier with particles being classified based upon the ratio of their electrostatic (charge) to drag (diameter) forces. Additionally, the resolution of the DMA is higher, typically able to differentiate particles within ~10% on diameter from vendor specifications advertising particle size ranges from 2 nm to 1 μm that are highly variable based upon the flow rates and voltages used in the instrument. However, the ELPI has a much larger dynamic range, with vendor

Table 6.9 SiO_2 Aerosol Nanoparticles with d_{50} in nm and σ_g as Classified by the Nano-DMA and the Long-DMA at T_{furn} = 850 °C and Various Q_{pr}

Q_{pr} (cm^3/min)	Nano-DMA	Long-DMA
1	12.3 1.59	10.4 1.70
3	18.0 1.53	17.0 1.60
6		24.36 1.51
10	32.7 1.45	31.9 1.44
25	53.5 1.49	46.9 1.37
35		52.7 1.37
45		56.6 1.36
55		54.4 1.36
65		57.8 1.36
75		60.8 1.35

specifications advertising classification from 7 nm to 10 μm in 12 preset size bins for the model used in this NOSH Consortium. As seen in Figure 6.17, the ELPI and DMA can have good agreement with particle size and number concentration at very limited particle sizes. As observed, the DMAs offer greater resolution, particularly at $d_p < 100$ nm. However, the ELPI is useful as a screening tool to gather information on broad particle size distributions.

6.3.1.2.3 CNC and AE

The condensation nucleus counter (CNC), also known as a condensation particle counter (CPC) or ultrafine condensation particle counter (UCPC) are instruments that operate on the principle of flowing aerosol particles through

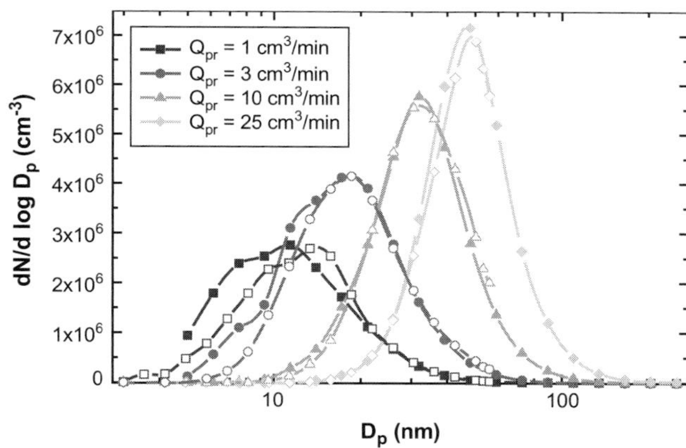

FIGURE 6.16 *Particle Size Distribution Comparisons Between the Nano-DMA (Open) and the Long-DMA (Solid) for Four Different SiO_2 Aerosol Nanoparticle Distributions.*

a supersaturated environment and allowing vapors to condense onto the aerosol particles by controlling the supersaturation ratio and the temperatures of the different zones. Once activated and with vapor present, these particles continue to grow to sizes where they can be optically detected. Several commercial instruments are currently able to detect particles >3 nm at a concentration of $<1 \times 10^5$ particles/cm^3.

The aerosol electrometer (AE) is another aerosol detector that measures the amount of charge carried by an aerosol as it deposits onto a well-insulated feature connected to a sensitive electrometer. By knowing the charged

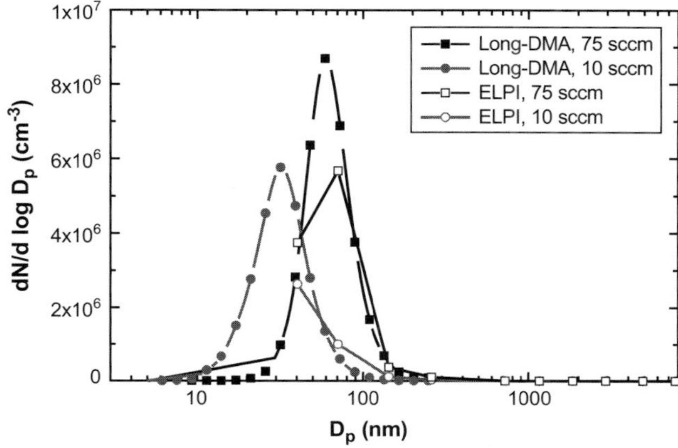

FIGURE 6.17 *Comparison Between the Long-DMA and the ELPI for Two SiO_2 Aerosol Nanoparticle Distributions.*

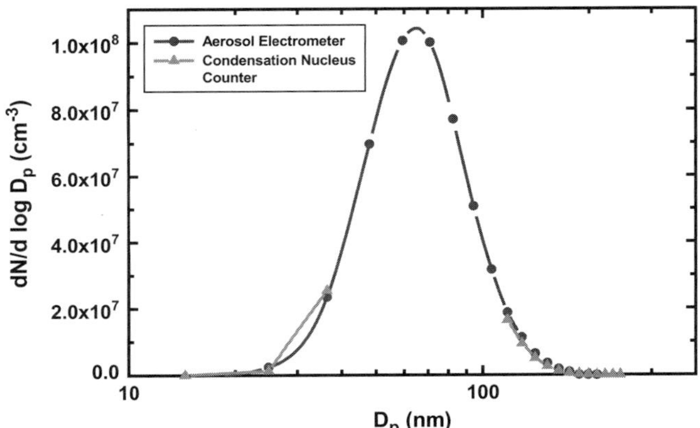

FIGURE 6.18 *Comparison of the CNC and AE Detector Response for One SiO_2 Aerosol Nanoparticle Distribution.*

frequency as a function of particle diameter for a classified, monodisperse aerosol, the number concentration can be determined. Due to the electrometer noise limitations, typical concentration ranges for the aerosol at the operating conditions used by the NOSH Consortium are $\sim 1 \times 10^3 – 1 \times 10^9$ particles/cm^3. Thus, the CNC is used to measure more dilute aerosols where $<1 \times 10^5$ particles/cm^3 and the AE is used to measure the more concentrated aerosols $>1 \times 10^3$ particles/cm^3. As seen in Figure 6.18, acceptable agreement between the two detectors is observed in the region of overlap between 1×10^3 and 1×10^5 particles/cm^3. Admittedly, by diluting aerosol, the operating concentration of the CNC could be expanded, but this activity was not a priority or a need for the NOSH Consortium to characterize detector performance or response.

6.3.1.3 Aerosol chamber

One of the major needs in the NOSH Consortium was to develop an understanding of how aerosol nanoparticles behave as a function of time. The primary goal of this study was to determine whether and how quickly aerosol nanoparticles can be transported from one location to another and whether they remain as nanomaterials over time and under various ambient conditions. The reason for this need is that currently existing containment and control procedures are largely designed to protect in the >100-nm size range. However, if nanomaterials are able to be transported throughout these environments as nanomaterials, the effectiveness of these current containment and control procedures must either be verified for nanoparticles <100 nm or new methods for reducing inhalation exposure risk to nanoparticles must be developed (Warheit, 2004; Pritchard, 2004; National Nanotechnology Initiative, 2007). If, on the other hand, aerosol nanoparticles have sufficiently short lifetimes and are not readily transported through environments as nanomaterials, these findings will be useful in focusing efforts on controlling environments near nanoparticle sources.

For the purposes of the NOSH Consortium, aerosol nanoparticle behavior over time was focused on particle diameters <100 nm. Thus, if aerosol nanoparticles agglomerated to sizes larger than 100 nm, they were considered to be lost from the aerosol since current containment systems are documented as being able to protect in the >100-nm size range. Several mechanisms for aerosol nanoparticle behavior were identified within the interests of the NOSH Consortium. These included rate of dispersion and extent of particle loss, either through growth to $d_p > 100$ nm via coagulation with other aerosol particles or through attachment to fixed surfaces. Aerosol chambers of different internal volumes and materials of construction were fabricated for these studies. Pictures of the two Lucite® aerosol chambers in the SiO_2 aerosol nanoparticle system with internal volumes of ~1.5 L (bottom) and 15 L (top) can be seen in Figure 6.19.

A wide variety of parameters investigated (in addition to aerosol chamber volume) are shown in Table 6.10.

Rate of dispersion was largely determined by examining the difference between when an aerosol nanoparticle sample was introduced into the chamber and when the aerosol nanoparticle sample exited the aerosol chamber as a function of particle diameter. An example can be seen in

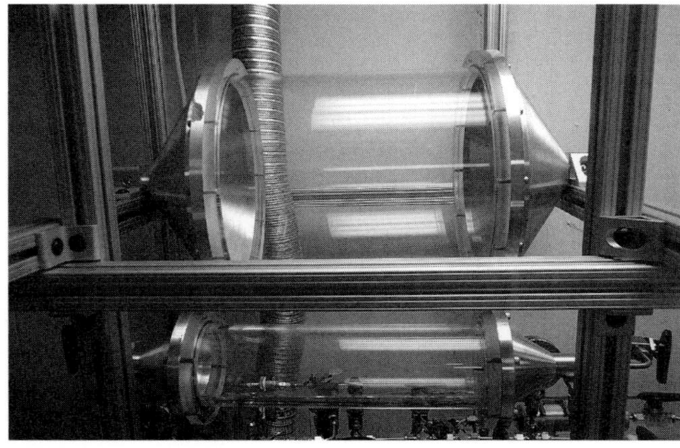

FIGURE 6.19 *Lucite® Aerosol Chambers Designed to Investigate Aerosol Behavior as a Function of Time for Various Process Conditions.*

Table 6.10 Variables Examined in the Aerosol Chamber Studies to Investigate Aerosol Behavior as a Function of Time

- Particle size distribution
  - $d_{50} = 10$, 30, and 60 nm
- Surface area of fixed surfaces
  - No insert in aerosol chamber
  - Insert in aerosol chamber
- Particle number concentration
  - No $= 1 \times 10^8$ particles/cm^3
  - No $= 1 \times 10^6$ particles/cm^3
  - No $= 1 \times 10^3$ particles/cm^3
- Chamber size
  - 1.5 L
  - 15 L
- Materials of construction
  - Aerosol chamber
  - Inserts
- Air flows
  - Stagnant
  - Movement
- Aerosol nanoparticle chemistry
- Particle charge

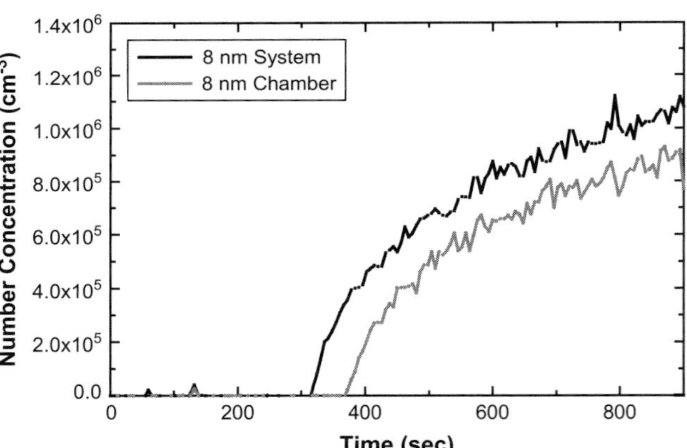

FIGURE 6.20 *Rate of Diffusion is Estimated from Time Series Plots that Compare Aerosol Concentration at Fixed Diameters Though the System Control and the Aerosol Chamber as a Function of Time.*

Figure 6.20. The time difference between the system and the control was used to estimate the rate of diffusion of particles of known d_p, taking into account the residence time of the aerosol and gas in the aerosol chamber.

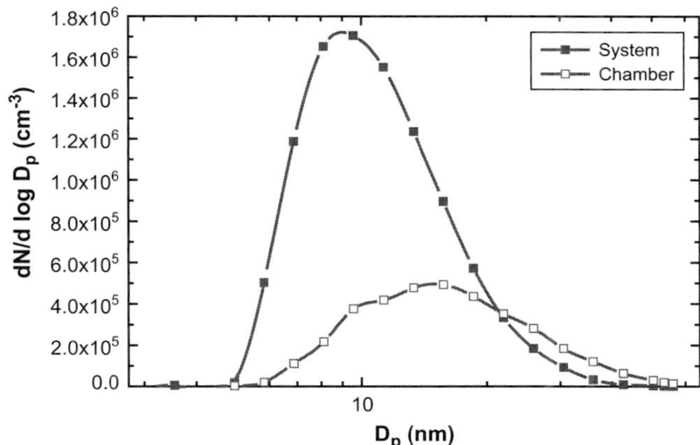

FIGURE 6.21 *Particle Size Distributions can be Used to Estimate Particle Loss Due to Attachment to Fixed Surfaces and to Coagulation with Other Aerosol Particles as well as Estimate Particle Growth Due to Coagulation.*

The extent of particle loss was assessed by comparing the aerosol particle size distribution entering the aerosol chamber and the particle size distribution exiting the aerosol chamber as a function of several process and experimental parameters. Representative particle size distributions are shown in Figure 6.21 below, illustrating loss of smaller particles due to a combination of loss to fixed surfaces (decrease in number concentration at a fixed d_p) and loss to coagulation with other aerosol particles (decrease in number concentration at a fixed d_p) and creation of larger particles (increase in number concentration at a fixed d_p).

To date, the aerosol chamber studies are underway and the final results will be published at a later date. However, preliminary data are shown for several variables tabulated above, including chamber volume, air flow, and inserts.

6.3.1.3.1 % Loss efficiency

For purposes of the aerosol chamber discussion, % Loss Efficiency (% LE) as a function of particle diameter is defined in Equation 2 as

$$\%\,\mathrm{LE}(d_p) = \frac{N_{\mathrm{enter}}(d_p) - N_{\mathrm{exit}}(d_p)}{N_{\mathrm{enter}}(d_p)} \times 100\,\% \qquad (2)$$

where $N_{\mathrm{enter}}(d_p)$ is the number concentration of particles of size d_p entering the aerosol chamber and $N_{\mathrm{exit}}(d_p)$ is the number concentration of particles of size d_p exiting the aerosol chamber. When % LE = 100%,

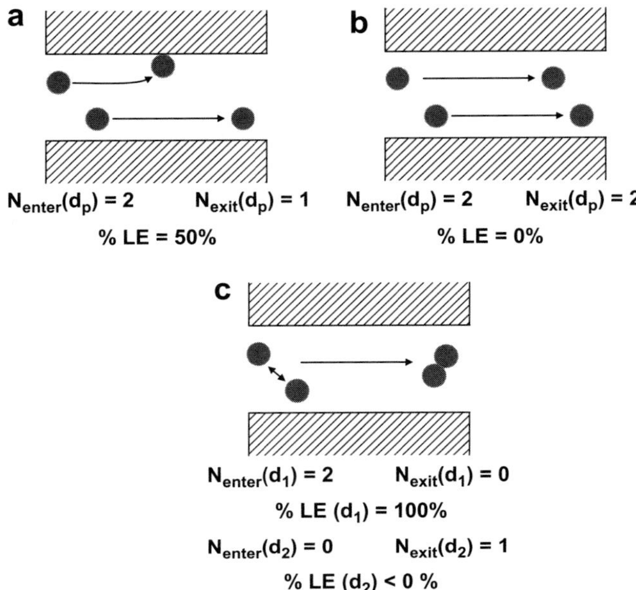

FIGURE 6.22 *(a) Particle Loss Due to Fixed Surface Attachment and No Creation of Additional Particles. (b) No Particle Loss Due to Fixed Surface Attachment and No Creation of Additional Particles. (c) No Particle Loss due to Fixed Surface Attachment, Particle Loss Due to Coagulation, and Particle Creation Due to Coagulation.*

$N_{\text{exit}}(d_p) = 0$, when % LE $= 0\%$, $N_{\text{enter}}(d_p) = N_{\text{exit}}(d_p)$, and when % LE $< 0\%$, $N_{\text{exit}}(d_p) > N_{\text{enter}}(d_p)$. Thus, a negative % LE indicates the creation of new particles within the aerosol chamber, most likely from coagulation of smaller particles. For purposes of this discussion, no assumptions are made about the fate of individual nanoparticles and no aerosol nanoparticles are tracked through the chamber to understand their specific fate. Only the number concentrations at a specific d_p of the entering and exiting locations in the aerosol chamber are recorded. Representative fates of aerosol nanoparticles in the aerosol chamber and the impact on the % LE calculation are shown schematically in Figure 6.22a, b, and c.

6.3.1.3.2 Aerosol chamber volume

As seen in Figure 6.23, by increasing the volume of the aerosol chamber, the % LE increases across all particle sizes. Across each chamber volumes, decreasing d_p increases the % LE, meaning that smaller particles are either lost to collisions with the fixed surfaces of the aerosol chamber or to coagulation with other particles and are not replaced. Similarly, larger particles

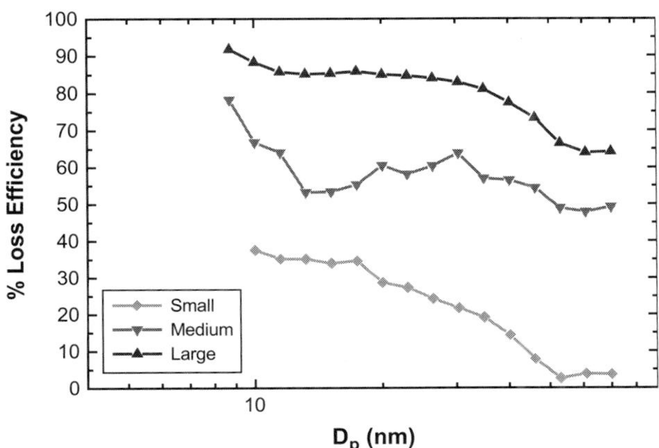

FIGURE 6.23 *% Loss Efficiency for Different Aerosol Chamber Internal Volumes.*

may also be lost to collisions with the wall or with collisions between other aerosol particles, but they can be replaced by collisions of smaller particles to produce the larger particle sizes. In this system, larger particles can be created by collisions between smaller particles, but smaller particles cannot be created by collisions of larger particles.

6.3.1.3.3 Air flows

An example of % LE due to mixing within the aerosol chamber can be seen in Figure 6.24. In the laminar flow condition, particle losses across all particle sizes ~40% for $d_p < 60$ nm and begin to decrease $d_p > 60$ nm, indicating growth in the number of particles with $d_p > 90$ nm due to collisions with smaller particles. By increasing the air flow in the aerosol chamber by adding a fan that operates at low speed (and does not create particles during operation), the % LE increases to ~60% at $d_p < 60$ nm and the negative % LE (creation of particles) decreases more rapidly at $d_p > 80$ nm, indicating that the air mixing may be inducing more particle collisions at the small sizes (higher losses) to produce more larger particles (negative % LE values).

6.3.1.3.4 Inserts and orientation

Inserts are used to increase the internal surface area of the aerosol chambers without dramatically reducing the internal volume. Pictures of the 15 L aerosol chamber Lucite® inserts are shown in Figure 6.25.

The hypothesis being tested with the inserts is that by increasing the surface area, the opportunities for particle losses due to collisions with these fixed surfaces will be increased and, thus, the % LE should be higher with

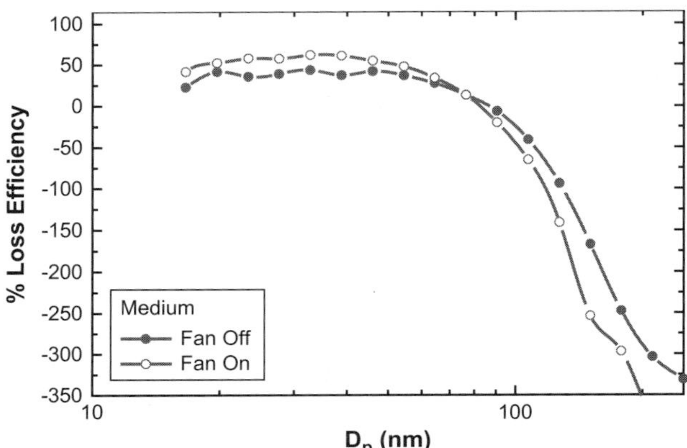

FIGURE 6.24 *% Loss Efficiency for Stagnant and Low Mixed Environments in the Aerosol Chamber.*

inserts. Several remarks can be made about Figure 6.26. In all cases, the % LE increases as d_p decreases. The presence of inserts increases the % LE from 15-40% (depending upon d_p) with no inserts to ~40-75% (depending upon d_p) with inserts. However, the presence of inserts is not the only variable that impacts % LE. By changing the orientation of the inserts from parallel to the aerosol flow to perpendicular to the aerosol flow, a dramatic increase in % LE is observed for particles $d_p < 40$ nm. Additionally, the perpendicular inserts also appear to increase the formation of particles $d_p > 50$ nm, presumably to

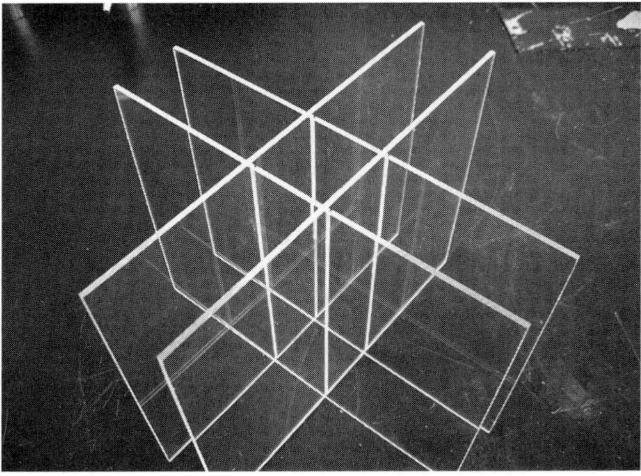

FIGURE 6.25 *Lucite® Inserts are Used to Increase Internal Surface Area While Approximately Maintaining the Internal Aerosol Chamber Volume.*

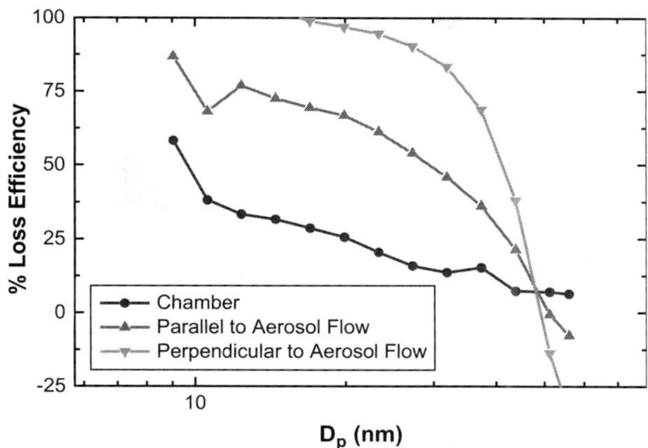

FIGURE 6.26 *% Loss Efficiency for No Inserts, Parallel Inserts, and Perpendicular Inserts.*

coagulation of smaller particles as shown by the increased magnitude of the negative % LE at these larger particle sizes. Interestingly, in this example, nearly 100% of the aerosol particles $d_p < 20$ nm can be removed from the existing aerosol stream by placing an insert perpendicular to the entering aerosol stream.

As shown in the limited examples from the aerosol chamber results, much can be learned about the behavior of aerosol particles over time and many results can have direct implications for occupational safety and health. Work continues to progress in this area and results will be reported at a later date. The aerosol chamber results indicate that nanoparticles can be lost due to a variety of mechanisms and that changing aerosol flows from stagnant to mixed or introduction of physical structures can enhance losses of aerosol nanoparticles, particularly for particles with $d_p < 20$ nm.

6.3.2 Deliverable 2

6.3.2.1 Portable monitor needs from industry

One major and continuing need in industry is the ability to sample occupational environments for the presence or absence of aerosol nanoparticles. Although many sampling instruments exist for aerosol particles, many are either insensitive to nanomaterials, not robust or portable, or do not have the ability to differentiate aerosol nanomaterials from non-nanoscale materials.

As part of the NOSH Consortium, a list of desired attributes of the portable monitor from representatives of the entire membership was

Table 6.11 Desired Attributes in a Portable Aerosol Monitor

Desired attributes in an air sampling instrument	
High or medium priority attributes consistently important to all members	
■ Cost	■ ~$10,000 for daily management work ■ >$10,000 as a specialists tool with limit number per company
■ Ease of use	■ Be able to use the same resources used today to take samples ■ OK to send the instrument back to supplier once per year for maintenance ■ Would value a standard on-site aerosol calibration kit
■ Size	■ For 1st generation: toaster sized is acceptable ■ Hand held instrument ■ Ideally, would want instrument that could take personal breathing zone samples
■ Operating environment	■ Wide variety of particle chemistries ■ Wide concentration ranges ■ Insensitive to particle charge
Other attributes that are important to most members	
■ Explosion proof	■ Given that the instrument will need to function in potentially high dust situations, there must be an intrinsicially safe version available
■ Measurement units	■ Would like for the instrument to measure a parameter that correlates with health effects ■ Many members would also convert the result back to mass per unit volume
■ Resolution	■ At least 3 size bins in the 1-100 nm range
■ Sampling time	■ Able to take measurements in 5 min, 15 min, and 8-h time frames

Continued

Table 6.11 Desired Attributes in a Portable Aerosol Monitor—*cont'd*

Attributes that are important to consider	
	■ Able to transport the instrument by road or air
	■ Able to operate independently of main power
	■ Baseline drift < 5%
	■ An alarm at a set % of limit

prioritized and communicated. The tabulated desired attributes can be found in Table 6.11.

Internal NOSH Consortium's efforts to develop instrument concepts are underway and will be released once suitable designs are finalized. Simultaneously, external instrument manufacturers and academic researchers are making significant progress toward the development of portable instruments to address the needs of the NOSH Consortium membership and the NOSH Consortium membership continues to track advances made by external developers.

6.3.3 Deliverable 3

6.3.3.1 Motivation

Prudent practices for nanotechnology safety, health, and environmental issues recognize the importance of containment and control measures for exposure control. Measures to contain and control potential exposures to airborne nanoparticles should include good handling techniques and work practices, a wide variety of engineering controls (i.e., isolation of the hazard at the source and local exhaust ventilation) and personal protective equipments, such as protective clothing, gloves, and respiratory protection. Developing an understanding of filtration efficiency of filter media and improved methods to measure filtration efficiency as a function of aerosol properties as well as of exposure time will compliment the decision to institute filter media controls (i.e., respiratory protection) based on the results of risk assessment and risk management.

Literature sources are extensive for filter media and respirator efficiencies for aerosol particle filtration efficiencies. Martin and Moyer (2000) developed and refined methods that would later form the basis for the respirator certification test adopted by NIOSH that uses sodium chloride (NaCl) and dioctyl phthalate (DOP) for solid and liquid aerosol particles for filtration efficiency determination. The effects of filtration efficiency for NaCl and DOP with particular focus on examining effects of preloading the filter with aerosol particles prior to testing have been investigated (Fardi and Liu, 1991). From previous work, it has also been determined that not only do NaCl and DOP have different behaviors in filtration experiments, but the charge state of the aerosol itself is a critical parameter (Fissan et al., 1984; Ji et al., 2003). More recently, the effect of sampling method and measurement of charged and neutralized monodisperse aerosols on filtration efficiencies of metal and polymeric filter media has been examined, as has the filtration efficiency as a function of particle diameter for charged and uncharged aerosols as a function of relative humidity (Kim et al., 2006) and silver nanoparticle penetration through commercial filter media (Kim et al., 2007). Although outside of the scope of the NOSH Consortium technical effort (but still highly relevant to occupational safety and health issues), filtration performance using a Manakin-based protocol with a sealed face fit has been examined with reports that charge neutralization of the aerosol is critical in evaluating respirator efficiency (Balazy et al., 2005). Differential mobility analyzers (DMA) have also been used to produce monodisperse aerosols of charged or neutralized aerosol particles (Kim et al., 2006) or charged and uncharged aerosol particles (Yun et al., 2007) that are then used to determine filtration efficiency of filter media to monodisperse aerosols. Specific filter media performance has been reported by numerous sources, including the effect of aerosol loading on the performance of Electret filter media (Barrett and Rousseau, 1998) and of HEPA filters exposed to submicron aerosol particles (Sinclair, 1976).

Current filter media testing protocols generate aerosol (typically NaCl or DOP) at a known particle size and size distribution and transport the aerosol to a test chamber in which a filter mask or cartridge is sealed in place, often with a wax or glue to prevent leakage around the filter. The filter efficiency is then calculated by dividing the total aerosol number concentration across all particle sizes that move across this box and penetrate through the filter media by the total aerosol number concentration measured upstream of the test chamber and filter media or by dividing the output aerosol number concentration by the input aerosol number concentration at selected particle diameters. For further information, please refer to the NIOSH Certification documents (NIOSH 2005a,b).

The technical portion of the NOSH Consortium filtration study focused on three areas where current aerosol filtration methods and instrumentation can be explored, including (1) isolating and quantifying particle losses due solely to aerosol particle interactions with filter media, (2) measuring the filtration efficiency of filter media to charged and reneutralized aerosol particles as a function of exposure time and of particle diameter, and (3) examining the filtration efficiency of polydisperse aerosols of industrially relevant particle chemistries.

In all filter media studies, aerosol particles are exposed to the filter media under investigation as well as to the internal structures of the filter units, including surfaces of chamber walls, materials of construction, and glues or waxes used to hold filter media in place. To quantify particle capture efficiencies due solely to the filter media, it is necessary to quantify particle losses due to factors other than aerosol nanoparticle interaction with filter media and to separate these losses prior to final calculations on filter media filtration efficiencies. Although diffusion losses may not be significant for larger aerosol particles, diffusion becomes more critical for aerosol nanoparticles, and thus, must be accounted for in any measurements that evaluate aerosol nanoparticle behavior. To address these issues, the NOSH Consortium filtration measurement system employs a dual neutralizer setup that can be integrated into the aerosol characterization system to evaluate differences in filtration efficiency of filter media to charged (i.e., as-generated) and neutralized (i.e., brought into a Boltzmann equilibrium charge distribution) aerosol particles across broad particle sizes. Based upon the number and location of aerosol neutralizers used in the procedure, the filtration behavior to charged and neutralized aerosol nanoparticles for filter media can be identified as a function of particle diameter and filter exposure time based upon a variety of situations described in detail.

In typical filter media testing, an aerosol neutralizer is used to enable electrostatic classification (and perhaps electrostatic detection) of the aerosol nanoparticles, either to verify that the desired particle size distribution is within specification or to generate a monodisperse aerosol for media exposure. A second neutralizer is used in some examples to produce a reneutralized aerosol following classification. This reneutralized monodisperse aerosol can then be exposed to electrostatic plates to remove all charged particles from a reneutralized aerosol to produce an uncharged monodisperse aerosol (Barrett and Rousseau, 1998). With a single neutralizer, depending upon its placement, the resulting data provide meaningful information on either charged or uncharged aerosol nanoparticle interactions with filter media, but not both. In some literature examples, however, the filtration efficiencies of charged and uncharged aerosol particles are erroneously assumed to be equivalent. In an important industrial example, Electret filters have been optimized to remove charged aerosol particles from gases. Therefore, filtration efficiency experiments in which only charged particle behaviors are being measured may very well show extremely good initial filtration efficiencies of these Electret filters to aerosol particles. The filtration efficiency of these same Electret filters to uncharged aerosols, however, cannot be assumed from the charged aerosol filtration efficiencies. In an occupational setting in which either the charge state of the individual aerosol particles is unknown or uncharged aerosol nanoparticles are present, an Electret filter may or may not provide the best protection despite the published filtration efficiencies being high. Thus, it is critical to know either (1) the charge distribution of the occupational aerosol or (2) the performance of a recommended filter media to both charged and uncharged aerosol particles in order to best protect occupational workers in environments that may contain charged, uncharged, or unknown charge distribution aerosols.

6.3.3.2 Filtration test methodology

To address this issue, this study employs two identical filter housings: one filter housing does not contain any filter media and functions to measure the control aerosol size distribution and one filter housing unit contains the filter media under test. With identical filter housing units, the effect of the filter media on the change in the particle size distribution and number concentrations can be determined independently of diffusion losses by comparing the particle size distributions between the empty and the filter media-containing housings.

This program utilized the SiO_2 aerosol nanoparticle reactor upstream of the filter measurement capability. Furthermore, this filtration setup incorporated (1) a dual housing capability for rapid determination of aerosol nanoparticle collection efficiency as a function of a time and of particle size distribution for a variety of filter media and (2) a dual neutralizer configuration that enables the determination of filtration behavior based upon charged and uncharged aerosol particles to broad particle size distributions. The experimental setup is shown as a diagram in Figure 6.27.

In this test method, flat sheet samples of filter media from commercially available filter masks are punch from the mask (Figure 6.28). These flat sheets are inserted into commercially available filter housings for testing under a variety of conditions.

6.3.3.2.1 Diffusion losses in tubing

Diffusion losses of aerosol nanoparticles due to internal surface area of filter housing units and associated tubing can be quantitated by comparing aerosol particle size distributions obtained from an aerosol that follows different paths within the reactor. As shown in Figure 6.29, the solid circle data is the particle

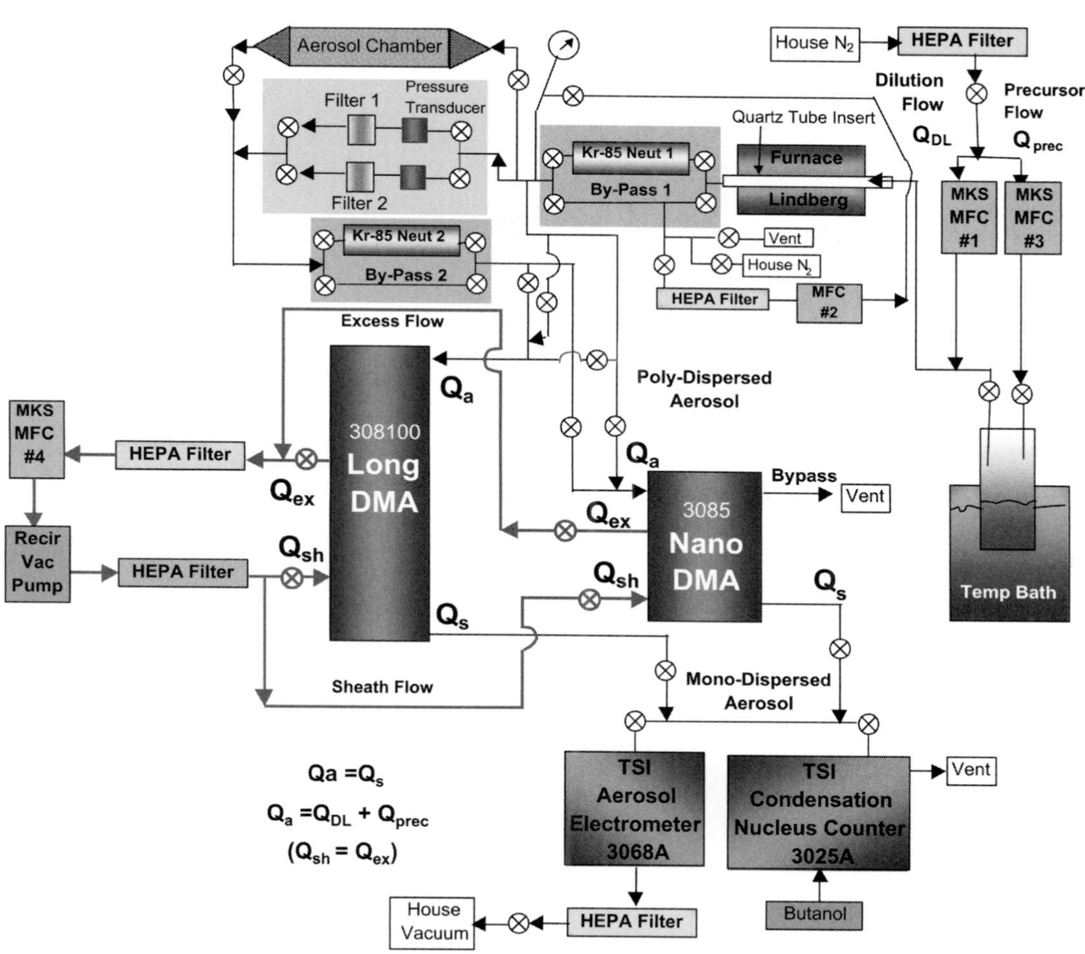

FIGURE 6.27 *Schematic of the SiO_2 Aerosol Nanoparticle Reactor, Including Classification and Detection, with Integrated Filtration Capabilities.*

size distribution from the aerosol going from N1 into the long-DMA and detected with the AE. This data represents the particle size distribution measured with the smallest internal volume within the aerosol system. The open circle data is the particle size distribution of the aerosol that follows the sequence N1, H1E, N2. The difference between these two particle size distributions is a measure of the particle loss as a function of diameter due to internal volume differences in H1E and N2 and the associated tubing. By changing the d_{50} of the original SiO_2 nanoparticle aerosol, one can measure the effect of diffusion losses for different particle diameters through the system (data not shown). When normalized, the resulting data is a quantitative

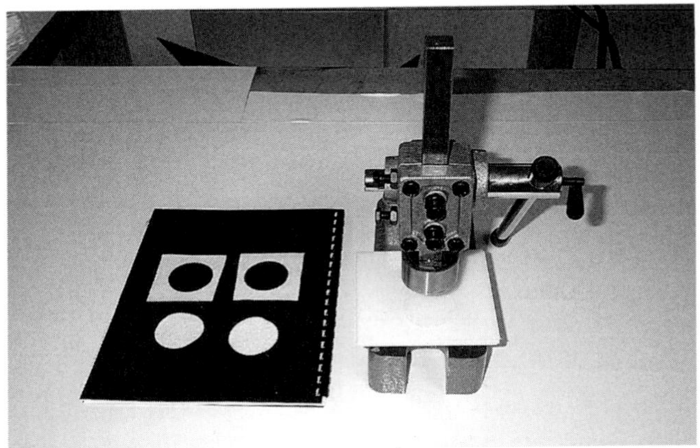

FIGURE 6.28 *A Punch was Used to Remove Flat Samples of Filter Media from Commercially Purchased Filter Masks to Enable Filter Media Characterization.*

measure of the diffusion losses as a function of particle diameter and number concentration that can be determined independently of the original particle size distribution. In this particular dataset in which the current system is purposefully designed to have minimal internal volumes, losses of ~15% are observed for particles 20 nm < d_p < 50 nm as seen in Figure 6.29. Below 20 nm, the resolution of the long-DMA (as discussed in Section 3.1.2.1 of this chapter) becomes less definitive as these flow configuration and, thus, can have more noise associated with the measured number concentrations.

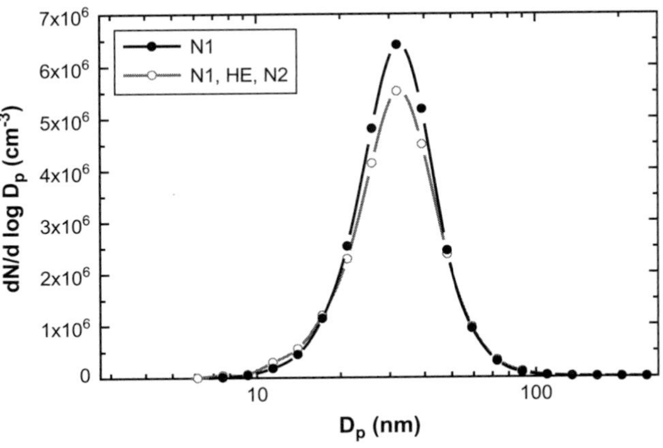

FIGURE 6.29 *Diffusional Losses of SiO_2 Aerosol Nanoparticles Due to Differences in Path Through the Aerosol System.*

6.3.3.2.2 Diffusion losses in filter housing

Diffusion losses of aerosol nanoparticles can be quantified for empty filter housings under various conditions and with different orientations. Assessing and understanding the diffusion losses associated with filter housing interior volumes is important for the following reasons. Filtration efficiency is commonly calculated using Equation 3 below:

$$\%\,\mathrm{FE}(d_\mathrm{p}) = \frac{[N_\mathrm{in}(d_\mathrm{p}) - N_\mathrm{out}(d_\mathrm{p})]}{N_\mathrm{in}(d_\mathrm{p})} \times 100\,\% \qquad (3)$$

However, Equation 3 assumes that the filter housing itself does not interact with the aerosol particles and that any losses of aerosol nanoparticles are due to the presence of the filter media. As previously seen in the aerosol chamber experiments, internal volumes and surface areas of aerosol structures can influence the % losses through those structures and the % LE can also become more pronounced as the particle diameter decreases. These results are verified by measuring the particle size distribution before and after filter housing units that do not contain filter media. Figure 6.30 shows the particle losses as a function of particle diameter through a filter housing unit that does not contain filter media. By comparing the particle size distribution through no filter housing versus through an empty filter housing, an understanding of the diffusion losses due to the internal structure of the filter housing can be identified. As a function of particle diameter and at these number concentrations, the % losses through an empty filter housing can approach >30% for particles <30 nm as measured by the long-DMA. From these results in

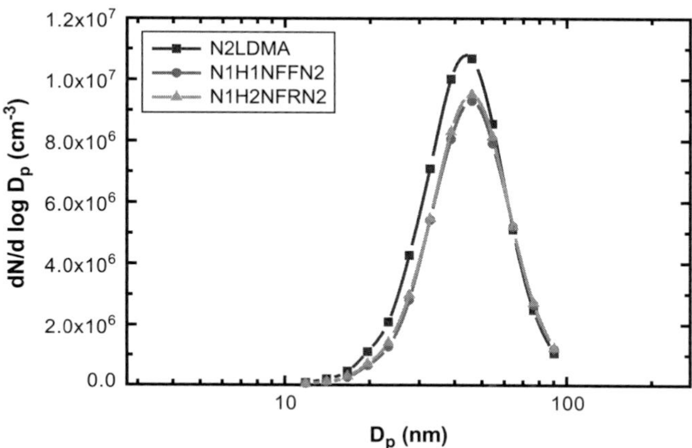

FIGURE 6.30 *Diffusional Losses of SiO_2 Aerosol Nanoparticles Due to Internal Volumes and Structures within Empty Filter Housings.*

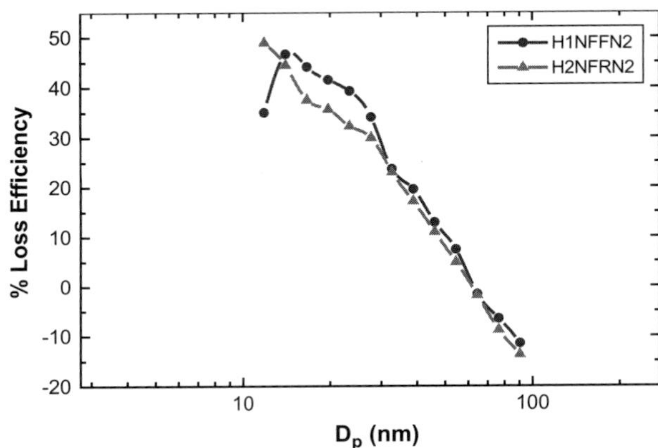

FIGURE 6.31 *% Loss Efficiency of SiO_2 Aerosol Nanoparticles Through Nominally Identical Filter Housings that Do Not Contain Filter Media.*

Figure 6.30, the % LE as a function of particle diameter is calculated in Figure 6.31. With a result similar to that observed in the aerosol chamber experiments, the % LE is seen to increase as the particle diameter decreases.

6.3.3.3 Measurement of filter media filtration efficiencies

6.3.3.3.1 Filtration efficiencies for dust masks and N95 filter media

Although the member companies did not use N95 and dust mask filter media in any process involving nanomaterials, the evaluation of dust mask and N95 filters was useful in the test methods development portion of this effort. Additional results will be disseminated via scientific manuscripts as they become available. With these filter media, certain trends can be observed in the filtration efficiency versus particle diameter as a function of exposure time. As an example, charge mechanisms in N95 filter media show different filtration efficiencies of charged and reneutralized SiO_2 aerosol nanoparticles as observed in comparing the charged aerosol nanoparticle filtration efficiencies in Figure 6.32a with the reneutralized aerosol nanoparticle filtration efficiencies as shown in Figure 6.32b. However, in these examples, the filtration efficiency is >95% as required for N95 filter media (NIOSH, 1996).

From Figure 6.32a and b, several observations can be made. First, the filtration efficiency to charged particles is higher than the filtration efficiency to reneutralized particles. Second, the filtration efficiency of charged particles is observed to decrease over time (data trend not observable in Figure 6.32a due to y-axis scale selection), whereas with the reneutralized particles, the filtration efficiency is often observed to increase over time.

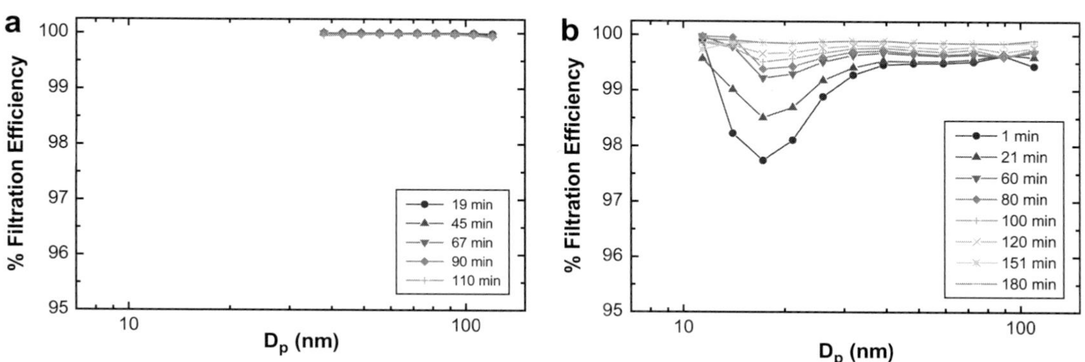

FIGURE 6.32 *(a) % Filtration Efficiency of Charged SiO_2 Aerosol Nanoparticles for N95 Filter Media. (b) % Filtration Efficiency of Reneutralized SiO_2 Aerosol Nanoparticles for N95 Filter Media.*

With a different vendor's N95 filter media shown in Figure 6.33a and b, filtration efficiencies to SiO_2 aerosol nanoparticles are extremely high for both charged (Figure 6.33a) and reneutralized (Figure 6.33b) particles when the particle size distribution is centered at $d_{50} \sim 10$ nm. In this N95 filter media, the filtration efficiency for charged particles is, again, higher than for reneutralized particles across all particle sizes. However, unlike the previous vendor N95 filter media shown in Figure 6.33a and b, this vendor filter media shown in Figure 6.33a and b does not demonstrate significant differences in the filtration efficiency as a function of exposure time when exposed to reneutralized SiO_2 aerosol nanoparticles.

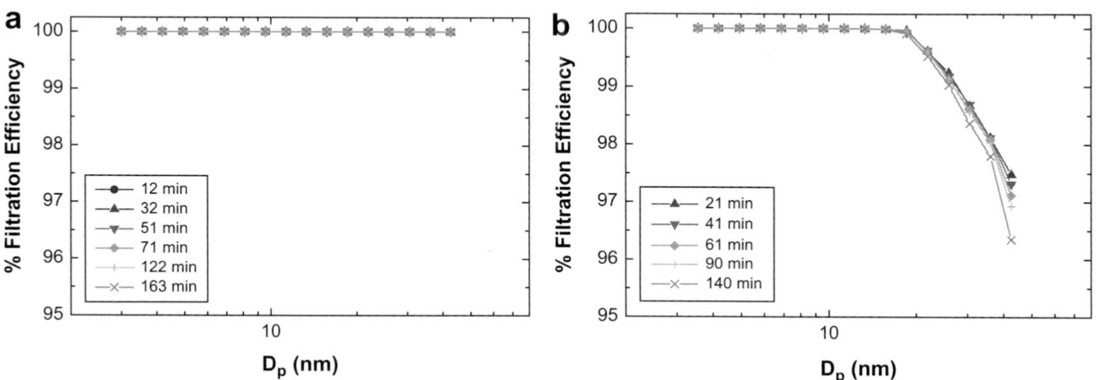

FIGURE 6.33 *(a) % Filtration Efficiency of Charged SiO_2 Aerosol Nanoparticles for N95 Filter Media. (b) % Filtration Efficiency of Reneutralized SiO_2 Aerosol Nanoparticles for N95 Filter Media.*

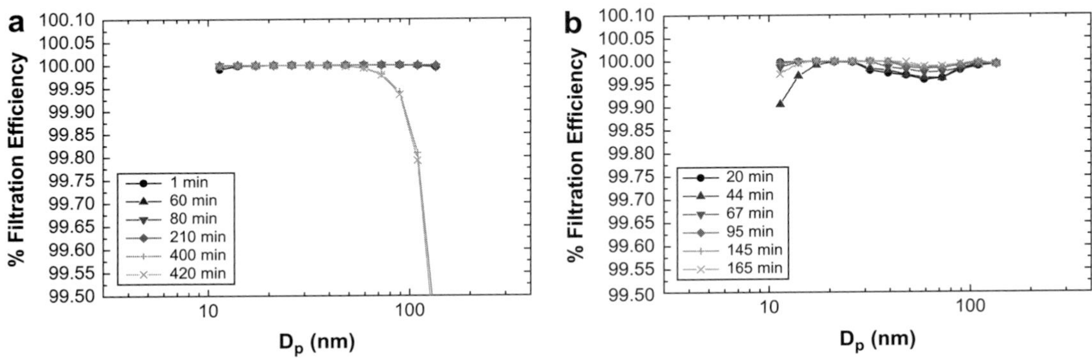

FIGURE 6.34 *(a) % Filtration Efficiency of Charged SiO_2 Aerosol Nanoparticles for N100 Filter Media. (b) % Filtration Efficiency of Reneutralized SiO_2 Aerosol Nanoparticles for N100 Filter Media.*

6.3.3.3.2 Filtration efficiencies for N100 and P100 filter media

For purposes of the NOSH Consortium, the measurement of commercially available N100 and P100 filter media upon exposure to aerosol nanoparticles was particularly significant, since these filter media are the ones commonly selected by the majority of the members in the NOSH Consortium since they are certified as having the highest filtration efficiency (>99.97%) by NIOSH certification test standards (13). For N100 and P100 filter media, measured, general trends in filtration efficiency decreasing for charged particles (see Figure 6.34a) and increasing for reneutralized particles (see Figure 6.34b) was reproduced. After prolonged testing, degradation in filtration efficiency is sometimes observed as shown in Figure 6.34a. With the exception of prolonged exposure testing (i.e., $t_{exposure} > 400$ min), these N100 filter media perform within the specified filtration efficiency levels as established by NIOSH for larger particle diameters.

6.4 PRESENTATIONS

One priority of the NOSH Consortium was to release information pertinent to occupational safety and health of nanoparticles via multiple outlets. This chapter fulfils part of these obligations. However, the dissemination of results and conclusions is also done through manuscripts submitted to peer reviewed journals and presentations at conferences and panel workshops. In many cases, the presentation materials of NOSH Consortium updates can be found online. The following information listed in Table 6.12 includes several conferences in which publicly released information on the NOSH

Table 6.12 Public Forums in Which Results from the NOSH Consortium have been Presented

- 2nd International Symposium on Nanotechnology, Occupational and Environmental Health, 2005
- American Association for Aerosol Research (AAAR) Annual Meeting, 2006
- International Aerosol Conference, 2006
- American Institute of Physics, Industrial Physics Forum, 2006
- American Institute of Chemical Engineers (AIChE), Health Effects of Nanoparticles, 2006
- Occupational and Environmental Health and Safety, 2006
- President's Council of Advisors on Science and Technology (PCAST), 2007
- 3rd International Symposium on Nanotechnology, Occupational and Environmental Health, 2007

Consortium to date has been shared. Additional information continues to be presented at conferences and forums and will be published in peer reviewed journals as appropriate.

6.5 TECHNICAL UPDATE COMMUNICATIONS FOR ADVISORY BOARD MEETINGS

For reference and for an indication of the technical priorities and program pace, broad technical topics discussed at each of the Advisory Board Meetings are tabulated in Table 6.13 below.

6.6 PHASE 2 FOCUS AND OBJECTIVES

As seen in Table 6.13 with the April 2, 2007 Advisory Board Meeting dedicated to Phase 2 topic discussions, the majority of the NOSH Consortium membership agreed to extend the scope of many of the objectives from the initial proposal based upon experimental results collected during the 18-month study. The additional experimental work was defined and work began on these objectives in July 2007 under Phase 2 of the NOSH Consortium. The objectives for Phase 2 are targeted for completion in October 2007 and are outlined in Table 6.14.

Table 6.13 Agenda Topics for Advisory Board Meetings Technical Updates

January 12, 2006

- SiO_2 aerosol nanoparticle reactor
- Filtration test method

April 11, 2006

- Nano-DMA and long-DMA evaluation and comparison
- Filtration studies on commercial dust mask and N95 filter media

July 11, 2006

- SiO_2 aerosol nanoparticle stability over multiple months
- CNC and AE detector evaluation
- Citric acid and silver aerosol nanoparticle synthesis
- Preliminary aerosol chamber design
- External communication with instrument vendors for Deliverable 2
- Filtration studies on commercial N100 filter media
- Laboratory tour of facilities in Wilmington, DE

October 18, 2006

- Aerosol chamber experimental plan and preliminary results
- Filtration studies on commercial P100

January 23, 2007

- ELPI evaluation and comparison with DMA
- PSL aerosol nanoparticle synthesis
- Aerosol chamber results
- SiO_2 vs. citric acid chemistry effects on commercial N95 filter media

April 2, 2007

- Phase 2 discussion with potential phase 3 concepts

June 27-28, 2007

- Final technical update
- Review of previous findings and accomplishments
- TiO_2 aerosol nanoparticle reactor
- Aerosol chamber results—extensive
- Portable aerosol monitor development and progress
- Extended time studies on N95, N100, and P100 filter media

Table 6.14 NOSH Consortium Phase 2 Scope Expansion and Objectives for Each Deliverable

Deliverable 1

- What commercially available materials are efficient getterers of aerosol nanoparticles?
    - Examine losses of charged and uncharged particles upon exposure to different materials of construction
- Aerosolization of bulk nanopowders
- Aerosolize montmorillonite clay using standard equipment at standard operating conditions
- Monitor particle size distribution and number concentration as a function of equipment settings
- Aerosolization of composite materials that contain embedded nanostructures
    - Can these materials produce aerosol particles at standard processing conditions?
    - Grinding, sanding, polishing, cutting
    - If aerosol particles are produced, quantify nanoparticle size distribution and number concentration with mechanical process parameters
- Introduction of ambient conditions into aerosol chamber
    - Currently use dry, particle-free nitrogen
    - Ambient room air may contain particles, humidity, etc that will influence aerosol nanoparticle behavior
    - Introduce $d_{50} \sim 0.5\ \mu m$ and $1.0\ \mu m$ particles
    - Introduce air with humidity ~0-85%
    - Introduce mixing into chamber via recirculation to simulate movement in ambient environment

Deliverable 2

- Continued efforts on portable monitor development

Deliverable 3

- Assess filtration efficiency performance
    - Role of particle chemistry
    - Can correlations be made between filtration efficiencies of SiO_2 vs. NaCl vs. citric acid vs. others?
    - How do NaCl/DOP materials compare to other particle chemistries?
    - Role of relative humidity
    - Under ambient working conditions
    - With entrained larger particles $\sim 0.5\ \mu m$, 25 °C and 50% relative humidity

6.7 SUMMARY

Although the results reporting is still under way, the NOSH Consortium has been viewed by a wide audience to be an excellent demonstration of the technical and professional progress that can be achieved as part of a successful collaboration between diverse and interested professionals. The fact that the NOSH Consortium was able to identify common goals, navigate through complex technical results, and find common ground to present findings to the technical community is a testament to the value of people working together to achieve exciting results.

The interactions and discussions between NOSH Consortium members raised the level of awareness of occupational safety and health related to nanotechnology, not only within their own companies, organizations, and government agencies as member representatives, but also increased the volume across broader organizations and remains one major success of the NOSH Consortium. The open discussion with instrument vendors and academic groups to highlight desired instrument features for a portable aerosol monitor, the creation of a stable SiO_2 aerosol nanoparticle reactor to enable additional occupational safety and health experiments, the development of aerosol chambers and protocols to begin assessing aerosol behavior over time, and the measurement of commercially available filter media to industrially relevant nanoparticle exposure aerosols remain some of the main successes of this collaboration.

Additionally, the NOSH Consortium was able to achieve the vast majority of its objectives, including the definition of synthesis methods for stable sources of aerosol nanoparticles of SiO_2, TiO_2, citric acid, silver, and PSL. The PSL particles were particularly important as a calibration standard for several aerosol instruments. The aerosol instrument characterization was successfully completed for numerous aerosol instruments, including the long- and nano-differential mobility analyzers, electrostatic-based impactor, aerosol chargers and neutralizers, and optical and electrostatic detectors.

Several aerosol chambers were designed and used to understand aerosol behavior over time with broad process and structural variables. Significant observations include evidence that aerosol nanoparticles $d_p < 20$ nm appear to suffer losses $\sim$50% (through agglomeration with other aerosol particles) such that they grow to particle sizes $d_p > 100$ nm, a size range in which current occupational health systems have shown to be effective in particle removal. External forces can further increase the particle loss through the aerosol chamber with the smallest particles $d_p < 20$ nm experiencing the highest particle losses.

The needs of a portable aerosol monitor were identified and prioritized by the broad NOSH membership and have been communicated to interested parties, including external instrument developers, though individual discussions, as well as through an instrument vendor workshop. External and internal efforts continue to focus on portable aerosol monitor concepts and designs since this need remains.

Versatile test methods to measure filtration efficiency of commercially available filter media to aerosol nanoparticle exposure were developed and used to measure filtration efficiencies of commercially available filter media. These test methods were designed to be able to distinguish filtration efficiencies as a function of particle size and of exposure time as well as of particle chemistry, particle charge, and extended time testing. In general, N95, N100, and P100 commercially available filter media perform within their specified filtration efficiency to aerosol nanoparticles $d_p < 100$ nm. In most cases, these filter media demonstrate excellent filtration efficiency to SiO_2 and citric acid aerosol nanoparticles. However, differences in filtration efficiency (initial and as a function of time) are observed for filter media upon exposure to charged (filtration efficiency decreases with time) and uncharged (filtration efficiency increases with time) particles. Prolonged usage beyond manufacturers recommended lifetimes of filter media may reduce the filtration efficiency, particularly if stored overnight.

Although the conclusion of the NOSH Consortium will not mean an end to the study of nanotechnology from an occupational safety and health perspective, it does conclude one chapter in this journey.

ACKNOWLEDGMENTS

The success of the NOSH Consortium is due entirely to the successful collaboration and participation of the entire NOSH Consortium membership, including DuPont, Procter & Gamble, Dow Chemical, Intel Corporation, Air Products & Chemicals, Inc, Degussa, Rohm & Haas, PPG, General Electric, Health and Safety Executive of the UK, Kimberly-Clark, Boeing, and the Department of Energy Office of Science.

The NOSH Consortium safety, legal, and management team, including Keith Swain, John Langworthy, Bruce Johnson, and Rick Bockrath, were integral to the early communication of the proposal, the acceptance and adaptation of the technical program, and the formation of the NOSH Consortium.

The NOSH Consortium technical team, including Bob Small, Erin McDermott, Jim Krajewski, and Tracey Rissman, were absolutely essential to the success of the technical program, the reduction of abstract proposals into experimental practice, and the thoughtful and thorough documentation of the experimental results.

REFERENCES

Aitken, R.J., Creely, K.S., Tran, C.L., 2004. An Occupational Hygiene Review. Institute of Occupational Medicine. Health and Safety Executive, Edinburgh, UK. Nanoparticles.

Balazy, A., Toivola, M., Reponen, T., Podgorski, A., Zimmer, A., Grinshpun, S.A., 2005. Manikin-based performance evaluation of N95 filtering-facepiece respirators challenged with nanoparticles. Ann. Occup. Hyg, 1–11.

Barrett, L.W., Rousseau, A.D., 1998. Aerosol loading performance of electret filter media. AIHA Journal 59, 532–539.

Biswas, P., Li, X., Pratsinis, S.E., 1989. Optical waveguide preform fabrication: silica formation and growth in a high-temperature aerosol reactor. J. Appl. Phys 65 (6), 2445–2450.

Bricard, J., Delattre, P., Madelaine, G., Pourprix, M., 1976. Detection of ultrafine particles by means of a continuous flux condensation nucleus counter. In: Liu, B.Y.H. (Ed.). Fine Particles. Aerosol Generation, Measurement, and Sampling. Academic Press, New York.

Camata, R.P., Atwater, H.A., Vahala, K.J., Flagan, R.C., 1996. Size classification of silicon nanocrystals. Appl. Phys. Lett. 68, 3162–3164.

Chen, D.-R., Pui, D.Y.H., Hummes, D., Fissan, H., Quant, F.R., Sem, G.J., 1998. Design and evaluation of a nanometer aerosol differential mobility analyzer (nano-DMA). J. Aerosol Sci. 29 (5/6), 497–509.

Ehrman, S.H., 1999. Effect of particle size on rate of coalescence of silica nanoparticles. J. Colloid Interface Sci 213, 258–261.

Fardi, B., Liu, B.Y.H., 1991. Performance of disposable respirators. Particle and Particle Systems Characterization 8, 308–314.

Fissan, H.J., Helsper, C., Thielen, H.J., 1983. Determination of particle size distributions by means of an electrostatic classifier. J. Aerosol Sci. 14, 354–357.

Fissan, H.J., Neumann, S., Schurmann, G., 1984. Electrostatic enhanced filtration. In: Proceedings of the First International Aerosol Conference. Minnesota, pp. 17–21.

Fuchs, N.A., 1963. On the stationary charge distribution on aerosol particles in a bipolar ionic atmosphere. Pure and Applied Geophysics 56, 185–193.

Hagen, D.E., Alofs, D.J., 1983. Linear inversion method to obtain aerosol size distributions from measurements with a differential mobility analyzer. Aerosol Sci. Technol. 2, 465–475.

Heim, M., Mullins, B.J., Wild, M., Meyer, J., Kasper, G., 2005. Filtration efficiency of aerosol particles below 20 nanometers. Aerosol Sci. Technol. 39, 782–789.

Holman, M., 2007. PCAST Agenda. 25 June. <www.ostp.gov/PCAST/pcast.html>.

Hoppel, W.A., 1978. Determination of the aerosol size distribution from the mobility distribution of the charged fraction of aerosols. J. Aerosol Sci. 9, 41–54.

Ji, J.H., Bae, G.N., Kang, S.H., Hwang, J., 2003. Effect of particle loading on the collection performance of an electret cabin air filter for submicron aerosols. Aerosol Science 34, 1493–1504.

Kim, C.S., Bao, L., Okuyama, K., Shimada, M., Niinuma, H., 2006. Filtration efficiency of a fibrous filter for nanoparticles. Journal of Nanoparticle Research 8, 215–221.

Kim, S.C., Harrington, M.S., Pui, D.Y.H., 2007. Experimental study of nanoparticles penetration through commercial filter media. Journal of Nanoparticle Research 9, 117–125.

Knutson, E.O., 1976. Extended electric mobility method for measuring aerosol particle size and concentration. In: Liu, B.Y.H. (Ed.), Fine Particles Aerosol Generation, Measurement, and Sampling. Academic Press, New York.

Knutson, E.O., Whitby, K.T., 1975. Accurate measurement of aerosol electric mobility moments. J. Aerosol Sci. 6, 453–460.

Kodas, T.T., Hampden-Smith, M.J., 1999. Aerosol Processing of Materials. Wiley Publishing, New York.

Li, X., Lin, Y., Chen, H., Roco, M.C., 1976–2004. 2007. Worldwide nanotechnology development: a comparative study of USPTO, EPO, and JPO patents. Journal of Nanoparticle Research 9 (6), 977–1002.

Liu, B.Y.H., Pui, D.Y.H., 1975. On the performance of the electrical aerosol analyzer. J. Aerosol Sci. 6, 249–264.

Liu, B.Y.H., Lee, J.-K., Mullins, H., Danisch, S.G., 1993. Respirator leak detection by ultrafine aerosols: a predictive model and experimental study. Aerosol Sci. Technol. 19, 15–26.

Lux Research, 2004. Revenue from nanotechnology-enabled products to equal IT and Telecom by 2014, exceed biotech by 10 times. <www.nanotech-now.com/news.cgi?story_id=06380>.

Martin, S.B., Moyer, E.S., 2000. Electrostatic respirator filter media: filter efficiency and most penetrating particle size effects. Appl. Occup. Environ. Hyg 15, 609–617.

Maynard, A.D., Kuempel, E.D., 2005. Airborne nanostructured particles and occupational health. Journal of Nanoparticle Research 7 (6), 587–614.

Nanosafe2, 2007. <www.nanosafe.org>.

National Institute of Occupational Safety and Health, 1996. NIOSH guide to the selection and use of particulate respirators certified under 42 CFR 84. NIOSH Publication No. 96-101, Cincinnati, OH.

National Institute of Occupational Safety and Health, 2004. NIOSH respirator selection logic. NIOSH Publication No. 2005-100 Cincinnati, OH.

National Institute of Occupational Safety and Health, 2005a. Determination of particulate filter penetration to test against solid particulates for negative pressure, air-purifying respirators standard testing procedure (STP). NIOSH Procedure No. RCT-APR-STP-0057, 0058, 0059. Cincinnati, OH.

National Institute of Occupational Safety and Health, 2005b. Determination of particulate filter penetration to test against liquid particulates for negative pressure, air-purifying respirators standard testing procedure (STP). NIOSH Procedure No. RCT-APR-STP-0051, 0052, 0053, 0054, 0055, 0056. Cincinnati, OH.

National Institute for Occupational Safety and Health, 2006. Approaches to safe nanotechnology: an information exchange with NIOSH (Version 1.1). NIOSH, 60 pp.

National Nanotechnology Initiative, 2007. What is nanotechnology? <www.nano.gov/html/facts/whatIsNano.html>.

National Nanotechnology Initiative, 2008. Budget request. <www.nano.gov>.

Okuyama, K., Huang, D., Seinfeld, J.H., Naoyuki, T., Yasuo, K., 1991. Aerosol formation by rapid nucleation during the preparation of SiO_2 thin films from $SiCl_4$ and O_2 gases by CVD process. Chemical Engineering Science 46 (7), 1545–1560.

Okuyama, K., Kousaka, Y., Tohge, N., Yamamoto, S., Wu, J.J., Flagan, R.C., et al., 1986. Production of ultrafine metal oxide aerosol particles by thermal decomposition of metal alkoxide vapours. AIChE Journal 32, 2010–2019.

Ostraat, M.L., Brongersma, M., Atwater, H.A., Flagan, R.C., 2005. Nano-engineered silicon/silicon dioxide nanoparticle heterostructures. Solid State Sciences 7, 882–890.

Ostraat, M.L., Swain, K.A., Krajewshi, J.J., 2008. SiO_2 aerosol nanoparticle reactor for occupational health and safety studies. J. Occup. Envir. Hyg. 5 (6), 390–398.

Pritchard, D.K., 2004. Literature review—explosion hazards associated with nanopowders. Document HSL/2004/12. Health and Safety Laboratory, Buxton, UK.

Project on Emerging Nanotechnologies, 2008. Nano-product inventory—analysis of on-line inventory. <http://www.nanotechproject.org/inventories/consumer/%3E%3B>.

Royal Society and Royal Academy of Engineering, 2004. Nanoscience and nanotechnologies: opportunities and uncertainties. RS-RAE, London.

Sinclair, D., 1976. Penetration of HEPA filters by submicron aerosols. J. Aerosol Sci. 7, 175–179.

Sinclair, D., Hoopes, G.S., 1975. A continuous flow condensation nucleus counter. J. Aerosol Sci. 6, 1–7.

Ten Brink, H.M., Plomp, A., Spoelstra, H., van de Vate, J.F., 1983. A high-resolution electrical mobility aerosol spectrometer (MAS). J. Aerosol Sci. 14 (5), 589–597.

Tsantilis, S., Pratsinis, S.E., 2004. Soft- and hard-agglomerate aerosols made at high temperatures. Langmuir 20, 5933–5939.

Wang, S.C., Flagan, R.C., 1990. Scanning electrical mobility spectrometer. Aerosol Sci. Technol 13, 230–240.

Ulrich, G.D., Riehl, J.W., 1982. Aggregation and growth of submicron oxide particles in flames. J. Colloid Interface Sci. 87 (1), 257–265.

Warheit, D.B., 2004. Nanoparticles: health impacts? Materials Today 7, 32–35.

Whitby, K.T., Liu, B.Y.H., 1968. Polystyrene aerosol-electrical charge and residue size distribution. Atmospheric Environment 2, 103–116.

Wiedensohler, A., 1988. An approximation of the bipolar charge distribution for particles in the submicron size range. J. Aerosol Sci. 19 (3), 387–389.

Xiong, Y., Akhtar, M.K., Pratsinis, S.E., 1993. Formation of agglomerate particles by coagulation and sintering—part II. The evolution of the morphology of aerosol-made titania, silica and silica-doped titania powders. J. Aerosol Sci. 24 (3), 301–313.

Yun, K.M., Hogan, C.J., Matsubayashi, Y., Kawabe, M., Iskandar, F., Okuyama, K., 2007. Nanoparticle filtration by electrospun polymer fibers. Chemical Engineering Science 62, 4751–4759.

APPENDIX

Nanoparticle benchmarking occupational HSE project proposal

Date: 10/6/2004

To: N and ethnology Health, Safety & Environment Colleagues

This is to invite you to participate in a collaboration to develop methodology that will support rapid safety clearance of nanotechnology.

Background

1. Commercial interest in nanotechnology is growing exponentially across a range of industries.
2. Many potential new users have little or no experience handling nanomaterials, which can have very different physical and chemical properties from normal conventional chemicals.
3. There is a high level of interest in nanotechnology in both the popular press and scientific literature. The general tenor is, "This technology offers major potential benefits but there is a lot we don't know from a human and environmental perspective. We need to close these knowledge gaps before moving ahead on a broad scale".

Net, strong Process Safety and Product Stewardship will be essential and miss-steps by a few practitioners could jeopardize the wider community's right to practice.

A group of four companies have benchmarked at the technical level. Our current experience is limited to upstream small bench scale work. We were interested in anticipating safety clearance needs if/when we proceed to large scale production of products involving nanotechnology. We identified 3 practical steps that would benefit this small group and, we believe, a much larger group of companies.

1. Build a test device to generate nano sized aerosols and measure aerosol behavior (solid in air) as a function of time – in particular rate of aggregation and speed of dispersion. Knowledge from this work will be critical for both consumer safety clearance and work place exposure control.
2. Develop a simple robust device to measure airborne concentration of nano-materials. This is needed to ensure work place controls are effective.

3. Develop a test to measure if/how much nanomaterials penetrate protective clothing.

One of the benchmark companies, DuPont, has the technical capability to do this work and has prepared the research proposal below.

We wish to engage other companies in this effort. This will share costs and, more importantly, help gain acceptance of and use of the work products we seek to develop. This in turns provides industry with tools for effective Process Safety and Product Stewardship.

If your company would like to participate in this work please contact Keith Swain or Gordon Peters. We are targeting the end of October 2004 to have a confirmed list of participants. Once we are clear on the participants we will meet as a group to finalize the proposal below.

Project Title: Nanoparticle Benchmarking Occupational Health. Safety & Environment

Project Start Date: Target start date of 1/3/2005

Project Abstract: This project will provide novel knowledge of workplace exposure monitoring capabilities and strategies with the design and development of portable aerosol monitoring instrumentation for conducting assessments of worker exposure to airborne engineered nanoparticles and nanomaterials. Additionally we will conduct studies to obtain knowledge of the barrier performance characteristics of various protective clothing fabrics to aerosols of nanoparticles or nanomaterials and provide the measurement capabilities as a service.

Project Deliverable/Objective:

1) **Development of a method to generate a well-characterized aerosol of solid nanoparticles in air and evaluate instrumentation to measure solid nanoparticles in air in the aerosol generation equipment.**

We will utilize an aerosol synthesis and characterization apparatus capable of studying aerosol behavior (e.g. rate of aggregation) and we will also evaluate aerosol instrumentation for measuring solid aerosol particle >3 nm. A standard tube furnace will be used to generate aerosol particles with controlled chemistries, including metals, oxides, and semiconductors. Baseline performance and efficiencies will be established with a RDMA due to the extended operation range of the instrument and the familiarity and experience with this instrument. An Electrostatic Detector will also be used for establishing baseline performance and efficiencies and obtaining comparative data. Particles will be detected optically with a condensation nucleus counter and electrically with a Faraday cup electrometer. Commercial DMAs (long and nano) will be evaluated and compared against the RDMA for performance, transmission efficiency, and particle range limitations. In order to relate this study to aerosol inhalation and lung deposition studies previously conducted and available in the literature, a MOUDI impactor will be evaluated to determine impactor performance, particularly < lum, and to develop correlations between impactor and DMA data. A dedicated and well-characterized aerosol generation and characterization unit will be designed and built to be transportable and stable in order to conduct experiments and exposure assessments in the workplace.

Nanoparticles that have already been formed and collected will be subsequently redispersed in air, although the resulting aerosol will largely consist of agglomerated particles. A small-volume fluidized bed will be used to redisperse the particulates, which will be extracted through an aspirator tube. The differential mobility analyzer will be used to determine particle size distribution under a set of standard operating conditions.

The tube furnace approach has been chosen because we believe it is the most versatile and inexpensive means of generating aerosols from solid, liquid, and gas precursors in inert or reactive environments More specifically, solids can be directly evaporated from the hot zone of a tube furnace, bubblers and atomizers can be used to introduce liquid vapors, and gases can be fed directly from cylinders. Once synthesized, the aerosol is characterized on-line through the use of 1) a differential mobility analyzer that classifies particles based upon the ratio of electrostatic and drag forces in the presence of an applied electric field or 2) an impactor that classifies particles based upon the ratio of inertal and viscous forces. Particle detection is accomplished through the use of a condensation nucleus counter. This system is capable of producing aerosol concentrations between 1×10^1 and 1×10^{10} particles/cm^3 at sizes between 3 nm–1.5 μm. Particles can be made into single spheres, rods (for example), or agglomerates. The accurate characterization of an aerosol requires that the aerosol is generated in situ with the characterization/detection equipment.

RDMA: Caltech, 3-1500 nm size classification–made into remote sensing systems for aircraft studies, has already been incorporated into portable aerosol characterization system.

Electrostatic Detector: TSI Corp, Model 3068A.

DMA: TSI Corp, model 3080, long-DMA, 100-1500 nm size classification TSI Corp, model 3085, nano-DMA, 3-150 nm size classification.

Neutralizer: TSI Corp, model 3077, Sealed source ^{85}Kr used to produce aerosol with Fuch's charge distribution–required for DMA classification.

Detector: TSI Corp, model 3025 CNC, detection range >2 nm, < 10^5 particles/cm – input aerosol can be diluted to extend aerosol generation rate. Typical flow rates ~ 1.5 LPM.

Faraday Cup Electrometer, capable of detecting individual ions, larger particle concentration detection range than CNC, limitation in that only charged particles are detected multiply charged particles are detected as multiple particles.

Impactor: MSP Corp, classification based upon inertial impaction, effective above ~1 μm, some new capabilities below l um that need to be verified. Use individual stages (approximately 3 stages/diameter decade) and collect impacted particles on filter paper, weigh filter paper. Method is much less accurate, has less resolution, and requires more time and/or higher particle concentrations in order to detect.

Milestone Dates & Descriptions (Projection based on target start date of January 2005)

April 2005: Report baseline performance data to project participants

June 2005: Report comparison data results for instrumentation to project participants

July 2005: Demonstrate portable generator and detector system for project participants

2) Develop an air sampling method that can be used on a day-to-day basis in R&D or manufacturing settings.

Objective: In order to develop an air sampling method that can be used on a day-to-day basis in R&D or manufacturing settings, a two-pronged approach will be utilized to develop two distinct aerosol exposure metrics: 1) Monitor aerosol exposure within a laboratory environment via an installed, although portable air sampler; and 2) monitor personal aerosol exposure for an individual throughout their daily routine via a small, wearable unit. To address 1), a "black box" aerosol characterization and detection unit will be built to be stable, transportable, and require minimal maintenance. To address 2), an academic collaboration will be initiated to develop and characterize personal air samplers for occupational employee exposure assessments to aerosols of engineered nanoparticles or nanomaterials.

Milestone Dates & Descriptions: (Projection based on target start date of March 2005)

April 2005: Share plans for academic collaboration with project participants

June 2005: Demonstrate portable air sampler effectiveness to project participants

January 2006: Explore partnership for commercial manufacturing of portable air sampler unit

March 2006: Provide wearable portable air sampler unit to project participants for evaluation

3) **Measure filtration or penetration/permeation and protection of protective clothing and materials with respect to specific engineered nanoparticles or nanomaterials. Provide measurement capabilities as a service.**

Background: Protective clothing, by definition, has been used to protect workers from exposures to chemicals and particulates. In assessing the barrier performance characteristics of various protective clothing fabrics following exposures to hazardous participates, we have previously demonstrated that flashspun polyethylene fabrics (i.e., Tyvek®) provided a twenty-fold enhanced penetration barrier when compared to competitive fabrics, such as spunbonded polypropylene composite fabric. Both fabrics were subjected to aerosols of chrysotile asbestos fibers and crystalline silica particles, both considered Class I human carcinogens by the International Agency for Research on Cancer. In the asbestos studies, the barrier effectiveness of the fabrics was determined by a morphometric election microscopy method. In the silica studies, an online instantaneous method for assessing barrier protection was developed by measuring particle penetration among the various fabric samples. In this regard, evaluations of particle penetration for each fabric type were made using particle counters to quantify the particle concentrations in the airstream both before and after exposure to the commercial fabric samples. Crystalline silica particles (particle size < 1 μm MMAD) were generated with a microdust feeder and dispersion nozzle. Assessment for each fabric type were made by measuring the penetration of crystalline silica particles (particle counter size range = 0.5 μm–10.0 μm MMAD) through the fabric materials by an online particle counter measuring system.

Although respiratory protective devices and protective clothing fabrics are generally considered to provide adequate protection for exposures to fine-sized particulates, it is unclear whether these are effective barriers for nanoparticulates, defined as particulates with particle sizes <100 nm. Unfortunately, the currently available methodologies utilized in industrial hygiene practices to measure particle exposures also may not be sufficiently sensitive to measure occupational or ambient aerosol concentrations, whether in terms of particle mass, particle numbers or surface area. Therefore, it will be critical to develop a sensitive system to assess the barrier effectiveness or permeation of protective clothing fabrics, filters and respirators.

Objective: Unfortunately, the system described above does not have the sensitivity to measure particles in the <100 nm size range. However, utilizing more sophisticated particle generation and counting equipment, we can develop a similar online direct method for assessing the barrier effectiveness of protective clothing fabrics to nanoparticle penetration. In this regard, we can provide a service to measure materials for particle filtration or permeation that will utilize fixtures designed to hold various filters or filter media, including clothing swatches or membranes. This test will measure the before and after filter aerosol concentration as a function of particle size, chemistry and of testing time, i.e., filter aging. The setup will include the following: The test nanoparticles will be generated through a neutralizer and the particle sizes and concentrations will be characterized using a differential mobility analyzer (DMA) in concert with a condensation nucleus counter (CNC) prior to the filter unit containing the fabric or HEPA filter sample to be tested. The airflow containing nanoparticles continues after encountering the filter and the nanoparticle characteristics will be characterized using a neutralizer, DMA and CNC. Therefore, we will have a before the filter particle count (and characterization) and an after the filter particle count and characterization. Thus, we will be able to calculate the barrier effectiveness of the fabric or filter to an aerosol of well-characterized nanoparticles. The equipment being utilized in this project is highly sensitive and can measure particles sizes as small as 3 nm.

In the first set of experiments, we will test the barrier effectiveness of fabrics to aerosols (singlets) of monodisperse silver nanoparticles or titanium dioxide nanoparticles – each <50 nm. Although this first set of experiments may not simulate the research or occupational environment, being more extreme than the normal laboratory atmosphere, wherein nanoparticles tend to aggregate into larger clusters, it will provide important information on the effectiveness of these fabrics or filters to the "worst case scenario" – i.e., aerosols of singlet nanoparticles.

In the second set of experiments, we will test the barrier effectiveness of fabrics to polydisperse nanoparticle aerosols – of nano TiO_2 and/or nano silver particles. This would provide a better simulation of the relevant occupational nano-environment – as the generated particles are likely to aggregate.

Thereafter experiments can be conducted to test the barrier effectiveness of fabrics to singlets and polydisperse nanoparticle aerosols from consortium members and others.

Milestone Dates & Descriptions: (Projection based on target start date of March 2005)

May 2005: Demonstrate setup for project participants

July 2005: Present results measuring specified clothing and materials to project participants

August 2005: Provide as a service

CHAPTER 7

Nanotechnology Risk Management and Small Business: A Case Study on the NanoSafe Framework[1]

Matthew S. Hull

(Preface written by David Rejeski, Director, Project on Emerging Nanotechnologies)

CONTENTS

PREFACE

At least 600 businesses work on nanotechnology in the United States, of which small firms or start-ups make up the majority. Small- and medium-sized businesses and laboratories face unique challenges; in particular, many indicate that they lack the resources and the necessary information to deal with nanotechnology environmental, health and safety (EHS) issues in the workplace. Studies continue to show that nanobusinesses need information and guidance in order to adequately manage potential EHS risks associated with nanotechnology.

We recognize that dealing with uncertain risks from engineered nanomaterials to human health and the environment is not an easy task. However, it is an important and critical one given that some of the properties of materials at the nanoscale may present harm to human health and the environment. As nanomaterial manufacturing expands, and companies—particularly small businesses—seek guidance to help them ensure their

[1] This chapter has been adapted from a report prepared for the Project on Emerging Nanotechnologies by M. Hull with permission from the original copyright holder, the Woodrow Wilson International Center for Scholars.

CONTENTS

processes and products are safe, the Project on Emerging Nanotechnologies sought to help fill this need with the development of a resource document on EHS risk management approaches and practices.

This document was written by Matthew Hull, one of the leading experts in this arena. In 2003, Mr. Hull initiated the concept of an integrated EHS approach for nanobusiness operations and shortly thereafter he persuaded his employer, a manufacturer of carbon nanomaterials, to pursue research to proactively minimize worker exposure to nanomaterials and consider life cycle impacts on nanomanufacturing. That effort resulted in the NanoSafe five-point program, a practical near-term risk management approach developed at the interface between industry, academia, and authoritative agencies such as the National Institute for Occupational Safety and Health (NIOSH). It encourages proactive engagement on environmental safety issues in the nanotechnology workplace within five components: (1) facility management, (2) product stewardship, (3) workforce protection, (4) environmental management, and (5) emerging technologies and strategies.

This chapter, a reproduction of the resource document delivered to the Project on Emerging Nanotechnologies, describes the NanoSafe framework and presents resources and information that can aid nanobusinesses. It is intended to serve as an information resource for small businesses and laboratories that are interested in developing their own proactive approaches for managing nanotechnology EHS risks. Managing risks earlier rather than later will not only protect workers and users of nanomaterials and nanoproducts, but will also help protect firms from potential liability or regulatory risks. In addition, proactive EHS programs enhance the public image of nanobusinesses to consumers (both individuals and other firms).

My colleagues and I hope this document will be a useful source of information for small businesses and laboratories interested in assuring the safety of their workers and users of their products.

David Rejeski

Director, Project on Emerging Nanotechnologies

7.1 INTRODUCTION

The availability of proven approaches to effectively manage workplace and environmental exposures to engineered nanoparticles is understandably limited due to the relative novelty of this emerging technology—there is simply not enough information currently available to justify either the need for or exclusion of specialized management strategies. Nevertheless, interest in nanotechnology and associated manufacturing and application of engineered nanoparticles has surged in recent years. As discussed elsewhere in this book, nanotechnology was incorporated into more than US $50 billion in manufactured goods in 2006 (Lux Research, 2007), and is projected to reach US $2.6 trillion, or about 15% of total global output, by 2014 (Lux Research, 2006). This growth, coupled with emerging studies cautioning that some engineered nanomaterials may have important toxicological consequences stemming from their small size, has created human and environmental health risks, either actual or perceived, that must be managed. Consequently, it is prudent for nanotechnology-related enterprises to adopt proactive "good practices" approaches to minimize any potential health and safety risks to employees, surrounding communities, and end-users of nanotechnology-based products (Royal Society and Royal Academy of Engineering, 2004).

Despite the obvious need for a long-term management plan for emerging nanotechnology environmental, health, and safety (EHS) risks, practical strategies that can be readily implemented in a range of facilities are needed in the near-term to manage the most pressing potential risks to human health and the environment. Without effective near-term strategies, the uncertainty of EHS risks associated with some engineered nanomaterials, such as carbon nanotubes or nanoscale silver particles, may pose challenges to widespread acceptance of emerging nanotechnologies in society.

As the field of nanotechnology continues to advance, stakeholders such as the companies that create and market nanomaterials have an unprecedented opportunity to proactively address and minimize risks, engage and educate the public, and ultimately, effectively develop and commercialize nanotechnologies whose societal benefits are found to outweigh their associated risks. To accomplish this, however, corporate stakeholders, particularly small and start-up businesses, must be convinced that they can address emerging EHS concerns without sinking their business in the process—e.g., small companies and young start-ups teetering on the brink of major product discoveries are highly limited with respect to the resources they can dedicate to proactive EHS management strategies. Thus, the purpose of this document is to provide an information resource—derived primarily from a US-based case study—targeted at small businesses with interests in nanotechnology as they attempt to navigate the complex and emerging nanotechnology EHS landscape. This chapter concludes with a brief summary of the unique EHS risk management challenges facing small nanotechnology businesses or laboratories and one strategy that has been proposed for overcoming them.

7.2 UNCOVERING EHS INFORMATION GAPS

The recent "Survey of Current Practices in the Nanotechnology Workplace" (Gerritzen et al., 2006) produced by the International Council on Nanotechnology (ICON) in collaboration with researchers from the University of California at Santa Barbara (UCSB) provides the most comprehensive information to date on the EHS management concerns expressed by key stakeholders working with nanomaterials. The report states that organizations cite a "lack of information" as the primary barrier to implementation of effective risk management strategies for emerging nanotechnology EHS risks. Consequently, these organizations seek "new information from scientific literature and governmental guidelines for help in assessing the risks related to their nanomaterials and the appropriate steps that should be taken to address them." The survey further declares that there is strong demand for "additional industry and governmental guidance in risk assessment and EHS practices."

In addition to the general need for more guidance and information, below is a list of several examples of specific EHS issues faced by companies and laboratories identified by the ICON/UCSB survey:

- Basing safety strategies on properties of bulk materials;
- Failure to monitor the workplace or environment for fugitive particle emissions; and
- Failure to provide formal guidance to downstream users on the safe handling and disposal of nanomaterials.

Other surveys have yielded results similar to those obtained through the ICON/UCSB work. For example, a survey of nano start-up firms in Connecticut and New York in 2006 revealed that a lack of information is a major barrier to implementing EHS approaches dealing with nanomaterials (Lekas et al., 2006). However, firms' perceived ability to proactively manage potential risks varied depending on company size, resources, and internal leadership on EHS issues. Overall, firms indicated a strong preference for receiving information on nanomaterial precautionary measures electronically and from a government source. Findings from a more recent survey, including in-depth interviews, of nano firms in New England states show that firms (both large and small) want technical environmental management assistance (Lindberg and Quinn, 2007). In addition, this study found that 80% of the large firms (as compared to 33% of the small- and micro-sized firms) were taking steps to manage potential risks in their materials and processes.

7.3 EHS MANAGEMENT AND SMALL BUSINESSES

One of the areas where the development of EHS management approaches may be both especially useful and challenging is in the segment of the nanotechnology community comprised primarily of small- and medium-sized businesses. These businesses comprise "some 90% of all the businesses in the world" and are "responsible for 50–60% of total employment" (United Nations Environment Programme, 2003). They also represent a large and growing segment of the commercial nanotechnology landscape (Gerritzen et al., 2006). In fact, among businesses investing in nanotechnology, small start-ups or university-led initiatives account for the majority of companies (Garrett, 2005). Despite their significant contribution to global economies, small businesses are often overlooked when it comes to the development of initiatives and strategies that specifically address their unique EHS management needs. With respect to the development of proactive EHS approaches, some of the challenges that small businesses face are summarized in Table 7.1 (United Nations Environment Programme, 2003). The same challenges encountered by small businesses with respect to managing EHS issues in conventional industries may also influence their ability to manage emerging nanotechnology EHS issues.

Given the unique challenges facing smaller organizations, some stakeholders have indicated that the development of management frameworks with specific provisions to assist small businesses investing in nanotechnology with addressing emerging nanotechnology EHS issues may be especially useful (Maynard, 2006; Small Times Magazine, 2007).

Table 7.1 Barriers to Adoption of Environmental and Social Responsibility in Small- to Medium-Sized Businesses (United Nations Environment Programme, 2003)
Insufficient technology, expertise, training and capital
Lack of initiatives tailored for small companies
Inadequate understanding of the business case for environmental and social responsibility
The need to deal with more pressing matters, such as upgrading the quality of technology, management, and marketing
Price competition
Limited consumer pressure

In 2005, the European NanoBusiness Association (ENA) released its survey of 142 European businesses (of which 18% were small- to medium-sized businesses) on their attitudes of the impact of nanotechnologies on their businesses, the role of regulation, and perceptions of nanotechnologies. When asked what needs to be studied with regard to nanotechnologies, the vast majority of respondents answered with health and environmental impacts (European NanoBusiness Association, 2005). Despite the clear support for additional work in this area, an extensive European survey of small nanotechnology businesses and start-up concerns revealed that environmental and social impacts of nanotechnology rank low among companies' concerns amidst other challenges (European Commission, 2005). The authors of this study concluded that "this shows that there is a lack of conscience/awareness on the potential risks of such aspects for the nanomaterial branch among [small- to medium-sized businesses]." However, this may also indicate that with a lack of information and so many uncertainties about risk, firms are focusing their efforts on other more certain aspects of business.

7.4 A PRACTICAL SMALL BUSINESS APPROACH

To address the need for a near-term nanotechnology EHS management paradigm designed specifically with small business concerns in mind this chapter describes a five-point management program focused on proactive minimization of nanotechnology EHS risks. This approach—referred to as the NanoSafe framework (Figure 7.1)—was developed at the interface between small business, academia, and NIOSH, and was first presented in 2005 at the International Conference on Nanotechnology Occupational Safety and Health in Minneapolis, MN (Hull et al., 2005). While several frameworks (Environmental Defense and DuPont Nano Partnership, 2007), principles (Coalition, 2007), standards (American Society for Testing and Materials International, 2005; International Standards Organisation, 2007), and codes of conduct (e.g., the Responsible NanoCode[2]) have recently been proposed for addressing emerging nanotechnology EHS risks, NanoSafe is unique in that aspects of the program were researched and developed within an actual small business nanomanufacturing facility, and thus were found to have practical relevance to a real-world setting. Other companies, particularly small- to medium-sized businesses and

[2] See Responsible NanoCode at: www.responsiblenanocode.org/.

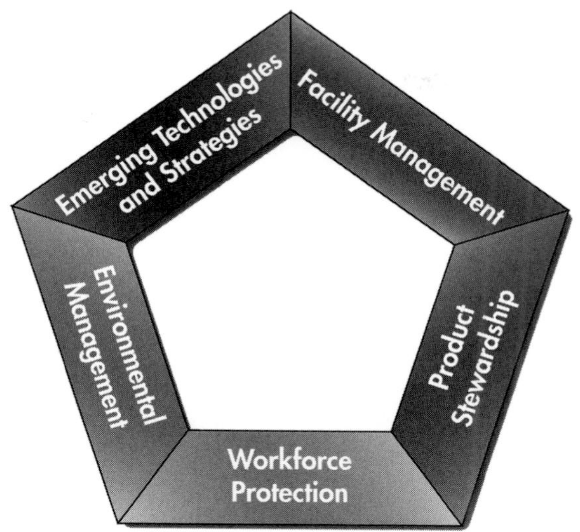

FIGURE 7.1 *NanoSafe: Conceptual five-point nanomaterials safety management approach stemming from collaboration among small business, government, and academia.*

laboratories, may find this information helpful as they prepare to balance the requirements of bringing nano-inspired products to market with ensuring the safety of their workforce, the general public, and the natural environment.

Table 7.2 summarizes the five elements of the NanoSafe framework, which arose from experience in working with engineered nanomaterials, as well as through discussions with federal and academic researchers investigating nanotechnology EHS issues. In a general sense, these five elements are thought to encompass many of the questions likely to face representatives of nanotechnology companies and research laboratories as they construct new manufacturing or R&D facilities, develop or launch new nanotechnology-based products, protect employees, manage releases of engineered nanoparticles to the natural environment, and finally, take steps to stay ahead of the nanotechnology EHS curve given the frequent emergence of new findings.

The sections that follow focus on key aspects of these five core elements of the NanoSafe management framework. These elements are intended to demonstrate a general organizational approach for how entities engaged in nanotechnology-related enterprises, particularly small- to medium-sized businesses, can take practical steps to proactively manage human and environmental, health, and safety risks. The information contained in this chapter is intended to provide other organizations, particularly small businesses and

Table 7.2 Five Primary Elements of the NanoSafe Approach Developed for Managing Nanotechnology EHS Risks in One Small Company

No.	Element	Rationale
1	Facility management	Uncertain risks place unique demands on facilities and facility managers. Specialized equipment, monitoring strategies, updated organizational structures, and revised working practices may be required.
2	Product stewardship	Any product poses an inherent risk to consumers and the environment. Ultimately, generators of these products are responsible for testing these materials to ensure their safety to consumers. Generators are also responsible for communicating possible hazards through accurate product labels and MSDS.
3	Workforce protection	Employees are on the "front lines" for exposures. Routine health surveillance may help identify and mitigate possible health risks to employees at the earliest stages. Workplace monitoring programs may be useful for characterizing exposures. New surveillance strategies and tools may be needed.
4	Environmental management	Environmental emissions (i.e., air, wastewater, solid wastes) from nanotechnology facilities may contain engineered nanomaterials. It is currently unclear what environmental risks are posed by such emissions. Proactive approaches to evaluating the properties of these emissions and/or managing them may be important for protecting public health and the natural environment. In the US, environmental regulatory policies are in place that apply to products and emissions containing engineered nanomaterials.
5	Emerging technologies and strategies	Given the frequent emergence of new findings and differing opinions on nanotechnology EHS issues, nanotechnology-related enterprises may consider participating in forums that facilitate the exchange of "lessons learned" and new information. In some instances, these lessons or even new tools created may have marketable value to others.

laboratories, with a first-tier information resource that may be of assistance as they develop their own nanotechnology-specific EHS risk management programs.

7.5 ELEMENT 1: FACILITY MANAGEMENT

7.5.1 Overview

The emerging nature of research findings and regulations pertinent to nanotechnology EHS may present unique challenges to safety managers of facilities where nanoscale materials are developed or otherwise handled. This is likely to remain the case until a universal "best practices" model or equivalent approach to facility management emerges. As evidenced by recent publications at the forefront of this dialogue (Royal Society and Royal Academy of Engineering, 2004; NIOSH, 2006; Maynard et al., 2006; Gerritzen et al., 2006; American Society for Testing and Materials International, 2007; BSI, 2007; EPA, 2007a; Environmental Defense and DuPont Nano Partnership, 2007), the establishment of such a model is a top priority on the agendas of many international organizations, including government agencies, and representatives from industry, academia, and non-government organizations (NGOs). As these international organizations continue to progress toward developing management practices based on sound science and thoughtful assessments of actual risks, individual entities engaged in nanotechnology-related activities have been encouraged to adopt their own practical strategies for identifying and managing EHS risks associated with their respective facilities and material handling practices.

7.5.2 A starting point for risk assessment: the OSHA Handbook for small business

The Occupational Safety and Health Administration (OSHA) developed the OSHA Handbook for Small Businesses (OSHA, 1996)[3] to assist small business employers with meeting the legal requirements imposed by, and under, the authority of the Occupational Safety and Health Act of 1970 (P.L.91-596) and to achieve an incompliance status voluntarily before an inspection performed pursuant to the Act.

Materials contained in the handbook are based on the federal OSHA standards and other requirements in effect at the time of publication, and on generally accepted principles and activities within the job safety and health field.[4]

One component of the OSHA Handbook for Small Businesses that may be particularly helpful to small- to medium-sized businesses engaged in nanotechnology-related activities as they start preparing a comprehensive

---

[3] Available online at: www.osha.gov/Publications/osha2209.pdf.

[4] **OSHA Disclaimer.** The booklet is not intended to be a legal interpretation of the provisions of the Occupational Safety and Health Act of 1970 or to place any additional requirements on employers or employees, but the material contained therein is expected to be useful to small business owners or managers and can be adapted easily to individual establishments. All employers should be aware that there are certain states (and similar jurisdictions) which operate their own programs under agreement with the U.S. Department of Labor, pursuant to section 18 of the Act. The programs in these jurisdictions may differ in some details from the federal program.

management plan for their nanotechnology facility is the OSHA Hazard Assessment Checklist. This checklist is designed to serve as a generic framework through which general industrial hazards may be identified. In its current form, the checklist may not necessarily identify any new workplace hazards created specifically by manufacturing and handling of engineered nanomaterials. However, with careful review, discussion among, and input from EHS professionals and individuals engaged in specific nanotechnology-related activities, the checklist may be helpful in identifying areas where additional considerations may be warranted for nanomaterials. Some example questions from the checklist are provided in Table 7.3. These questions were selected given their particular relevance to nanotechnology EHS information gaps. For example, how can a safety manager or an employer answer "yes" to questions regarding the adequacy of personal protective equipment (PPE), overall awareness of possible nanomaterial hazards, and/or Threshold Limit Value (TLV) or Permissible Exposure Limit (PEL) values for airborne contaminants given the current limited status of information industry-wide?

7.5.3 Comprehensive information on nano-specific risks and management strategies

Approaches to Safe Nanotechnology: An Information Exchange with NIOSH. One of the resources available for addressing emerging nanotechnology EHS issues at the facility level is the report: Approaches to Safe

Table 7.3 Example of Questions from the OSHA Hazard Assessment Checklist
Do you have a safety committee or group made up of management and labor representatives that meets regularly and report in writing on its activities?
Are you keeping your employees advised of the successful effort and accomplishments you and/or your safety committee have made in assuring they will have a workplace that is safe and healthful?
Has the employer been trained on personal protective equipment (PPE) procedures, i.e., what PPE is necessary for job tasks, when they need it, and how to properly adjust it?
Are employees aware of the hazards involved with the various chemicals they may be exposed to in their work environment, such as ammonia, chlorine, epoxies, caustics, etc.?
Are you familiar with the Threshold Limit Values or Permissible Exposure Limits of airborne contaminants and physical agents used in your workplace?

Nanotechnology: An Information Exchange with NIOSH.[5] As stated on the NIOSH Web page, the purpose of this document is as follows:

> *This document reviews what is currently known about nanoparticle toxicity and control, but it is only a starting point. The document serves as a request from NIOSH to occupational safety and health practitioners, researchers, product innovators and manufacturers, employers, workers, interest group members, and the general public to exchange information that will ensure that no worker suffers material impairment of safety or health as nanotechnology develops. Opportunities to provide feedback and information are available throughout this document.*

While NIOSH's Approaches to Safe Nanotechnology report does not provide mandated nanomaterial-specific recommendations for facility management, it does serve as one of the most trusted information resources currently available to assist safety managers with making rational decisions about risk minimization in their respective facilities.

To briefly demonstrate the utility of the Approaches to Safe Nanotechnology document, consider the following example question taken from the OSHA Hazard Assessment Checklist, as listed in the previous table. In this particular example, the checklist addresses threshold limit values (TLVs) or permissible exposure levels (PELs) of certain workplace contaminants.

> *Are you familiar with the Threshold Limit Values or Permissible Exposure Limits of airborne contaminants and physical agents used in your workplace?*

In most instances, TLVs or PELs have not been specifically determined for nanoscale materials as this is a time-consuming and resource-intensive process that cannot be readily undertaken by a small business. Nevertheless, these values are important for determining the effectiveness of engineering controls or the need for specific personal protective equipment (PPE) in the workplace. To address this information gap, NIOSH states the following on page 23 of its Approaches to Safe Nanotechnology:

> *In determining the effectiveness of controls or the need for respirators, it would therefore be prudent to consider both the current exposure limits or guidelines (e.g., PELs, RELs, TLVs) and the increase in surface area of the nanoparticles relative to that of particles for which the exposure limits or guides were developed.*

---

[5] Available online at: www.cdc.gov/niosh/topics/nanotech/safenano/.

As this example illustrates, facility safety managers may benefit from using the OSHA Handbook for Small Businesses and Approaches to Safe Nanotechnology documents together as complementing sources of information for instituting appropriate precautionary measures to deal with nanomaterial exposure within facilities.

While professional judgment remains a critical element of EHS decision-making, the general guidance issued by NIOSH through its Approaches to Safe Nanotechnology provides an important resource to facility safety managers tasked with ensuring the safety of workers in facilities where engineered nanomaterials are manufactured or otherwise handled. With this information, well-trained facility safety managers can make better informed EHS decisions in the workplace. Further, NIOSH periodically updates its Approaches to Safe Nanotechnology guidance to reflect significant recent progress in assessing and controlling exposures to engineered nanomaterials in the workplace.

American Society for Testing and Materials (ASTM) Standard Guide for Handling Unbound Engineered Nanoscale Particles in Occupational Settings. The ASTM recently published the ASTM E2535-07 Standard Guide for Handling Unbound Engineered Nanoscale Particles in Occupational Settings[6]. According to ASTM, this guide:

> *describes actions that could be taken by the user to minimize human exposures to unbound, engineered nanoscale particles (UNP) in research, manufacturing, laboratory and other occupational settings where UNP may reasonably be expected to be present.*

ASTM states that the intent of this document is to:

> *provide guidance for controlling such exposures as a cautionary measure where neither relevant exposure standards nor definitive hazard and exposure information exist.*

The ASTM guide provides detailed and methodical treatment of general issues related to controlling exposures to UNP in the workplace. Helpful features include terminology that is clearly defined at the beginning of the document and extensive discussion of the critical roles of management and a well-defined organizational structure when controlling workplace exposures to UNP. As the ASTM guide evolves, it would be helpful if later versions included information from specific case studies developed with input from nanomanufacturers.

[6] The document is available at: www.astm.org/Standards/E2535.htm.

British Standards Institute (BSI) Guide to Safe Handling and Disposal of Manufactured Nanomaterials. In January 2008, a UK-based team comprising SAFENANO, the Institute of Occupational Medicine, and the British Standards Institute (the UK National Standards body) published PD 6699-2:2007 Nanotechnologies – Part 2: Guide to Safe Handling and Disposal of Manufactured Nanomaterials.[7] According to a press release on the guide:

> *This document provides step-by-step guidance through the general approach to management of risks, information needs, hazard assessment, measurement of exposure, methods of control and disposal.*

In addition to the guide, BSI published eight other documents[8] offering guidance on nanotechnology-related issues. One of the most intriguing aspects of the BSI guide is its presentation of benchmark exposure levels for certain classes of engineered nanomaterials. Given that the reported benchmark exposure levels have not been subjected to the scientific rigor required for the establishment of such thresholds, the guide insists that their inclusion in the document is to provide pragmatic guidance only.

Environmental Defense and DuPont NANO Risk Framework. Environmental Defense and DuPont teamed up to develop a "comprehensive, practical, and flexible" framework intended for companies and organizations to evaluate and address potential nanomaterial risks.[9]

Some have argued that the framework may delay governments from establishing needed mandatory nanotechnology regulation (Civil Society-Labor Coalition, 2007) or set the EHS bar too high, especially for small companies; however, few can argue with the value of the comprehensive information, strategies, and case studies offered in this document. The framework is meant to guide a broad range of users working with nanomaterials on data gathering, assessing EHS risks, decision-making to reduce potential risks, and communicating that information.

7.5.4 Meeting resource needs through innovative partnerships

Throughout the process of developing a specific facility management strategy, it is likely that smaller entities will encounter situations where they require

---

[7] Available at: www.bsiglobal.com/en/Standards-and-Publications/Industry-Sectors/Nanotechnologies/PD-6699-2/Download-PD6699-2-2007/.

[8] Available at: www.bsigroup.com/nano.

[9] Available at: www.nanoriskframework.com.

resources beyond what they can readily provide on their own. These resources generally include access to expertise or equipment. In these situations, innovative partnerships may help provide necessary resources. The following sections describe the forms that some of these partnerships may take.

NIOSH Field Team. As part of its strategic research program on the occupational safety and health applications and implications of nanotechnology, NIOSH has formed an interdisciplinary field team of NIOSH researchers specifically focused on the area of nanotechnology (NIOSH, 2008a,b). The purpose of the team is to perform on-site assessments of processes, materials, control technologies, and potential occupational exposures to nanomaterials in participating nanotechnology workplaces. Participants in the program include research laboratories and companies who manufacture or otherwise handle engineered nanomaterials. The team is fully funded by NIOSH, and thus there is no monetary cost to participating companies and laboratories. However, participants are expected to invest a certain amount of time, availability, and level of facility access to support the team's efforts. Interested participants can contact NIOSH[10] to determine whether their facility fits with the team's stated objectives; a site visit will be arranged for qualifying participants. All data collected are communicated back to the participants and may be used in a general fashion to support NIOSH efforts to develop guidance on occupational safety and health implications of nanotechnology in the workplace. To maintain the participants' privacy, participants are not identified in any NIOSH documents disseminated publicly, without the permission of the participant.[11]

Universities, Government Laboratories. In addition to the NIOSH field team, a number of research groups from academia, government laboratories, and even industry may be interested in partnering with organizations engaged in nanotechnology R&D and/or manufacturing, to help fulfill obligations on research grants pertinent to EHS, or to enhance their service-providing capabilities to the emerging nanotechnology industry (in the case of some environmental consulting firms). These types of partnerships offer unique risks and rewards, but still may offer improved access to expertise and equipment resources needed to identify and manage EHS risks in nanotechnology facilities. Initiating an effective collaboration is usually a

[10] NIOSH Contact: Charles L. Geraci, Ph.D., CIH, Branch Chief, Education and Information Division and Nanotechnology Research Center, NIOSH, MS C-32, 4676 Columbia Parkway, Cincinnati, OH 45336, USA. Tel.: +1 513 533 8339; fax: +1 513 533 8230, Email: CGeraci@cde.gov.

[11] Additional information available at: www.cdc.gov/niosh/topics/nanotech/newsarchive.html#fieldteam.

facilities designed to "provide opportunities and support for multidisciplinary research among investigators from a variety of disciplines and from different research sectors, including academia, industry and government laboratories."[15] The tools and expertise available at such facilities, and others like them around the world, are critical to organizations with interests in nanotechnology, particularly small companies, as many of these resources cannot be readily accessed otherwise.

ICON EHS Database. One tool that may be especially useful for locating literature pertinent to EHS implications of engineered nanomaterials is the ICON Environmental, Health, and Safety (EHS) database.[16] The database contains summaries and citations for research papers that have specific relevance to nanotechnology and EHS. Users may also access full papers, but site registration or payment may be required for the majority of these articles.

7.6.3 Communicating product information effectively

To extract maximum value from voluntary product testing, producers must be able to communicate information about their products to consumers (as well as their own employees) in a clear and efficient manner. In general, chemical information is communicated in two primary forms: the material safety data sheets (MSDS) and product labels. According to the ICON/UCSB survey, "MSDS and personal interactions were the most commonly described methods for transmitting information of product stewardship. For safe use, manufacturers tended to provide MSDS as guidance" (Gerritzen et al., 2006).

Given the novelty or "prototype" form of many emerging nanotechnologies, as well as the questionable adequacy of some techniques used to quantify the physicochemical and/or toxicological properties of engineered nanomaterials, it is no small task for generators to obtain the information required to communicate information about their products and prototypes—not even the best labels or MSDS can communicate information you do not have. In response, some generators have created MSDS for their nanoscale products based on the properties of the bulk materials from which they were created (e.g., properties of graphite are used to describe single-wall carbon nanotubes). Some stakeholders (e.g., Balbus, 2005) have spoken out in clear opposition to this approach, suggesting that it has not been validated and may misrepresent certain size-associated properties of nanoscale materials.

---

[15] More information is available at: www.nano.gov/html/centers/home_centers.html.

[16] The database is available at: icon.rice.edu/research.cfm.

Despite the increased challenges facing generators of nanotechnology-based products, generators ultimately remain responsible for both determining and communicating any hazardous properties of their products to end-users. The sections immediately following summarize the perspectives of two U.S. federal agencies involved in evaluating and communicating product hazards as well as some of the tools and guidelines applied during this process.

The CPSC and Nanotechnology Products. The Consumer Product Safety Commission (CPSC) is the U.S. federal agency "charged with protecting the public from unreasonable risks of serious injury or death from more than 15,000 types of consumer products under the agency's jurisdiction." The CPSC protects consumers primarily from products that pose fire, electrical, chemical, or mechanical hazards.

A recent report co-authored by a CPSC staff member concluded that "if a substance is considered "hazardous," then the Federal Hazardous Substances Act (FHSA) requires cautionary labeling to address the principal hazard presented by the product and instructions for safe use, handling and storage of the product" (Thomas et al., 2006). If a substance is determined to be hazardous and the label deemed inadequate to protect public health and safety, then the CPSC can ban the substance.

According to the CPSC, manufacturers are responsible for determining whether their products are "hazardous substances" and for ensuring that such products are labeled as required by the FHSA. The CPSC report states a "hazardous substance" is defined using the following criteria:

> *The definition of a hazardous substance under the FHSA is risk-based and the regulation addresses both acute and chronic hazards. To be considered a "hazardous substance" under the FHSA (15 U.S.C. § 1261 (f)(1)(A)), a consumer product must satisfy a two-part definition:*
>
> *First, the substance (or mixture of substances) must be toxic under the FHSA, or present one of the other hazards enumerated in the statute.*
>
> *Second, it must have the potential to cause "substantial illness or substantial personal injury during or as a proximate result of any customary or reasonably foreseeable handling or use." Therefore, exposure and the likelihood of risk must be considered in addition to inherent toxicity when assessing whether a product meets the definition of a hazardous substance under the FHSA.*

OSHA and the Hazard Communication Standard. OSHA is the foremost regulatory body in the United States charged with ensuring that safe working conditions are provided for American workers. A major component of OSHA's efforts on this front is focused on ensuring that hazards are communicated clearly to the individuals who may be affected by them. The following statement regarding "hazard communication" was taken from the OSHA website[17] and summarizes requirements under OSHA's Hazard Communication Standard:

> *In order to ensure chemical safety in the workplace, information must be available about the identities and hazards of the chemicals. OSHA's Hazard Communication Standard (HCS) requires the development and dissemination of such information:*
>
> *Chemical manufacturers and importers are required to evaluate the hazards of the chemicals they produce or import, and*
>
> *Prepare labels and material safety data sheets (MSDSs) to convey the hazard information to their downstream customers.*
>
> *All employers with hazardous chemicals in their workplaces must have labels and MSDSs for their exposed workers, and train them to handle the chemicals appropriately.*

MSDS and Product Labels. The OSHA Hazard Communication Standard (HCS) incorporates a three-pronged approach to communicating hazards posed by materials:

- Labels on containers;
- Development of material safety data sheets (MSDS); and
- Employee training.

While employee training is usually limited to communicating information along the manufacturing chain, the importance of product labels and MSDS frequently transcend the boundaries of the workplace.

Product labels, though brief, are the most immediate source of information. Nevertheless, since the label is attached to the product container, it is typically accessible whenever the product is being used. Labels are snapshots used to remind product users of any potential hazards and to point out resources for more information (e.g., MSDS, Websites).

MSDS are typically as comprehensive as a product label is brief. They provide a "one-stop shopping source for everything you might need or want to know about a chemical." Given the diversity of the audience for which MSDSs are intended, they must provide a broad array of information.

[17] Available at: www.osha.gov/SLTC/hazardcommunications/index.html.

In particular, MSDS "must be useful to the safety and health professionals deciding what controls to use, the first aid or medical treatment to provide, and the precautionary measures to follow" (OSHA, 2004).[18]

As noted above, OSHA requires chemical manufacturers and importers to obtain or create an MSDS for each hazardous chemical they produce or import and maintain those MSDS in the workplace.[19] OSHA also points out that "producers of chemicals may be subject to "failure to warn" suits that can have significant financial implications."

7.6.4 Voluntary reporting schemes

Currently, it is unclear whether and to what extent businesses and laboratories working with nanotechnologies should report the nature of their nanotechnology-specific activities (e.g., types and quantities of nanomaterials generated, working practices, etc.) to state or federal regulatory agencies. One approach that has been considered is the implementation of voluntary reporting schemes that permit the exchange of information between regulators and entities engaged in nanotechnology activities. In general, these programs do not replace existing legislation; rather, they are intended to offer flexibility in the nature of information exchanged so that a moderate level of oversight can occur without unnecessarily hindering nanotechnology research. Two of these programs—the UK Voluntary Reporting Scheme for Engineered Nanoscale Materials and the U.S. EPA Nanoscale Materials Stewardship Program—are summarized in the sections that follow.

UK Voluntary Reporting Scheme for Engineered Nanoscale Materials. The UK Voluntary Reporting Scheme for Engineered Nanoscale Materials program[20] was initiated in September 2006 (DEFRA, 2008). The program is run by the UK Department for Environment, Food and Rural Affairs (DEFRA), in conjunction with other government departments and agencies. The aim of the program is to obtain from anyone involved in the manufacture or use of engineered nanomaterials information that provides "an indication of those nanomaterials which are currently in development or production." This information is expected to assist legislators with aligning

---

[18] More information on MSDS available at: www.osha.gov/pls/oshaweb/owadisp.show_document?p_table=STANDARDS&;p_id=10099#1910.1200(g).

[19] More information available at: www.osha.gov/.

[20] More information on the UK Voluntary Reporting Scheme for Engineered Nanoscale Materials is available at the following web-link: http://www.defra.gov.uk/environment/nanotech/policy/.

resource allocation and policy-making with relevant industry and consumer needs. The program recognizes the potential sensitivity of certain commercial business information and thus offers flexibility in the types of information that can be provided under the voluntary scheme.

EPA Nanoscale Materials Stewardship Program. EPA has implemented a voluntary Nanoscale Materials Stewardship Program (NMSP) under the Toxic Substances Control Act (TSCA), which is intended to "complement and support its efforts on new and existing nanoscale materials."[21] EPA indicates that, based on the outcomes of an extensive review process, the general components of the Stewardship Program could include:

- Assembling existing data and information from manufacturers and processors of existing chemical nanoscale materials;
- Encouraging the development of test data needed to provide a firm scientific foundation for future work and regulatory/policy decisions; and
- Identifying and encouraging the use of a basic set of risk management practices in developing and commercializing nanoscale materials.

Currently, EPA is working with stakeholders to develop the Stewardship Program as well as the means for implementing it. In July 2007, the agency solicited comments on its latest concept paper (EPA, 2007b) for the development of the NMSP, on information collection activities for the voluntary program (EPA, 2007c) program, and on the inventory status of nanoscale substances under TSCA (EPA, 2007d).[22]

EPA intends to encourage participation in the NMSP by individuals or entities that manufacture, import, modify, or use engineered nanoscale materials in the manufacture of a product. EPA indicates that information gathered through the Stewardship Program will be used to support further development of TSCA, specifically as it relates to nanoscale materials. This includes determining "any regulatory actions that may be needed to protect human health and the environment."[23]

---

[21] Available at: www.epa.gov/oppt/nano/.

[22] These documents and forms are posted at: www.epa.gov/oppt/nano/nmspfr.htm.

[23] Information on the Nanoscale Materials Stewardship Program available at www.epa.gov/oppt/nano/.

7.7 ELEMENT 3: WORKFORCE PROTECTION

7.7.1 Overview

Currently, over 800 entities engaged in nanotechnology research and development or manufacturing exist in the U.S. alone (PEN, 2007).[24] This includes commercial firms as well as government and university laboratories. In addition, it is estimated that there are at least 20,000 individuals working worldwide in nanotechnology today (NNI, 2007).

One approach for preventing adverse health effects to workers is occupational health surveillance. According to NIOSH, occupational health surveillance involves the "tracking of occupational injuries, illnesses, hazards, and exposures." Surveillance approaches include assessments of both individual- and group/population-based activities. Data obtained from health surveillance programs are used to "guide efforts to improve worker safety and health, and to monitor trends and progress over time."

Tracking occupational injuries, illnesses, hazards, and exposures has been an integral part of NIOSH since its creation by the Occupational Safety and Health Act in 1970. NIOSH complements important statistical or surveillance activities carried out by other federal agencies (including the Bureau of Labor Statistics, the Occupational Safety and Health Administration, the Mine Safety and Health Administration, and the National Center for Health Statistics), state governments, and private sector groups.[25] NIOSH's surveillance efforts include:

- Analyzing and interpreting existing data;
- Undertaking data collection efforts to fill gaps in surveillance data;
- Providing support to state agencies to conduct occupational surveillance and associated prevention efforts;
- Funding and conducting research on surveillance methods; and
- Working with federal, state, and private sector partners to improve occupational health surveillance.

---

[24] **Note:** These numbers are drawn from publicly available lists compiled by the Project on Emerging Nanotechnologies; the actual number of entities working in nanotechnology is likely to be much higher.

[25] Information available at: www.cdc.gov/niosh/topics/surveillance.

7.7.2 Elements of baseline and routine health surveillance in nanotechnology facilities

Health surveillance programs are carried out to prevent illness when there is knowledge about both the possibility of an exposure to a health hazard and the health effects caused by that exposure and tests available to detect those effects (Nasterlack et al., 2007). Successful surveillance programs involve assessing needs, setting program goals and defining the target population, choosing testing modalities, collecting and interpreting data to benefit individuals and groups of workers, intervening based on results, communicating results, and evaluating the program (Harber et al., 2003).

Currently, it is unclear whether employee health surveillance strategies geared specifically for workers involved in the manufacturing or integration of engineered nanomaterials are necessary. Some have argued in favor of some form of proactive health surveillance program, while others have questioned whether such programs can be justified given added costs and privacy concerns. Still, others are unclear exactly what components would comprise such a program since there are no clear biomarkers and/or health outcomes established around which to base an exposure assessment specific for engineered nanomaterials. The uncertainties about adverse effects from nanomaterial exposure present a challenge to designing and implementing a health or medical surveillance program in the nanotechnology workplace (Kosnett and Newman, 2007).

Much the same as with establishing effective parameters for workplace monitoring programs, researchers are investigating candidate indicators of human health impacts associated with engineered nanomaterials for surveillance purposes (Nasterlack et al., 2007; Kosnett and Newman, 2007). Testing parameters discussed in the literature and at recent conferences present a number of pros and cons. Nasterlack et al. (2007) conclude that none of the effect parameters proposed for nanoparticle-exposed employees, including heart rate variability, blood-clotting parameters, pro-inflammatory cytokines, are specific or sufficiently validated as individual health risk indicators. Some also require equipment that is not routinely available. Other parameters (e.g., ECG, chest X-ray, and pulmonary function) are useful diagnostic tools, but only when health effects are known, which is not yet the case for nanomaterial exposure (Nasterlack et al., 2007).

Kosnett and Newman (2007) point out the limitations of applying other parameters (e.g., spirometry, chest X-ray) in the nanotechnology workplace; however, they suggest that other parameters (e.g., serum biomarkers, imaging, and exercise oximetry) may serve as potential future modalities for pulmonary testing. This chapter does not intend to comment on which of these measurements are most appropriate for nanotechnology facilities. Given the existing constraints in developing surveillance programs and potential ethical issues of employee screening (as highlighted by Schulte and Salamanca-Buentello, 2007), some researchers have proposed the development of nanotechnology worker exposure registries.

As noted in its Approaches to Safe Nanotechnology report (NIOSH, 2009),[26] NIOSH is currently developing guidance for occupational health surveillance for nanotechnology, which should continue to serve as a useful and up-to-date resource for workplaces.

7.7.3 Workplace monitoring

Workplace monitoring typically accompanies health surveillance programs and is intended to relate certain parameters measured at a facility with observed human health outcomes (e.g., particulate levels measured relative to worker respiratory function). While many monitoring programs have been instituted at workplaces around the world, it is currently unclear as to which measurements are most critical in facilities where engineered nanomaterials are manufactured or otherwise handled. Researchers are actively working to identify these parameters (e.g., Maynard and Kuempel, 2005; Oberdörster et al., 2007; Maynard, 2007; Maynard and Aitken, 2007; Wittmaack, 2007), but a global consensus on these parameters has not yet been reached. In the meantime, resources are available to assist nanotechnology developers with establishing their own workplace monitoring programs. Perhaps the most well-known of these resources is the NIOSH field team (see earlier section), given their extensive background in workplace monitoring programs in general, and particulate/aerosol measurements in particular.

While the world awaits a standardized workplace monitoring program, some of the nanomaterial parameters to consider monitoring in the workplace—as reported in the literature and at recent conferences—include particle number, particle size distribution, surface area, chemistry or reactivity, solubility, shape, and mass concentration.

As discussed in Maynard and Aitken (2007), different situations will require different material attributes—whether surface area, mass, or particle number concentration—to be measured; the paper recommends measuring all three where possible. The idea of a universal aerosol sampler enabling the collection of personal exposure to all three of these metrics is explored in this paper and in the Nature paper on the safe handling of nanotechnology written by 13 distinguished nanotechnology experts (Maynard et al., 2006).

[26] Available at: www.cdc.gov/niosh/topics/nanotech/safenano/.

7.8 ELEMENT 4: ENVIRONMENTAL MANAGEMENT

7.8.1 Overview

Knowledge on engineered nanoparticles and their interaction with the natural environment is inadequate (Colvin, 2003). Researchers have acknowledged that nanoscale contaminants dispersed in air, sediment, and aqueous media may possess unique physical and chemical properties that ultimately could influence their fate, transport, transformation, and bioavailability in the environment (Masciangoli and Zhang, 2003). Despite the general lack of information regarding nanoparticle interaction with the environment, studies have suggested that some engineered nanomaterials are toxic in aquatic bioassays (e.g., Oberdörster, 2004) and biological systems (e.g., Derfus et al., 2004; Warheit et al., 2004). Some nanomaterials, such as hydroxylated C_{60} fullerenes and surfactant-modified carbon nanotubes, can have enhanced mobility in simulated groundwater systems (Lecoanet et al., 2004). These initial findings coupled with the rapid expansion of the field of nanotechnology have stimulated further research into the human and environmental effects of engineered nanoparticles. Elsewhere in this book, Santamaria and Sayes (2009) provide a more comprehensive and up-to-date review of ecotoxicological and toxicological studies with engineered nanomaterials.

7.8.2 Thinking beyond the workplace

Beyond the EHS issues encountered in the nanotechnology workplace, the potential exists for some nanomanufacturing processes to inadvertently release free nanoparticles into the environment through air emissions, discharged process water, commercial use, or disposal in solid waste streams. However, it remains unclear whether environmental releases of nanomaterials pose any actual EHS risks. This uncertainty has created challenges for U.S. federal agencies, such as the U.S. Environmental Protection Agency (EPA), charged with protecting human health and the environment. As indicated from the following statements issued on the EPA nanotechnology topic webpage,[27] the lack of conclusive information has hindered the development of specific regulatory policies pertinent to nanotechnology EHS:

> *At this early stage of development of nanotechnology, there are few detailed studies on the effects of nanoscale materials in the body or the environment. Early results are also inconclusive, and it is clear that*

[27] Available at: www.epa.gov/oppt/nano/nano-facts.htm.

> *it is not yet possible to make broad conclusions about which nanoscale substances may pose risks.*
>
> *There is a need for more information to assess the potential environmental, health, and safety impacts for most engineered nanoscale materials. Such information is important because EPA needs a sound scientific basis for assessing and managing unreasonable risks that may result from the introduction of nanoscale materials into the environment.*

Despite current data gaps, some environmental agencies may have existing laws and regulations, such as noted below by EPA, that provide them with authority to regulate engineered nanomaterials.

> *Many nanoscale materials are regarded as "chemical substances" under the Toxic Substances Control Act (TSCA). This law provides EPA with a strong framework for ensuring that new and existing chemical substances are manufactured and used in a manner that protects against unreasonable risks to human health and the environment. For example, EPA requires manufacturers of new chemical substances to provide specific information to the Agency for review before manufacturing chemicals or introducing them into commerce. EPA can require reporting or development of information to assess existing chemicals already in the marketplace. Additionally, EPA can take action to ensure that those chemicals that pose an unreasonable risk to human health or the environment are effectively controlled.*[28]

7.8.3 The concept of life cycle assessment

Life cycle-based assessment practices have been proposed as a means for helping to identify and manage unique EHS issues occurring throughout the product life cycle—from research and development, through production, commercial application, and ultimately to disposal.

Recently, a report issued by the Woodrow Wilson International Center for Scholars Project on Emerging Nanotechnologies and the European Commission reviewed the topic of nanotechnology and life cycle assessment (WWICS and European Commission, 2007). That document noted the following:

> *One approach that can improve our understanding of the possible impacts of nanotechnology is Life Cycle Assessment (LCA). This*

[28] Nanotechnology under the Toxic Substances Control Act www.epa.gov/oppt/nano/ (accessed November 27, 2007).

comprehensive analysis tool can be used to evaluate how a product or material—from the start of production through end-of-life—affects ecosystems and human health. LCA is already widely used internationally by scientists, engineers, and product designers in universities and businesses. If applied in the nanotechnology realm, the tool has the potential to guide researchers, policymakers, and companies as they seek to realize the commercial and practical benefits of a nanoproduct, while avoiding potential risks.

The UK Royal Society and The Royal Academy of Engineering (2004) also stressed the importance of using LCA as a tool to better understand the tradeoffs in environmental benefits and risks from nanotechnologies in its seminal 2004 report.

A lengthy discussion on LCA is beyond the scope of this chapter.[29] Rather, the intent is to introduce nanotechnology developers to the concept of examining the full impact potential of their products and to search for appropriate alternatives where possible. Even if a full LCA is not completed for each product, life cycle thinking (similar to product stewardship) about potential impacts should be incorporated into product design.

7.8.4 U.S. Environmental regulatory policy

On July 25, 2006, the American Bar Association (ABA) Section of Environment, Energy, and Resources (SEER) released a comprehensive review of the core federal environmental statutes pertinent to nanotechnology (ABA SEER, 2006). The review resulted in detailed briefing documents on six environmental statutes and a briefing document on innovative governance mechanisms. Collectively, these documents identify key legal and regulatory issues EPA can

[29] For more information on LCA, a few useful resources include:

EPA, 2006. "Life Cycle Assessment: Principles and Practice." Prepared by Scientific Applications International Corporation for the National Risk Management Research Laboratory, Office of Research and Development, U.S. Environmental Protection Agency. EPA/600/R-06/060. May. Available at: www.epa.gov/nrmrl/lcaccess/lca101.html.

Graedel, T.E., and B.R. Allenby, 2003. Industrial Ecology. Second Edition. Pearson Education, Inc.: Upper Saddle River, New Jersey. Chapters 15–17.

ISO 14040:2006: Environmental management – Life cycle assessment – Principles and framework. International Organization for Standardization (ISO). Available at: www.iso.org/iso/catalogue_detail?csnumber=37456.

35ISO 14044:2006: Environmental management – Life cycle assessment – Requirements and guidelines. International Organization for Standardization (ISO). Available at: www.iso.org/iso/iso_catalogue/catalogue_tc/catalogue_detail.htm?csnumber=38498.

be expected to encounter as it considers how best to address issues likely to arise in connection with nanotechnology. EHS personnel as well as legal counsels involved with nanotechnology facilities may find it helpful to review the briefing documents to determine initial applicability to their respective organizations. When necessary, specialized legal perspectives may be needed to help further assess compliance with applicable as well as emerging regulations.

The ABA SEER briefing documents provide the first comprehensive, scholarly review of the core federal environmental statutes with a view toward assessing the utility of each in addressing the legal and regulatory issues pertinent to EPA's jurisdiction presented by nanotechnology. In general, the papers concluded that the core environmental statutes were found to provide EPA with sufficient legal authority to address adequately the challenges EPA is expected to encounter as it assesses the enormous benefits of and potential risks associated with nanotechnology. Specifically, the ABA SEER briefing papers found the following:

- The existing environmental statutes of TSCA, RCRA, CAA, and FIFRA apply to nanomanufacturing and associated products and/or wastes;
- Other environmental statutes may apply or may soon apply to nanomanufacturing. These include CERCLA, CWA, and other new approaches customized specifically for nanomanufacturing facilities (EMS/Innovative Regulatory Approaches);
- Under TSCA, EPA has expansive authority to regulate nanomaterials, including the authority to require health and environmental testings; collect production, health, and environmental information about nanomaterials; and promulgate rules regulating, and even prohibiting, the manufacture, processing, distribution, and use of nanomaterials;
- Under RCRA, EPA has authority to regulate discarded wastes that might include nanoscale materials; and
- Under CAA, EPA has authority to regulate air emissions.

The Project on Emerging Nanotechnologies has also produced comprehensive analyses of the environmental statutes and their ability to deal with nanotechnology.

For instance, in EPA and Nanotechnology: Oversight for the twenty-first century, former EPA assistant administrator for policy, Davies; sets out an agenda for creating an effective oversight system as nanotechnology advances (Davies, 2007). He also suggests ways that the EPA can improve its ability to provide adequate oversight for nanotechnology and other emerging twenty-first century challenges. The nanotechnology industry also has an important role to play in this process. Davies recommends that industry members take part in dialogues with other stakeholders to discuss the optimal form of nano oversight.

The report, Where Does the Nano Go? End-of-Life Regulation of Nanotechnologies, by Linda K. Breggin and John Pendergrass of the Environmental Law Institute explores nanomaterial and nanoproduct end-of-life issues within the existing regulatory frameworks of the RCRA and the CERCLA (Breggin and Pendergrass, 2007). The authors point out that EPA must make key decisions about how to apply these statutes to nanotechnology waste to ensure adequate oversight for these technologies. However, the report notes that the agency lacks much of the data on human health and ecotoxicity that form the basis for such determinations, creating some tough challenges ahead in EPA's decision-making process. The report also calls on firms that manufacture nanomaterials, investors, and insurers to consider the new kinds of liabilities and environmental risks that may emerge as a result of the release and disposal of waste nanomaterials into the environment.

7.9 ELEMENT 5: EMERGING TECHNOLOGIES AND STRATEGIES

7.9.1 Overview

The fifth element of the NanoSafe framework provides an overarching perspective and strategy for conducting business in the face of both uncertainty and change. Given the dynamic and evolving nature of the nanotechnology EHS landscape, tools and strategies created to address risks identified and/or perceived today may require considerable modification in the future. Certainly, this is true of any rapidly advancing high-technology field, but as the research community has only recently begun to focus specifically on nanotechnology EHS issues, it is likely that new research findings could propel risk management approaches into unanticipated directions spanning from strict regulation to no regulation. The more probable scenario, however, is likely somewhere in between. Maintaining links to emerging information either on the Web or through conference attendance may help nanotechnology entities remain updated on the most recent findings.

7.9.2 Five grand challenges

Maynard et al. (2006) summarize five grand challenges for research on nanotechnology risk that the authors—an assemblage of international experts on the subject—believe must be met if the technology is to reach its full promise. This article is particularly valuable in that it describes key areas where nanotechnology EHS information is either currently limited or where new tools and approaches are needed (see article for a list of important target dates for meeting these challenges). The article provides insight into at least a few areas where developments may be especially critical. Thus, stakeholders may wish to pay careful attention to developments in these areas. For example, a company working with nanotechnologies and undertaking workplace monitoring for nanoscale particles may need to ask themselves periodically: "am I using the latest and most effective instruments to perform my workplace exposure measurements?"

7.9.3 Technology development partnerships

As indicated in the Maynard et al. (2006) publication, progress in nanotechnology is pushing the limits of instrumentation available to assess environmental exposure to nanomaterials. Thus, in certain instances nanotechnology facility managers may find that they require tools or strategies not addressed by existing safety technologies or approaches. In these situations, technology development partnerships between organizations requiring new tools and strategies to manage emerging nanotechnology EHS risks and developers of advanced instrumentation technologies may help marry possible solutions with specific needs. As mentioned previously in this document, there are many risks and rewards associated with such partnerships, but when managed appropriately, they may yield important advancements in developing next-generation EHS management tools.

7.9.4 Nanotechnology EHS meetings

Attending and participating in conferences, seminars, and workshops is one way to learn about and share strategies for managing nanotechnology-specific EHS risks. Over the past few years, there have been a number of key meetings that have fostered the dialogue required to catalyze partnerships among key stakeholders. Ultimately, this type of dialogue may help facilitate management practices that are both effective and attainable. Conferences and symposia on nanotechnology in general and nanotechnology EHS in particular emerge frequently. Appendix A lists several resources for obtaining information on meetings and events relevant to emerging findings in nanotechnology EHS.

7.9.5 Key organizations

Several organizations have been established to address emerging nanotechnology EHS issues. Nanobusinesses may wish to take part in one or more of these groups as a way of sharing best practices and staying abreast of new nanomaterial information. Appendix B lists several examples of these organizations.

7.9.6 Resources for emerging information

A number of newsletters and publications are available to provide the latest findings on nanotechnology EHS issues. Appendix C lists several examples of these publications.

7.10 SUMMARY AND CONCLUSIONS

Recent studies have shown that information gaps pose the greatest challenge to nanotechnology firms' identification and successful management of nanotechnology environmental, health, and safety (EHS) risks. This chapter was intended to help nanotechnology entities, particularly small businesses, to close these gaps. Key findings and conclusions for each of the five core elements of the NanoSafe approach are summarized in the sections that follow.

7.10.1 Facility management

Uncertain risks place unique demands on facilities and facility managers. Specialized equipment, monitoring strategies, updated organizational structures, and revised working practices may be required. To develop comprehensive EHS management plans, facility managers may start by consulting the "OSHA (Occupational Safety and Health Administration) Handbook for Small Businesses". The OSHA Handbook contains a useful "Hazard Assessment Checklist" that addresses a broad range of potential hazards in the workplace. While the checklist is not intended to be "nano-specific", readers will find that many elements of the list are useful for uncovering emerging nanotechnology EHS risks in the workplace. To consider checklist questions in the context of nanotechnology-specific risks, safety managers can consult references such as "Approaches to Safe Nanotechnology: An Information Exchange with NIOSH (the National Institute for Occupational Safety and Health), and the Environmental Defense-DuPont Nano Risk Framework." Such resources provide comprehensive and specific information to assist EHS personnel with making informed decisions regarding the management of emerging nanotechnology EHS risks.

More recent resources provided by ASTM International and the British Standards Institute contain useful information as well. In areas where significant questions remain, companies may wish to establish partnerships with groups such as the NIOSH Field Team, university and government laboratories, or qualified EHS consultants.

7.10.2 Product stewardship

Any product—nanotech-enabled or otherwise—poses inherent risks to consumers and the environment. Ultimately, generators of these products are responsible for testing these materials to ensure their safety to consumers. Generators are also responsible for communicating possible hazards through accurate product labels and MSDS.

Resources are available to assist entities with taking steps to identify, quantify, and manage potential risks of products to employees, consumers, and the environment. Some of these resources include the Nanoparticle Information Library maintained by NIOSH; collaborations with universities and government laboratories; the National Nanotechnology Initiative (NNI)-mandated National Nanotechnology Characterization Centers; and the International Council on Nanotechnology (ICON) Nanotech EHS Reference Database.

Entities developing and commercializing nanotechnology products should consider "Product Stewardship" approaches integrating Life Cycle Assessment. These strategies may help developers identify and manage risks from the earliest stages of product conceptualization to disposal and/or recovery/reuse.

Comprehensive stewardship efforts assist generators with characterizing their products and ultimately, determining possible hazards to consumers and the natural environment. Information obtained by the generator and/or third parties can then be conveyed to workers and consumers through product labels and MSDS. Care should be taken to avoid characterizing the properties of a given nanoscale material simply based on the properties of the same material at the bulk-scale, as any such claims should be supported by data.

According to U.S. federal agencies such as the CPSC and OSHA, generators of nanotechnology-based products are ultimately responsible for determining and communicating potential hazards associated with their products. Resources and guidelines are available to assist generators with this process.

Voluntary stewardship programs are one approach that has been taken by Federal governments in the UK and U.S. to address emerging nanotechnology EHS risks.

7.10.3 Workforce protection

Employees working in nanotechnology facilities are on the "front lines" for exposures to engineered nanomaterials. Routine health surveillance may help identify and mitigate possible health risks to employees at the earliest stages. Workplace monitoring programs may be useful for characterizing exposures. New strategies and tools for health surveillance and workplace monitoring may be needed.

The nanotechnology workforce is growing and thus opportunities for exposure to engineered nanomaterials are increasing—particularly in workplaces where these materials are generated and handled. To ensure worker safety amidst uncertain nanotechnology EHS risks, health surveillance strategies should be considered. Such strategies are effective for identifying and tracking health problems attributable to workplace operations. Since its inception, NIOSH has played an important role in the development and refinement of occupational health surveillance programs. Workplace monitoring typically is incorporated into an employee health surveillance program, as it helps quantify and track physicochemical parameters that may be linked to employee health outcomes.

Quantifying employee health before the employee begins a particular job function provides a baseline health profile to which future health screens may be compared. In this regard, the coupling of baseline and periodic health screens may help identify potential health hazards at their earliest and most correctable stages. The specific elements of employee health surveillance and/or monitoring programs for the nanotechnology workplace are evolving.

7.10.4 Environmental management

Environmental emissions (i.e., air, wastewater, solid wastes) from nanotechnology facilities may contain engineered nanomaterials. It is currently unclear what environmental risks are posed by such emissions. Proactive approaches to evaluating the properties of these emissions and managing them may be important for protecting public health and the natural environment. In the US, environmental regulatory policies are in place that apply to products and emissions containing engineered nanomaterials.

While initial safety concerns focus primarily on potential human health hazards in the workplace, it is important for nanotechnology facility operators to consider downstream implications of emerging nanotechnologies on surrounding communities and the natural environment. Facility managers may consider mapping their manufacturing processes and laboratory handling procedures to identify potential release scenarios in air emissions, process water, and solid waste streams. For organizations with sufficient resources, efforts may be taken to modify processing steps or implement control technologies to reduce or eliminate unintended environmental emissions.

Many nanotechnology organizations are unclear as to how current state and federal environmental regulations relate specifically to nanotechnology. Studies have shown that many existing environmental statutes (the Toxic Substances Control Act, the Resource Conservation and Recovery Act, the Clean Air Act, and the Federal Insecticide, Fungicide, and Rodenticide Act) apply to nanomanufacturing and associated products and/or wastes. Other environmental statutes may apply or may soon apply to nanomanufacturing. These include the Comprehensive Environmental Response, Compensation and Liability Act, the Clean Water Act, and other new approaches (Environmental Management Systems/Innovative Regulatory Approaches) customized specifically for nanomanufacturing facilities.

Comprehensive life cycle assessment approaches (i.e., cradle-to-grave) may help identify, mitigate, and communicate possible environmental hazards associated with engineered nanomaterials and nano-enabled products.

7.10.5 Emerging technologies and strategies

Given the frequent emergence of new findings and differing opinions on nanotechnology EHS issues, organizations may consider participating in forums that facilitate the exchange of "lessons learned" and new information.

A distinguished group of international experts published a paper describing "Five Grand Challenges" for nanotechnology EHS research. These challenges represent key areas where information is limited, yet especially critical. Given the significance of emerging technologies and strategies in these five areas, EHS professionals may wish to familiarize themselves with the current status, trends, and implications of research under way in these areas.

Many organizations, particularly small laboratories and start-up companies, lack the resources to effectively implement robust and forward-looking EHS management approaches. For these organizations, technology development partnerships may be an effective means for accessing expertise and equipment. Moreover, at this early stage of development, new strategies and tools developed through such partnerships may improve the safety of emerging nanotechnologies and thereby possess marketable value. These organizations may also wish to take advantage of a number of key resources and activities that can provide emerging and practical information on managing EHS issues.

ACKNOWLEDGMENTS

The Woodrow Wilson International Center for Scholars (WWICS) funded the preparation and distribution of the original report on which this chapter is based. Special thanks are owed to Deanna Lekas, Dave Rejeski, Andrew Maynard, Alex Parlini, and Evan Michelson of the Project on Emerging Nanotechnologies for their extensive assistance in compiling and editing the report. In addition, intellectual contributions of the following individuals contributed greatly to the content of this chapter: Chuck Geraci, Mark Hoover, and Vladimir Murashov of NIOSH; Linsey Marr of Virginia Tech; Nora Savage of EPA; and Jeffrey Steevens, Alan Kennedy, and Igor Linkov of US Engineer Research and Development Center (ERDC).

REFERENCES

American Bar Association, Section of Environment, Energy, and Resources, 2006. Section Nanotechnology Project Briefing Papers. ABA SEER, Washington, DC.

American Society for Testing and Materials International, 2007. Standard Guide for Handling Unbound Engineered Nanoscale Particles in Occupational Settings. Document ASTM E2535–07.

Balbus, J. 2005. Protecting Workers and the Environment: an Environmental NGO's Perspective. In: Platform Presentation at the Second International Symposium on Nanotechnology and Occupational Safety and Health. Minneapolis, MN.

Breggin, L.K., Pendergrass, J., 2007. Where Does the Nano Go? End-of-Life Regulation of Nanotechnologies. Document PEN 10, Prepared for the Project on Emerging Nanotechnologies, Woodrow Wilson International Center for Scholars.

British Standards Institute, 2007. Nanotechnologies – Part 2: Guide to Safe Handling and Disposal of Manufactured Nanomaterials. Document BSI-PD6699–2.

Civil Society-Labor Coalition, 2007. Civil Society-Labor Coalition Rejects Fundamentally Flawed DuPont-ED Proposed Framework. An Open Letter to the International Nanotechnology Community at Large.

Coalition, 2007. Principles for the Oversight of Nanotechnologies and Nanomaterials. Coalition led by the International Center for Technology Assessment.

Colvin, V., 2003. The potential environmental impacts of engineered nanomaterials. Nature Biotechnology 21, 1166–1170.

Davies, J.C., 2007. EPA and Nanotechnology: Oversight for the 21st Century. Document PEN 09, Prepared for Project on Emerging Nanotechnologies, Woodrow Wilson International Center for Scholars.

Department of Environment Food and Rural Affairs, 2006. UK Voluntary Reporting Scheme for Engineered Nanoscale Materials. DEFRA, London.

Derfus, A., Chan, W., Bhatia, S., 2004. Probing the cytotoxicity of semiconductor quantum dots. Nano Letters 4 (1), 11–18.

Environmental Defense and DuPont, 2007. Nano Risk Framework. EDF, New York.

Environmental Protection Agency, 2007a. Nanotechnology White Paper. Available at: http://es.epa.gov/ncer/nano/publications/whitepaper12022005.pdf.

Environmental Protection Agency, 2007b. Concept Paper for the Nanoscale Materials Voluntary Program under TSCA. Office of Pollution Prevention and Toxics, Environmental Protection Agency.

Environmental Protection Agency, 2007c. Supporting Statement for an Information Collection Request. Office of Pollution Prevention and Toxics, Environmental Protection Agency.

Environmental Protection Agency, 2007d. TSCA Inventory Status of Nanoscale Substances – General Approach. Office of Pollution Prevention and Toxics, Environmental Protection Agency.

European Commission, 2005. European Survey on Success Factors, Barriers and Needs for the Industrial Uptake of Nanomaterials in SMEs. EC, Brussels.

European NanoBusiness Association, 2005. The 2005 European NanoBusiness Survey. ENA, Brussels.

Garrett, D., 2005. Opinion: Stars Aligning for Nano Offerings. Small Times Magazine, 28 October.

Gerritzen, G., Huang, L., Killpack, K., Mircheva, M., Conti, J., 2006. A Survey of Current Practices in the Nanotechnology Workplace. Prepared for the International Council on Nanotechnology (ICON), 13 November.

Harber, P., Conlon, C., McCunney, R.J., 2003. Occupational medical surveillance. In: McCunney, R.J. (Ed.), A Practical Approach to Occupational and Environmental Medicine. Williams and Wilkins, Philadelphia.

Hull, M.S., Hoover M., Wilson, S., 2005. Assessing an emerging technology in practice. Presentation given at the Second International Symposium on Nanotechnology and Occupational Health, Minneapolis.

International Standards Organisation, 2007. Workplace Atmospheres—Ultrafine, Nanoparticle and Nano-structured Aerosols—Inhalation Exposure Characterization and Assessment. Document ISO/TR 27628.

Kosnett, M.J., Newman, L.S., 2007. Medical Surveillance for Nanomaterials. Presentation given at the 135th Annual Meeting of the American Public Health Association, Washington, DC.

Lecoanet, H.F., Bottero, J.Y., Wiesner, M.R., 2004. Laboratory assessment of the mobility of nanomaterials in porous media. Environmental Science and Technology 38, 5164–5169.

Lekas, D., Lifset, R., Rejeski, D., 2006. Nanotech Startup Concerns, Information Needs, and Opportunities to Proactively Address Environmental, Health, and

Social Issues: Focus on Firms in Connecticut and New York. Master's Project completed at Yale's School of Forestry and Environmental Studies.

Lindberg, J., Quinn, M., 2007. A Survey of Environmental, Health and Safety Risk Management Information Needs and Practices among Nanotechnology Firms in the Massachusetts Region. Department of Work Environment and the Lowell Center for Sustainable Production, University of Massachusetts Lowell. Prepared for the Project on Emerging Nanotechnologies.

Lux Research, 2006. The Nanotech Report™: Investment Overview and Market Research for Nanotechnology. Lux Research Inc., New York.

Lux Research, 2007. Profiting from International Nanotechnology, Report Press Release: Top Nations See Their Lead Erode. Lux Research Inc., New York.

Masciangoli, T., Zhang, W.X., 2003. Environmental technologies at the nanoscale. Environmental Science and Technology 102A, 01 March.

Maynard, A.D., Kuempel, E.D., 2005. Airborne nanostructured particles and occupational health. Journal of Nanoparticle Research 7 (6), 587–614.

Maynard, A.D., 2006. Testimony to the U.S. House of Representatives Committee on Science. Hearing on: Research on Environmental Safety Impacts of Nanotechnology: What are the Federal Agencies Doing? 21 September.

Maynard, A.D., Aitken, R.J., Butz, T., Colvin, V., Donaldson, K., Oberdörster, G., Philbert, M.A., Ryan, J., Seaton, A., Stone, V., Tinkle, S.S., Tran, L., Walker, N.J., Warheit, D.B., 2006. Safe handling of nanotechnology. Nature 444, 267–269.

Maynard, A.D., 2007. Nanotechnology: The next big thing, or much ado about nothing? Annals of Occupational Hygiene 51, 1–12.

Maynard, A.D., Aitken, R.J., 2007. Assessing exposure to airborne nanomaterials: current abilities and future requirements. Nanotoxicology 1 (1), 26–41.

Nasterlack, M., Zober, A., Oberlinner, C., 2007. Considerations on occupational medical surveillance in employees handling nanoparticles. International Archives of Occupational and Environmental Health 81 (6), 721–726.

National Institute for Occupational Safety and Health, 2006. Approaches to Safe Nanotechnology: An Information Exchange with NIOSH (Version 1.1). NIOSH, 60 pp.

National Institute for Occupational Safety and Health, 2008a. The Nanotechnology Field Research Team Update. NIOSH Publication No. 2008-120. Available at: www.cdc.gov/niosh/docs/2008-120/.

National Institute for Occupational Safety and Health, 2008b. NIOSH Nanotechnology Field Research Effort. NIOSH Publication No. 2008-121. Available at: www.cdc.gov/niosh/docs/2008-121/.

National Nanotechnology Initiative, 2007. Frequently Asked Questions. National Nanotechnology Initiative Available at: www.nano.gov/html/res/faqs.html.

Oberdörster, E., 2004. Manufactured nanomaterials (Fullerenes, C_{60}) induce oxidative stress in brain of juvenile largemouth bass. Environmental Health Perspectives 112, 1058.

Oberdörster, G., Stone, V., Donaldson, K., 2007. Toxicology of nanoparticles: a historical perspective. Nanotoxicology 1 (1), 2–25.

Occupational Health and Safety Administration, 1996. OSHA Handbook for Small Businesses. Safety Management Series. OSHA 2209. Available at: www.osha.gov/Publications/osha2209.pdf.

Occupational Health and Safety Administration, 2004. Hazard Communication in the 21st Century Workplace. OSHA. Available online at: www.osha.gov/dsg/hazcom/finalmsdsreport.html.

Project on Emerging Nanotechnologies, 2007. Putting Nanotechnology on the Map Available at: www.penmedia.org/maps/mappage.html.

Royal Society and Royal Academy of Engineering, 2004. Nanoscience and Nanotechnologies: Opportunities and Uncertainties. RS-RAE, London.

Santamaria, A., Sayes, C., 2009. Nanotox. In: Hull, M.S., Bowman, D.M. (Eds.), Nanotechnology Risk Management. Elsevier, London, pp. 3–47.

Schulte, P.A., Salamanca-Buentello, F., 2007. Ethical and Scientific Issues of Nanotechnology in the Workplace. Environmental Health Perspectives 115 (1), 5–12.

Small Times Magazine, 2007a. SOCMA's new coalition represents SME nano developers to government. Available at: www.smalltimes.com/articles/.

Small Times Magazine, 2007b. Educating Small Tech Revolutionaries. Available at: www.smalltimes.com/articles/.

Thayer, A., 2007. Nanoproliferation. Chemical and Engineering News 85 (15).

Thomas, T., Thomas, K., Sadrieh, N., Savage, N., Adair, P., Bronaugh, R., 2006. Research strategies for safety evaluation of nanomaterials, part VII: evaluating consumer exposures to nanoscale materials. Toxicological Sciences 91 (1), 14–19.

United Nations Environment Programme, 2003. Big challenge for small business: sustainability and SMEs. Available at: http://www.uneptie.org/media/review/vol26no4/IE26_4-SMEs.pdf.

Warheit, D.B., Laurence, B.R., Reed, K.L., Roach, D.H., Reynolds, G.A.M., Webb, T.R., 2004. Comparative pulmonary toxicity assessment of SWNTs in rats. Toxicological Sciences 77, 117–125.

Wittmaack, K., 2007. In search of the most relevant parameter for quantifying lung inflammatory response to nanoparticle exposure: particle number, surface area, or what? Environmental Health Perspectives 115, 187–194.

Woodrow Wilson International Center for Scholars and European Commission, 2007. Nanotechnology and Life Cycle Assessment: A Systems Approach to Nanotechnology and the Environment. Available at: www.nanotechproject.org/111/32007-life-cycle-assessment-essential-to-nanotech-commercial-development.

APPENDIX A FOR NANOTECHNOLOGY RISK MANAGEMENT AND SMALL BUSINESS: A CASE STUDY ON THE NANOSAFE FRAMEWORK

Matthew S. Hull

NANOTECHNOLOGY EHS MEETINGS

Attending and participating in conferences, seminars, and workshops is one way to learn about and share strategies for managing nanotechnology-specific EHS risks. Over the past few years, there have been a number of key meetings that have fostered the dialogue required to catalyze partnerships among key stakeholders. Ultimately, this type of dialogue may help facilitate management practices that are both effective and attainable. Conferences and symposia on nanotechnology in general and nanotechnology EHS in particular emerge frequently. The sections that follow summarize examples of resources that typically provide the latest information on meetings and events that may be of interest to small businesses with interests in nanotechnology.

a. Nanowerk: Nanotechnology Conferences and Events

- **Link:** www.nanowerk.com/phpscripts/n_events.php
- **About:** This resource provides a hyper-linked database of upcoming nanotechnology conferences and symposia. The database is searchable by month and city.

b. ICON Events Page

- **Link:** http://icon.rice.edu/eventsother.cfm
- **About:** This resource offers a database of current and archived events with an emphasis on nanotechnology EHS. The database is searchable by date. Additional coverage of events specific to the International Council on Nanotechnology is provided.

c. The Project on Emerging Nanotechnologies Events Page

- **Link:** www.nanotechproject.org/events/
- **About:** This resource provides links to upcoming PEN events and major international activities with a strong emphasis on EHS.

APPENDIX B FOR NANOTECHNOLOGY RISK MANAGEMENT AND SMALL BUSINESS: A CASE STUDY ON THE NANOSAFE FRAMEWORK

Matthew S. Hull

KEY ORGANIZATIONS

Several organizations have been established to address emerging nanotechnology EHS issues. Businesses with interests in nanotechnology may wish to take part in one or more of these groups, as a way of sharing best practices and staying abreast of new nanomaterial information. A few examples of these organizations are provided below:

a. SOCMA (Synthetic Organic Chemical Manufacturers Association)

- **Link:** www.socma.com
- **About:** The Synthetic Organic Chemical Manufacturers Association is a preeminent trade organization that caters to industrial scale manufacturers. SOCMA has nearly 275 members across several industries that include small specialty suppliers to large multinational corporations. The organization serves to promote innovative, yet safe and environmentally responsible chemical production methodologies. Recently, SOCMA formed a new coalition for start-ups and small businesses developing and manufacturing nanoscale materials.

b. ANSI (American National Standards Institute)

- **Link:** www.ansi.org
- **About:** The American National Standards Institute serves as the collective governing body with regard to product or service standardization. The institute is responsible for the oversight, development, and implementation of thousands of guidelines and accepted norms across countless businesses ranging from electronic devices, to energy delivery systems, to dairy and livestock products. ANSI has a Nanotechnology Standards Steering Panel, as well as the U.S. Technical Advisory Committee (TAG) for participation in the development of international standards at the level of the International Organization for Standardization (ISO).

c. ASTM International

- **Link:** www.astm.org
- **About:** ASTM International (formerly known as the American Society for Testing and Materials) is a voluntary standards development organization that assists in the guidance and quality of product development and integration. The organization functions on a global scale and addresses the standardization needs of the global economy. ASTM technical committee E56 addresses nanotechnology issues.

d. BSI (British Standards Institute)

- **Link:** www.bsigroup.com/britishstandards
- **About:** BSI British Standards is the UK's National Standards Body, recognized globally for its independence, integrity, and innovation in the production of standards and information products that promote and share best practice. BSI works with businesses, consumers, and government to represent UK interests and to make sure that British, European, and international standards are useful, relevant, and authoritative.

e. ILSI (International Life Sciences Institute)

- **Link:** www.ilsi.org
- **About:** The International Life Sciences Institute serves as a global forum in which issues pertaining to food safety, consumer health, and bodily nutrition are addressed by individuals from the academic, government, and scientific communities. The ILSI mission is to improve the understanding of the aforementioned issues by fostering area-specific programs and building collective information resources on these issues.

f. ISO (International Organization for Standardization)

- **Link:** www.iso.org
- **About:** The International Organization for Standardization is a global standard-setting body that is comprised of nearly 198 countries, and establishes industrial and commercial standards. These standards are used in manufacturing, products, and services to ensure efficiency, safety, and quality. Additionally, ISO standards serve to ensure consumer and environmental product safety. ISO Technical Committee 229 addresses issues for nanotechnologies.

g. NanoBusiness Alliance

- **Link:** www.nanobusiness.org
- **About:** The NanoBusiness Alliance is the industry association for the emerging nanotechnology industry. Through its extensive network of leading start-ups, Fortune 500 companies, research institutions, NGOs, and public–private partnerships, the Alliance shapes nanotechnology policy and helps accelerate the commercialization of nanotechnology innovations. The NanoBusiness Alliance has offices in New York, Chicago, Washington, DC, and Connecticut.

APPENDIX C FOR NANOTECHNOLOGY RISK MANAGEMENT AND SMALL BUSINESS: A CASE STUDY ON THE NANOSAFE FRAMEWORK

Matthew S. Hull

RESOURCES FOR EMERGING INFORMATION

A number of newsletters and publications are available to provide the latest findings on nanotechnology EHS issues. A few examples of these publications are provided below:

a. NIOSH Safety and Health Topic: Nanotechnology

- **Link:** www.cdc.gov/niosh/topics/nanotech/
- **About:** NIOSH is the leading federal agency conducting research and providing guidance on the occupational safety and health implications and applications of nanotechnology. This research focuses NIOSH's scientific expertise, and its efforts, on answering the questions that are essential to understanding these implications and applications. The Website includes details of the NIOSH nanotechnology research program strategy and accomplishments, the Nanoparticle Information Library, and the Web-based Approaches to Safe Nanotechnology: An Information Exchange with NIOSH.

b. Woodrow Wilson International Center for Scholars, Project on Emerging Nanotechnologies

- **Link:** www.nanotechproject.org
- **About:** The Project on Emerging Nanotechnologies, an initiative of the Woodrow Wilson International Center for Scholars and The Pew Charitable Trusts, collaborates with researchers, government, industry, NGOs, policymakers, and others to look long term, to identify gaps in knowledge and regulatory processes, and to develop strategies for closing them. The Project provides independent, objective knowledge, and analysis that can inform critical decisions affecting the development and commercialization of nanotechnologies.

c. International Council on Nanotechnology (ICON)

- **Link:** icon.rice.edu
- **About:** ICON is an international, multi-stakeholder organization whose mission is to develop and communicate information regarding potential environmental and health risks of nanotechnology, thereby fostering risk reduction while maximizing societal benefit. ICON activities include an online journal, an EHS bibliography, reports and user surveys, and also a new GoodWiki pilot initiative to share ideas about good handling practices for nanotechnologies.

d. Nanowerk

- **Link:** www.nanowerk.com
- **About:** Nanowerk.com is a nanotechnology and nanosciences portal developed and maintained by Honolulu-based Nanowerk LLC.

e. SAFENANO

- **Link:** www.safenano.org
- **About:** The Safenano Initiative is a venture by the Institute of Occupational Medicine (IOM). The initiative was designed to help industrial and academic communities to quantify and control the risks to their workforce, as well as to consumers, to the general population and to the environment, through both information provision and consultancy services.

f. NANOSAFE2

- **Link:** www.nanosafe.org
- **About:** The overall aim of NANOSAFE2 is to develop risk assessment and management for secure industrial production of nanoparticles.

g. NanoSafe Australia

- **Link:** www.rmit.com.au/NANOSAFE
- **About:** The NanoSafe Australia network is a group of Australian toxicologists and risk assessors, who have formed a research network to address the issues concerning the occupational and environmental health and safety of nanomaterials.

h. NanoRegNews

- **Link:** www.nanoregnews.com
- **About:** NanoReg is a professional services firm specializing in the regulation of the products of nanotechnology. The NanoReg Report is published by NanoReg to provide current information on government regulations and environmental, health, and safety issues related to the production and use of nanoscale materials throughout the nanotechnology value chain.

i. Nanotechwire

- **Link:** www.nanotechwire.com
- **About:** Nanotechwire provides nanotechnology news from various global sources.

j. Nanotechnology Law Report

- **Link:** www.nanolawreport.com
- **About:** Nanotechnology Law Report is produced by Porter Wright Morris & Arthur LLP's nanotechnology practice group. The blog is dedicated to providing up-to-date information and commentary on the intersection of nanotechnology and the law.

k. Nanoforum

- **Link:** www.nanoforum.org
- **About:** Nanoforum is a pan-European nanotechnology network funded by the European Union (EU) under the Fifth Framework Programme (FP5) to provide information on European nanotechnology efforts and support to the European nanotechnology community. On the Nanoforum Website, all users (whether they are members of the public, industry, R&D, government, or business communities) can freely access and search a comprehensive database of European nanoscience and nanotechnology (N&N) organizations, and find out the latest on news, events, and other relevant information (including education tools, further training, jobs, and other EU projects). In addition, Nanoforum publishes its own specially commissioned reports on nanotechnology and key market sectors, the economical and societal impacts of nanotechnology, as well as organizing events throughout the EU to inform, network, and support European expertise.

l. InterNano

- **Link:** www.internano.org
- **About:** InterNano is an open-source online information clearing house for the nanomanufacturing research and development (R&D) community in the United States. It is an initiative of the National Nanomanufacturing Network (NNN). InterNano is supported by the Center for Hierarchical Manufacturing through a grant from the National Science Foundation. It is designed to provide the nanomanufacturing community with an array of tools and collections relevant to its work and to the development of viable nanomanufacturing applications, including descriptions of nanomanufacturing processes and features for describing EHS controls and good practices.

CHAPTER 8

A Case Study of a Nanoscale-Research Facility Safety through Design and Operation

John R. Weaver

CONTENTS

This chapter presents a philosophy and methodology for designing safety into nanotechnology facilities, using Birck Nanotechnology Center (BNC) at Purdue University as a case study. While the actual designs described are specific to the BNC, they can be easily translated into a wide variety of nanotechnology facilities. The principles employed are universal and therefore directly applicable to the design of these facilities.

When considering nanotechnology safety, the initial thoughts center on dealing with the nanomaterials used or fabricated in the facility. In actuality, the primary concerns in this type of facility are the "raw materials" used in the processes. These materials range from pyrophoric, detonable gases to hazardous biological materials. This chapter provides both a thought process and specific guidance on methods for dealing with this variety of hazard.

In reviewing this chapter, the reader will see a particular application of designing a facility to enable safe practices during operation. By using this approach, operational controls can be eased and a far safer environment achieved.

8.1 THE BIRCK NANOTECHNOLOGY CENTER FACILITY

The Birck Nanotechnology Center is a large university research facility located in Discovery Park on the campus of Purdue University in West Lafayette, Indiana. The overall building is 286,000 assignable square feet and was specifically designed for interdisciplinary collaborative research in nanotechnology, with cleanroom and laboratory areas purposely designed to support the specialized equipment necessary for this type of research. Planning for the facility began in 2001 and the facility was considered fully

Nanotechnology Environmental Health and Safety

operational in 2006. Both building and operational systems have been modified during the initial years of building operation.

Safety was a major consideration from the early design concepts of the building. In addition to occupant-safety considerations, this is a public facility, which school groups and community neighbors tour on a regular basis. Additionally, the building is located immediately adjacent to a married-student housing complex and two childcare facilities (Figure 8.1).

Unlike traditional department-owned facilities—generally containing a mixture of classrooms and laboratories—this facility operates across department lines, housing researchers from 35 schools and departments, from Forestry to Electrical and Computer Engineering. There are no classroom facilities in the building.

Users of the facility fall into two general classes, residents and non-residents. There are approximately 200 resident users of the facility—students and post-docs who maintain an office in the building. In addition, there are approximately 50 non-resident users who perform research in the building on an intermittent basis. Additionally, approximately 50 faculty members have either primary (single-person) or secondary (shared) offices in the building. The varied backgrounds of these faculty and students create a special challenge from an environmental health and safety (EH&S) standpoint. The entire operation is supported by an engineering staff of 25 people as well as 11 business office and secretarial staff.

Safety training was developed to support the variety of people working in the facility as well as those who come into the facility intermittently.

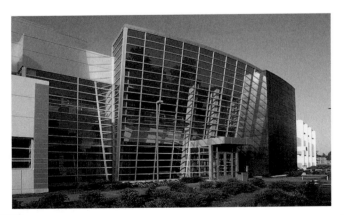

FIGURE 8.1 *The Birck Nanotechnology Center is located in Discovery Park on the campus of Purdue University. While part of the main campus, facilities in Discovery Park are all interdisciplinary rather than owned by individual departments.*

Residents of the facility who do not use the cleanroom and laboratory facilities—theoretical researchers, secretaries, business office personnel, and similar groups—receive basic training regarding the materials in use in the facility, the alarm systems, and emergency response procedures. People using the laboratories and/or cleanroom—residents and non-residents—receive more intense training that is customized to the areas of the facility they will be using. As an example, a training matrix was developed for laboratory users. The matrix indicates the laboratory number on one axis and the required training on the other axis. An "x" indicates that this training is required before the user is allowed access to that laboratory. If a laser of Class 3B or above is present in the laboratory, laser training is required. If the laboratory has a fume hood—acid or solvent—fume hood training is required. Once the required training has been completed, the User ID card is activated to allow them into the laboratory.

Specialized training was also developed for maintenance personnel working in the facility and emergency responders including fire, police, emergency medical technicians (EMTs), and outside contractors. Included in all training programs is a "sunset clause" indicating the expiration of training (and therefore access) and refresher courses. Additionally, an annual all-user safety and operations meeting is held—attendance is mandatory.

The facility consists of two distinct areas. The office and laboratory area is a "B" rated occupancy containing offices, conference rooms, and laboratories. The laboratories are designed specifically for the type of research that is being supported—biological laboratories (BSL-1 and BSL-2+),[1] deposition/epitaxy laboratories, laser/nanophotonics laboratories, surface-analysis laboratories, electron-microscopy laboratories, etc.

The 25,000-square-foot BNC cleanroom, the Scifres Nanofabrication Laboratory, consists of a nanofabrication cleanroom joined to a 2500-square-foot pharmaceutical-grade cleanroom. Pass-through units allow materials to be passed between the cleanrooms without breaking cleanliness protocol. Personnel, however, must exit one cleanroom and re-gown in the appropriate cleanroom garments before entering the other cleanroom.[2] This portion of the facility is an "H" rated occupancy.

While the "B" occupancy rating reduces the quantity of chemicals that can be present in the laboratory areas, it is a much less restrictive rating than

---

[1] Biosafety levels are defined by the Center for Disease Control and Prevention (CDC) in the handbook Biosafety in Microbiological and Biomedical Laboratories (BMBL). See: www.cdc.gov.

[2] The fabrication cleanroom uses an ISO 3 compatible GORE-TEX garment system while the biocleanroom uses a disposable garment system.

the "H" rating of the cleanroom. This significantly reduces design and construction costs, and the resultant reduction in chemicals enhances the safety of the laboratory areas.

A significant complexity related to EHS is the diversity of the research. While many nanotechnology facilities concentrate on two or three major thrust areas, the BNC has eight (Figure 8.2).

Within these thrust areas are a wide variety of research activities. Research in nanoelectronics includes the development of transparent integrated circuits and transistors fabricated on graphene layers. Nanoelectromechanical systems (NEMS) research ranges from implantable biomedical devices to sensors that are located within jet engines to measure bearing temperatures. Nanophotonics work includes the development of metamaterials—materials not found in nature—that have negative refractive indexes, actually causing objects to become invisible. Fundamental research is also underway to understand deposition and growth processes, allowing changes to those processes and the novel materials they produce.

The 21,000 square feet of BNC laboratories are arranged as laboratory modules on an 11-foot × 22-foot grid, with the facility containing 88 modules in four wings. Each laboratory consists of one or more modules, with the largest laboratory being a seven-module laboratory. Utilities are run along the outside walls of the laboratories and multiple-module laboratories have overhead service carriers on 11-foot centers. Each wing contains two rows of laboratories with an intervening service galley. These service galleys contain all utilities needed in the laboratories as well as vacuum pumps, chillers, and other equipment that would cause vibration, electromagnetic interference (EMI), or acoustic noise in the laboratory (Figure 8.3).

BNC Major Thrust Areas
Nanoelectronics and microelectronics
Nanofabrication of NEMS and MEMS devices
Nanophotonics
Materials growth and deposition
Bio-nanotechnology
Nanoscale metrology
Electronic characterization
Theory and computation

FIGURE 8.2 *The diversity of research in the BNC results in special challenges to EH&S.*

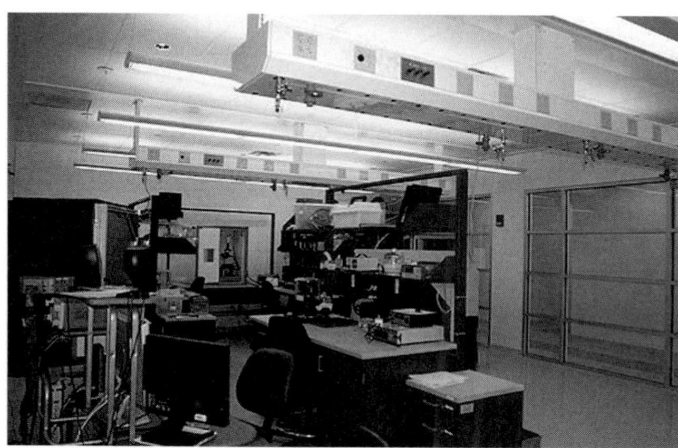

FIGURE 8.3 *A three-module laboratory in the Birck Nanotechnology Center. The multiple-module design fosters multiple users on similar projects, thus enhancing the potential of collaborative research.*

The cleanroom has three levels: a fifteen-foot-tall subfab that is separated from the airflow path, the cleanroom level, and an air-handling deck housing the makeup and recirculation air handlers (Figure 8.4).

The subfab is a utility distribution and cleanroom support level that is located immediately beneath the cleanroom. The use of a subfab allows the installation of contamination-producing support equipment, such as vacuum pumps and chillers, outside of the cleanroom airflow path, and provides a location for the distribution of inert gases. A major advantage in the use of a subfab is the ease of modification of utilities. Changes can be made in utility distribution systems in the subfab, and the new utility runs can penetrate the cleanroom floor to the area needed. This reduces the cost of making utility modifications and increases the flexibility of the facility (Figure 8.5).

From an EH&S perspective, the subfab has a very high intrinsic value. This restricted space is off-limits to all but the most highly trained personnel in the facility—the engineering staff and the maintenance staff—thus providing a physical barrier to prevent "adjustments" by less-trained personnel.

The cleanroom level has above-the-ceiling air-distribution boxes, an ULPA-filtered ceiling and a perforated raised floor that stands two feet above the concrete waffle slab. ULPA (Ultra Low Penetration Air) filters provide 99.999 percent efficiency on 100 nm particles, as compared to HEPA (High Efficiency Particle Air) filters which provide 99.97 percent efficiency on 180 nm particles. ULPA filters are generally used in facilities with cleanliness levels below ISO Class 4 (formerly Class 10).

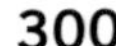

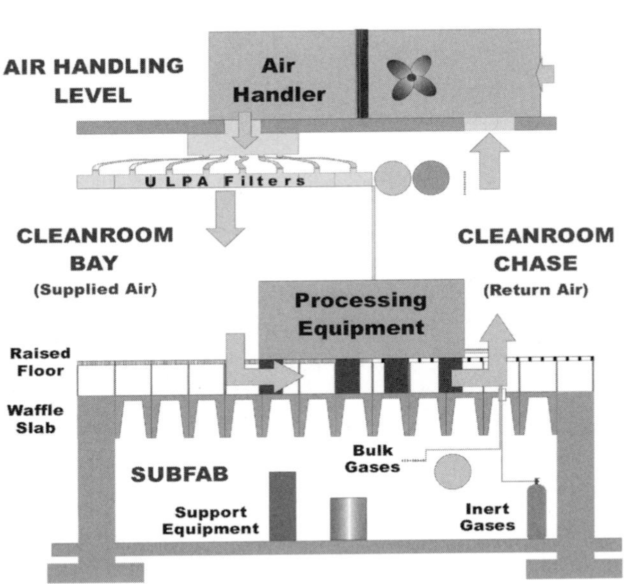

FIGURE 8.4 *Section view of the cleanroom. The subfab is at grade, with the cleanroom on the second floor and the air-handling deck on the third floor.*

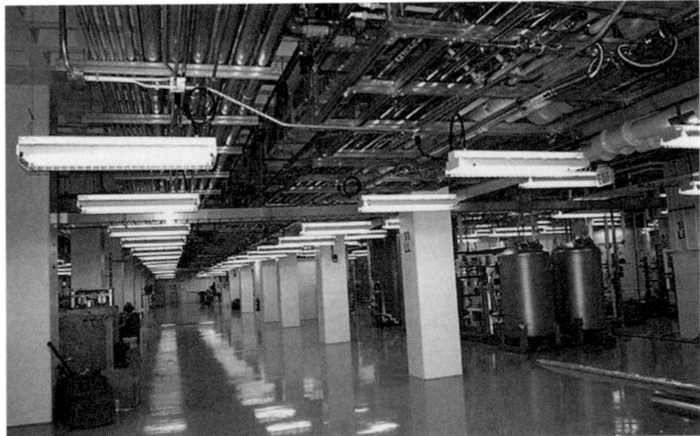

FIGURE 8.5 *The subfab is located immediately below the BNC cleanroom, and provides a location for support equipment and utility distribution. This area is not part of the cleanroom airflow stream.*

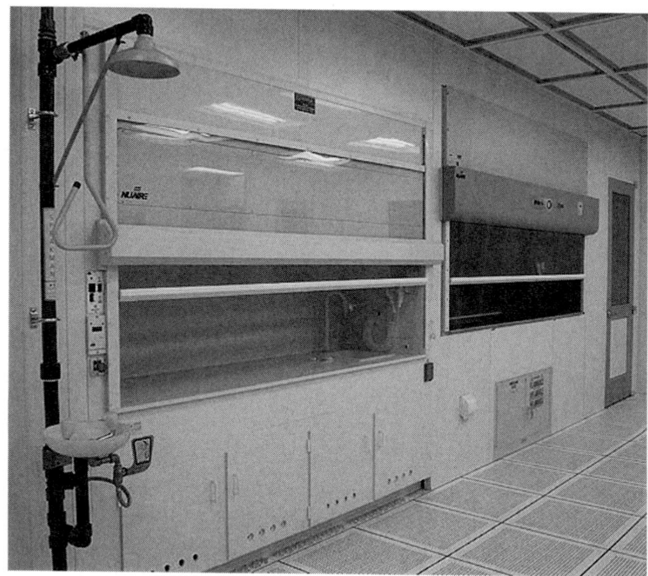

FIGURE 8.6 *Acid and solvent fume hoods bulkhead mounted in the BNC cleanroom. Bulkhead mounting equipment allows the separation of the operational side of the equipment (shown) from the maintenance side of the equipment, accessible through the cleanroom chase.*

The interior of the cleanroom utilizes a bay-chase design, with air supplied in the ceiling of the bays and returned through the chases. Equipment is bulkhead mounted through the chase wall, with the operational side of the equipment accessible to the cleanroom and the maintenance side of the equipment accessible from the chase (Figure 8.6).

Forty-five percent of the cleanroom operates at ISO Class 3 (formerly known as Class 1), forty percent at ISO Class 4, and fifteen percent at ISO Class 5. The vibration level in the cleanroom is within NIST A levels, extremely quiet for a second-floor cleanroom.

8.2 SAFETY CONSIDERATIONS

As with any large, multi-floor facility, the BNC has general safety concerns related to electrical hazards, fall protection, confined-space entry, and similar hazards. While all of these hazards were addressed in the design of the facility, only the specialized hazards related to a high-technology research facility will be addressed in this chapter. For example, the design of tie-off points throughout the facility was critical for the safe repair of equipment, but this is a standard consideration in all facilities and so is not included here.

Operational factors in the Birck Nanotechnology Center provide significant challenges in terms of the safety of those working in the facility. Most significantly, there is a wide range of hazardous materials used in the facility. Hazardous chemicals in gaseous, liquid, and solid forms range from highly toxic materials to pyrophoric and detonable gases. Active biological species in the BSL-2+ category, such as anthrax and *Escherichia coli* (e-coli), are also in use. Additionally, nanoscale materials—many with indeterminate toxicity levels—are generated and used in the facility. These include carbon nanotubes and nanowires created by physical vapor deposition and graphene films created by epitaxial deposition. Physical hazards are also a major consideration. Optical systems with Class 3B and Class 4 lasers are present in several areas of the facility. Electron microscopes, analytical equipment, and electrical-testing equipment use very high voltages and sometimes high currents. Test equipment using high magnetic and electrical fields, such as a Hall-effect measurement system using an 8 T magnet, provides hazards to personnel with pacemakers and/or other sensitive devices. Finally, the use of liquid helium and liquid nitrogen presents thermal hazards to people working in the vicinity of those systems.

Complicating the use of these materials and physical hazards is the diversity of technical backgrounds of the researchers. The strength of the facility is in its collaborative character, but this places biologists in roles where they are working with semiconductor gases and electrical engineers using BSL-2+ agents. The depth of knowledge regarding the handling of these diverse materials is often lacking.

Another complicating factor is the round-the-clock operation of the facility. Graduate students often "go nocturnal"—a significant amount of research in the facility is performed between midnight and 5:00 AM. The cultural diversity of the researchers is also a factor in the implementation of safety programs. English is a second language to many researchers, and a trainer—generally a member of the engineering staff—may be unsure whether a new researcher has fully understood the material presented. Additionally, different cultures have varied attitudes toward obeying rules and reporting mistakes or accidents. Finally, the very creativity that makes graduate students excel often falls at odds with following rules.

8.3 DESIGNING IN SAFETY

Safety issues are best addressed during the design phase of a project. By designing safety systems into the facility and by considering the safety aspects of all the design considerations, engineering controls can be used to ensure safety rather than relying on operational controls. For example, fixed barriers are designed into systems rather than requiring the use of personal protective equipment. Another example would be the use of card-access security systems to restrict access to potentially hazardous locations.

Implementing these controls during the design phase of a building, a process or a product is the key. Early implementation allows for the use of more effective control schemes, as the designer is not constrained by existing architecture, machinery, or processes. Additionally, it is much more cost effective to implement controls early in the design cycle than to retrofit existing systems or place construction change orders. The National Institute for Occupational Safety and Health (NIOSH) Prevention through Design (PtD) initiative is based on these principles. Though the PtD initiative was developed well after the design of the BNC, the BNC is considered a prime example of the PtD concept.

A one-sentence summary of the design goal of the BNC is to "Make it easier to do it the safe way!" If building, process, and product designs comprehend safety principles in their early-design stages, controls can be built in that lead people to safe operation. Conversely, if doing something the safe way is awkward and/or difficult, there will always be a temptation to perform the task in a less-safe manner (Figure 8.7).

The importance of incorporating safety in the design of a facility must be supported through manpower. At the BNC, a senior safety engineer was assigned to the user team to assist in this process. A certified industrial hygienist and highly experienced safety professional was assigned at the early-design stages and became the facility Safety Manager when operations commenced. It was also the responsibility of the BNC Engineering Staff to ensure that the best safety practices were designed into the facility. The Facility Manager was involved from the early planning stages and was

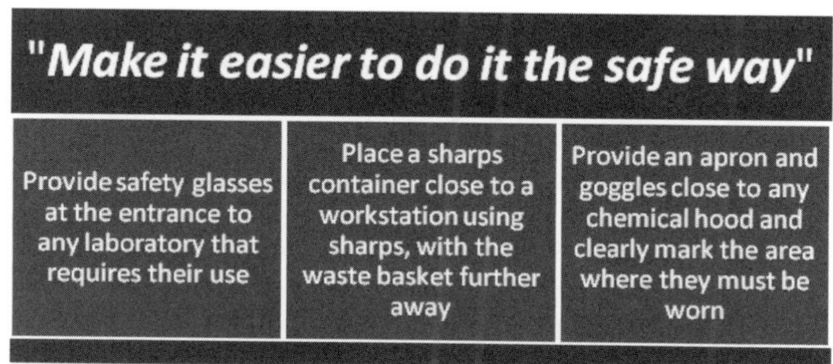

"Make it easier to do it the safe way"
Provide safety glasses at the entrance to any laboratory that requires their use
Place a sharps container close to a workstation using sharps, with the waste basket further away
Provide an apron and goggles close to any chemical hood and clearly mark the area where they must be worn

FIGURE 8.7 *The principles of Prevention through Design used in the design of the BNC can be summed up by the phrase "Make it easier to do it the safe way."*

heavily involved throughout the design process. He had extensive safety experience as well as cleanroom design and operational experience, and was a principal member of the National Fire Protection Association (NFPA) 318 Committee—Fire Standard for Cleanroom Manufacturing Facilities. Finally, faculty who would be working in the facility provided strong technical support.

The implementation of the BNC design follows the following principles. First, the designers must identify safety hazard "potentials" in the early planning stages of the facility. A thorough hazard assessment of facilities, processes, raw materials, finished products, and byproducts must be completed and updated as more information is obtained. The hazard assessment is a living document that is constantly updated during the design process.

An example of a hazard assessment would be the installation of a Class 3B laser for a laser-assisted deposition system. The laser uses fluorine gas which must be changed periodically, it uses high-voltage power supplies for its operation, and it produces hazardous light levels when the system is open for maintenance. Once identified, each of these hazard potentials was addressed during the facility design. The fluorine gas hazard was mitigated using concentric tubing, exhausted enclosures, and monitoring. The voltage hazards were addressed using appropriate lockout/tagout points designed into the laboratory, and the laser hazards were mitigated by door-lock controls, lockout/tagout points, and cubbies for laser glasses at the laboratory entrances.

The hazard identification process involves the use of cross-disciplinary teams working together. Faculty, staff, and maintenance personnel provide the bulk of the input, but other disciplines, such as housekeeping, can also provide valuable insight. The teams generally are led by a safety professional who works to extract information from the various groups and coalesce it into a usable format.

Each potential then becomes an opportunity to design engineering controls to mitigate the risk. Depending on the complexity of the design solution, costs ranged from nominal to relatively expensive systems, such as the door interlocks that block the laser when a door is opened. It is difficult to generalize on the cost of the engineering controls because of this wide variation.

The use of procedural controls should be avoided and considered as the "last resort" if appropriate engineering controls cannot be designed into the facility, process, or product. An example of the use of personal protective equipment (PPE) in lieu of engineering controls would be the use of a fume hood. While the hood has appropriate engineering controls such as a monitored exhaust flow and a physical barrier (the sash), the separation of the user from the chemicals is incomplete. The sash must be raised to allow the pouring of chemicals into a beaker and the user must reach into the hood to work with the samples being reacted. Therefore, the engineering controls do not provide adequate protection to the user. PPE, consisting in this case of goggles, gloves, and a coat-apron, is required.

Like the hazard assessment, these engineering controls are updated as new information becomes available and as the design process continues. This new information may be as a result of research reported in journals and at conferences or may be as a result of changes in codes and best practices. It is the role of the technical staff—safety and process—to keep up with these changes. As the design process continues, new information may be gleaned from the basis of design that the A&E constantly updates and from the design details that emerge from the developing documentation. It is the role of the technical staff and safety staff to review all of these information sources and update the hazard assessment accordingly. Changes in the hazard assessment will always foster a review of the control plan.

These principles were used throughout the design process. A thorough hazard analysis was completed and hazard potentials were continuously reviewed. Since the highest potentials were in the fabrication portions of the facility, the cleanroom facility was designed utilizing the best practices used in the design of a semiconductor manufacturing facility. In addition to following applicable building codes, non-mandatory codes were applied where appropriate. For example, NFPA 318 Standard for the Protection of Semiconductor Manufacturing Facilities was applied to the cleanroom areas of the BNC. Even though that code is not mandatory for research facilities, NFPA 318 provides the best practices for dealing with the types of materials that would be used in the facility. For this reason, there was full support for the implementation of these practices in the building design process. Best practices were also gleaned from Semiconductor Equipment and Materials International (SEMI), the Santa Clara Toxic Gas Model Ordinance, and documents from the Semiconductor Environmental Safety and Health Association (SESHA).

Best practices from the pharmaceutical industry were applied in the design of the biological areas, such as the separation of bacterial laboratories from cell-culture laboratories. Handwashing stations—completely hands-free—were built into the entrance and exit areas of the BSL-2+ laboratories. Ultraviolet (UV) sanitization lights were incorporated into the room design, with appropriate door interlocks and window coverings. Full-exhaust biosafety cabinets were accommodated for all biohazard work.

A world-renowned pharmaceutical company reviewed designs and offered methods of incorporating safe practices for the biocleanroom facility.

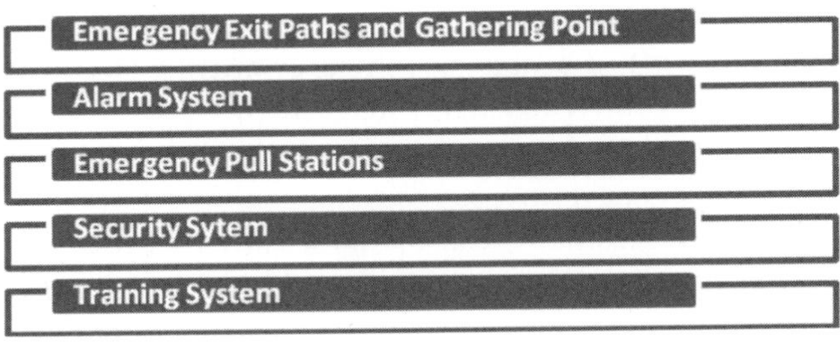

FIGURE 8.8 *Five Major Areas of Building Control.*

The biological laboratories made use of Center for Disease Control and Prevention (CDC) standards, such as the BMBL mentioned previously, and designed-in engineering controls to minimize hazards.

At the time, the National Institute for Occupational Safety and Health (NIOSH) guide to the use of nanoscale materials was not published; therefore it was not available as a resource. Today, that would be a prime document to use during the facility design process.

Finally, the facility was designed in full compliance with Purdue University safety and environmental practices. A new program of certification[3] of laboratory facilities at Purdue had just been initiated by the internal Purdue EH&S organization, Radiological and Environmental Management (REM), and the principles of this program were designed into the BNC.

Five major areas of overall building controls were considered. The design of emergency exit paths to quickly and easily route people away from hazardous areas during an evacuation was integrated into the building design and coupled with a plan to allow the gathering of evacuated personnel in a protected, indoor location. All plans were considered based on worst-case scenarios, such as the evacuation of personnel at 3:00 AM during a bitter Indiana winter. Also designed into the system was a swipe-in/swipe-out card access system for the cleanroom to allow emergency responders to gauge whether any personnel were left in the cleanroom following an evacuation—a potential rescue situation (Figure 8.8).

Alarm systems were designed to ensure that there was a clear understanding of what actions are required for given situations. A voice-over announcement system was implemented that contains various context-sensitive prerecorded messages that tell personnel—in short, simple terms—what to do in a given situation. For example, a hazardous gas alarm

[3] This program was originally called "indemnification," with the name later changed to "certification." The program evaluates engineering and procedural controls and audits the compliance to stated policies. Once achieved, an annual recertification is required.

initiates the evacuation horns and strobes and is accompanied by the message: "The toxic gas monitoring system has detected a leak. Please evacuate the building immediately."

The voice-over message moves the reaction to an emergency away from the memory of the person in the facility when the alarm occurs. This attempts to prevent situations where people flee outside the building when the tornado alarm sounds—leaving them in a far more vulnerable condition. In the BNC, the tornado alarm is accompanied by voice-over text that instructs occupants to seek appropriate shelter areas within the facility. Note that it is important to consider the natural disaster potentials in the area of the facility being constructed. With the BNC being located in the Midwest, tornados are a significant problem while earthquakes are not. The building emergency plans must comprehend these local factors.

Emergencies are often discovered by personnel working in the facility, not by the trained responders. To minimize hazards and shorten reaction time to emergency situations, emergency evacuation pull stations are located throughout the facility. Triggering these alarms shuts down hazardous gas inputs into the building and announces an evacuation.

A key element is the building security system. As was previously mentioned, the BNC is a public building on a major university campus. It has three daycare facilities in proximity to the building and the facility is located amidst a housing complex. Additionally, tour groups of kindergarten to grade 12 (K-12) classes and outside community groups are frequently in the building. These situations make the development of a building security system with appropriate access controls vital in maintaining a safe environment in the facility.

Maintaining the safety of these groups is twofold. First, the security system must be designed to keep these groups in the public areas of the facility, away from the research work. Second, the design of the alarm system gives specific direction as to what to do in the event that the alarm sounds. This, coupled with building-orientation training for tour guides, promotes a safe evacuation of the facility should the need arise.

A careful review of potentially hazardous areas of the building was integrated with a review of personnel who needed access to non-public areas of the building. This evolved into a set of access levels based on access needs and training requirements. A combination of card-access levels and issuance of keys was used to allow and deny access, as appropriate.

Programming of the card access system for access to the cleanroom and laboratories also allowed for denial of access on expiration of training or in disciplinary situations. A collection of preset conditions allows for appropriate responses to emergencies, such as requiring card-access to the building during an external campus violence incident, such as the Virginia Tech shootings. During emergency evacuations, access to external building doors is via key access only—card access is disabled. At the same time, all interior card-access doors unlock to provide easy access by emergency personnel. Access to the public areas of the facility is also limited to normal business hours—when these areas are generally occupied by BNC personnel.

The security system for the facility is a combination of card-access levels and the issuance of keys. The public areas of the building are open during normal business hours, 7:00 AM to 6:00 PM. During these hours, people may enter the atrium areas, the cleanroom viewing aisle, the conference rooms, and the rest rooms. Outside of these hours, access to these areas is limited to those who have gone through any level of BNC training. Once the training has been received, the individual's BNC identification card is activated, allowing access through three sets of outside entrance doors. Offices can be reached through these public areas and are individually locked. They are not part of the card-access system, so individual keys are issued for office access.

The second level of access is the laboratories and cleanroom, dependent on the training matrix described previously. Once the entrance requirements have been met, the BNC identification card is activated for the appropriate area. The cleanroom is a scan-in/scan-out system such that the cleanroom population is always known. The laboratories are scan-in only.

The third level of access is "all doors, all the time." This is granted only to engineering staff and maintenance staff and allows access to restricted areas such as the subfab. It also grants access to all laboratories in the facility.

Key access to exterior building doors is granted to the engineering staff and select other individuals who need this level of access. This allows entry to the building in all conditions, including a power outage or emergency situation. It also allows access to all exterior doors, not just those with card-access capability.

There are two levels of key-access to interior doors. One master key allows access to all interior doors except offices, the other includes office access. The former is issued to all technical staff members, the Director and the Managing Director. The latter is only issued to the Facility Manager, the Building Manager, and the Emergency Response Team.

Closely coupled with the security system is the training system. All building occupants must attend training sessions, the extent of which depends on the desired access levels. Office-only residents—secretarial, business-office, computational personnel, and non-laboratory faculty—receive a short-training course covering building emergency response. Completion of this training program allows the issuance of an office key and after-hours public-area access. Faculty members who are resident in the facility and supervise students who work in the laboratories or cleanroom receive a more extensive level of training. Students, post-docs, and faculty who actually work in the laboratories and cleanroom receive significantly more extensive training. Specialty programs for emergency responders (fire department, EMTs, police), housekeeping personnel, maintenance personnel, engineering staff, and similar groups have also been developed and are presented as needed to those groups. In each case, access is dependent on the completion of the training program.

To develop the training plan for the BNC, a list of categories of people to be trained was developed, beginning with those who will simply reside in the facility through those who will be designing equipment installations. Once this exhaustive list was developed, the various groups were analyzed for similarity of need in an attempt to minimize the number of courses to be developed and taught. In addition, a hierarchy of courses was developed to prevent duplication of material presented to any individual group. This manifested itself in a set of prerequisites for the more in-depth courses. Ultimately, this led to several independent training courses for specialized groups and a set of progressive courses for user groups. The users take whichever courses in the matrix are appropriate to their usage of the facility (Figure 8.9).

In addition to those shown above, specialty laboratory training would be required depending on the laboratory. These specialty courses would include laser safety, X-ray safety and biosafety levels one and two. To prevent the

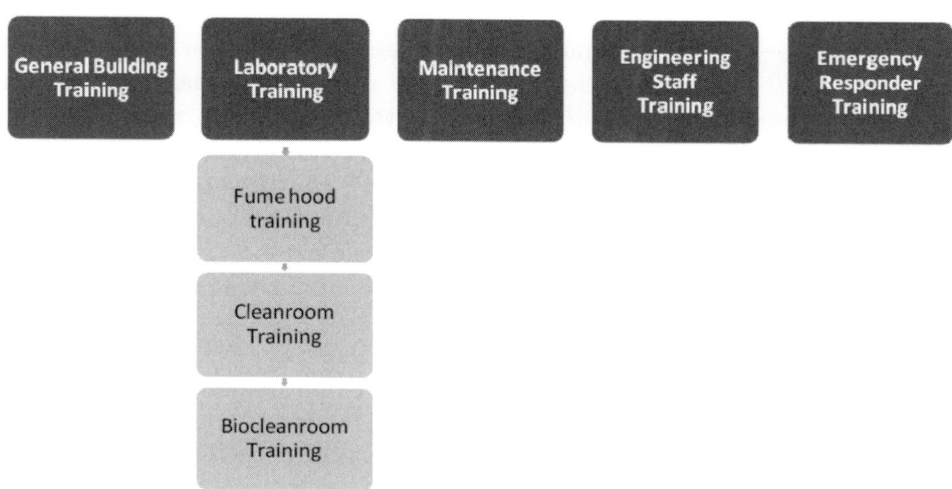

FIGURE 8.9 *The hierarchy of training in the BNC. The tracks are based as an analysis of the types of training needed by various groups who enter the facility.*

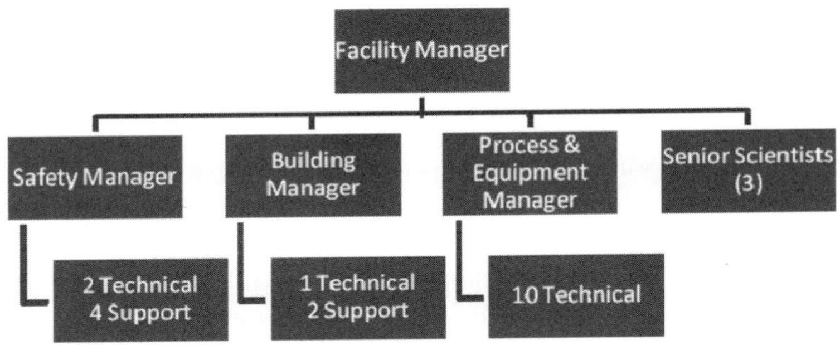

FIGURE 8.10 *The organizational structure of the BNC Operations group. The importance of safety is stressed by the reporting relationships and staffing levels.*

duplication of effort, those specialty classes already taught at the university were incorporated into the training matrix.

Once the user completes the training required for access, he/she can schedule specific equipment training. This training is taught by the engineer responsible for the equipment and includes all safety and operational issues involved in equipment usage. Depending on the complexity of the equipment, this training can range from one hour to several days.

The importance of supporting safe design through appropriate manpower—numbers and technical competence—during design and construction was mentioned previously, but it is equally important to continue the strong technical support with safety as a priority during operation. The BNC provides that support by dividing the operations organization into three parts: Safety, Infrastructure, and Process & Equipment. A senior-level technical manager runs each of these groups, providing their "hands" and technical expertise as well as managing the engineers and support personnel in their respective groups. The organization of the technical staff is shown in Figure 8.10.

The Safety Manager has overall responsibility for safety within the facility, but each member of staff has that responsibility as well. In addition to being included in the job description of each staff member, it is also included as part of their rating in their annual performance evaluation. This sends a tangible message that safety is a priority in this facility.

Safety responsibility is divided among the staff through technical expertise as well. An engineer supporting vacuum systems has over 20 years of experience in the semiconductor-gases industry and is the coordinator for all gas-safety issues. An engineer supporting epitaxial systems has a strong computer background and supports the toxic gas monitoring system functions. These are just two examples of the shared responsibility for safety issues among the staff.

Identification of Hazard Potentials in the BNC

The Birck Nanotechnology Center uses a number of hazardous materials and contains additional physical hazards due to its processing characteristics. The mitigation of standard building hazards was left to the architects—they have ample experience in these areas—but the more specialized hazards were considered by the user group. These were divided into three major categories: chemical hazards, biological hazards, and physical hazards. These were put in a matrix with their status in their life cycle—incoming materials, products, byproducts, and effluents. In the chemical category, the state of the materials was also considered—solid, liquid, or gaseous chemicals. The following chart outlines the three hazard categories (Figure 8.11).

Of particular interest were the gaseous raw materials. They range from pyrophoric/detonable gases to simple asphyxiants, with different precautions necessary for each category. Of highest concern are the pyrophoric and detonable gases such as silane. Germane, a highly toxic and pyrophoric gas, is also of significant concern. Three flammable gases are in use: hydrogen, dichlorosilane, and methane. Finally, a number of highly toxic gases, such as arsine, provide significant hazard potential.

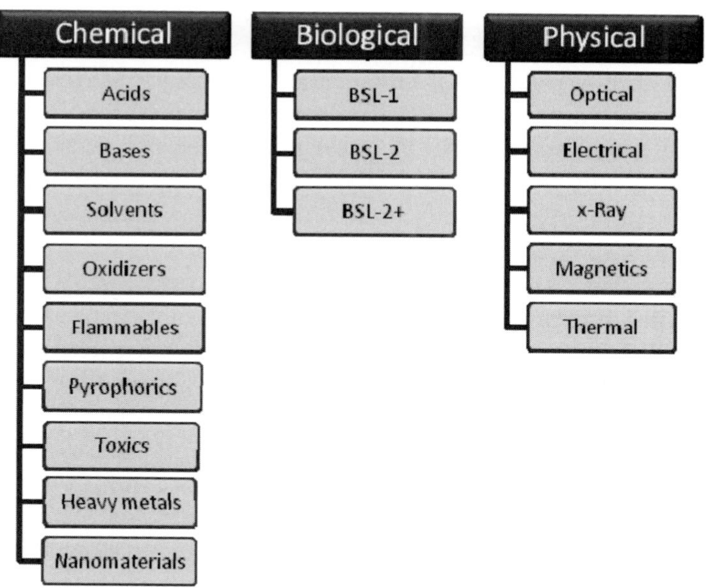

FIGURE 8.11 *The hazardous–material categories in the BNC. Each of the noted materials could be in solid, liquid, or gaseous phase.*

There is little agreement on the hazards of nanomaterials, but a conservative approach to nanomaterial safety was taken. Nanomaterials used in the BNC are either bonded to surfaces or used in liquid solutions. This greatly reduces the potential for exposure through inhalation, but engineering controls were also implemented. The primary engineering control used is containment—physical barriers and ventilation—to separate the nanomaterials from the general laboratory environment. All work is performed in a glove box or fume hood, exhausted outside the laboratory. In addition, the laboratories use "single pass" air—all air is exhausted, none returned to the laboratory.

To further mitigate risk, respirators—fitted by the safety department—are worn by those working in laboratories where nanomaterials are grown or deposited. Gloves are also worn by workers in the nanomaterial laboratories, and those using a fume hood (as opposed to a glove box) must wear further PPE—coat-apron and goggles for an acid hood, lab coat and goggles for a solvent hood.

8.4 DESIGNING IN SAFETY—KEY EXAMPLES (FIGURE 8.12)

8.4.1 Gas hazard mitigation design

Most of the hazards present in a nanotechnology facility relate to areas that are well understood in specific industries. It is the bringing together of different technical backgrounds that underscores the need for cross-disciplinary safety information. The designs shown in this example are standard in most semiconductor fabrication facilities, but are not necessarily applied to nanotechnology facilities using the same, or similar, incoming materials. The application of these known technologies is a critical element in the design of a facility using nanoscale materials.

The mitigation of gas hazards was chosen as the example of the overall safe-design concepts used in the BNC. The safety program at the BNC has a clear hierarchy: Prevention → Monitoring → PPE. The goal is to provide prevention programs that consist of engineering controls to eliminate or minimize the hazard. Where these controls are not 100% effective, monitoring systems provide a secondary safeguard, alerting occupants when a potentially hazardous situation occurs. Finally, PPE serves as a final barrier between the hazard and the individual (Figure 8.13).

Prevention is the first priority in the mitigation of gas hazards. The first step is to control access to vulnerable areas. A card-access system was

Chemical Hazards
- Separate dock
- Secure staging areas
- Special distribution path
- Spill containment
- Emergency exhaust
- Gas detection and monitoring
- Personal protective equipment
- Emergency response consideration

Physical Hazards
- Laboratory security system
- Specialized training prior to access
- Door interlocks for laser laboratories
- Warnings and signs
- Personal protective equipment

Biological Hazards
- Laboratory security system
- Specialized training prior to access
- Negative-pressure laboratories
- HEPA filters in all outgoing air
- Personal protective equipment/easily identifiable

FIGURE 8.12 *Examples of several designs used to mitigate hazards within the BNC.*

developed to separate public spaces from spaces with potential hazards. These potential hazard areas were then classified by access needs and hazard level. For example, very few people needed access to the gas-cylinder delivery cage. This was protected by a distinct lock and key that was accessible to very few individuals. This was also the case for the gas distribution rooms and a further safeguard with a separate key was designed for the gas cabinets—they provide a high vulnerability point. Camera systems also record the presence of people in those areas to protect against tampering and to document suspicious activities. These have proven fairly effective and have been looked upon favorably by most users. The cameras have been used to clarify an event and "clear" a user in the past, setting the tone for a positive response to their presence.

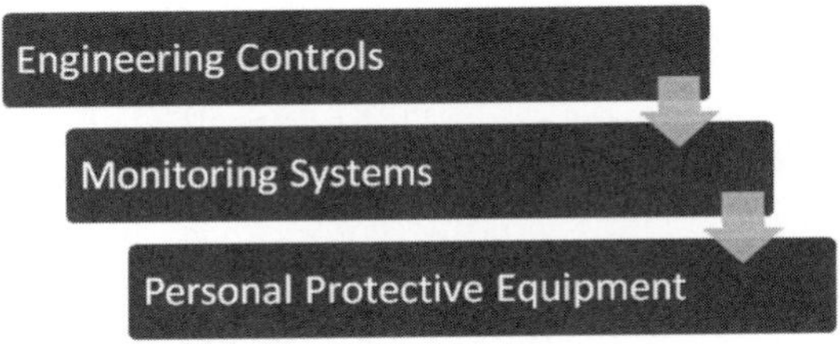

FIGURE 8.13 *Safety hierarchy utilized in the design and operation of the BNC.*

The separation of the hazardous materials dock from the general delivery dock removes the hazard of a shared delivery space. People handling heavy or bulky items are not attempting to operate next to people handling hazardous gas cylinders or glass bottles of acids. Those operating on the hazardous materials dock are aware of the sensitivity of that area and behave accordingly. Likewise, people handling routine deliveries and/or large equipment need not be concerned that they are sharing dock area with hazardous materials. This separate dock area also contains an area for the outdoor staging of incoming and outgoing gas cylinders. Codes and best practices highly recommend the staging of these cylinders in an outdoor area, and this location provides security, weather protection, and isolation from routine traffic.

For pyrophoric and detonable gases, further protection is necessary. Calculations, supported by experimentation, have determined that a distance of twelve feet from a silane detonation provides ample degradation of the overpressure wave for human safety. To mitigate the hazards, a special bunker was constructed with three poured concrete walls, a blow-out wall, and a blow-out roof. Inside this structure are located the gas cabinets for all pyrophoric and/or detonable gases, with a sixteen-foot safety zone created beyond the blow-out wall. The bunker has a locked, explosion-proof door that provides access to a very small number of trained individuals. The gas-cabinet controllers are remote from the bunker, located on the opposite side of the poured-concrete wall. This allows the engineer to be in a safe location while performing purging operations (Figure 8.14).

For non-pyrophoric/detonable hazardous gases, two gas rooms were constructed. These rooms are accessed from the hazardous material area, but are distinct rooms opening off that area. This provides two levels of security as access to the hazardous material area is limited and a distinct key is needed to access the gas rooms. Each hazardous gas is located inside a gas cabinet within the gas room, with a maximum of two gas cylinders per cabinet. Cylinders sharing a single cabinet must be compatible gases and of like

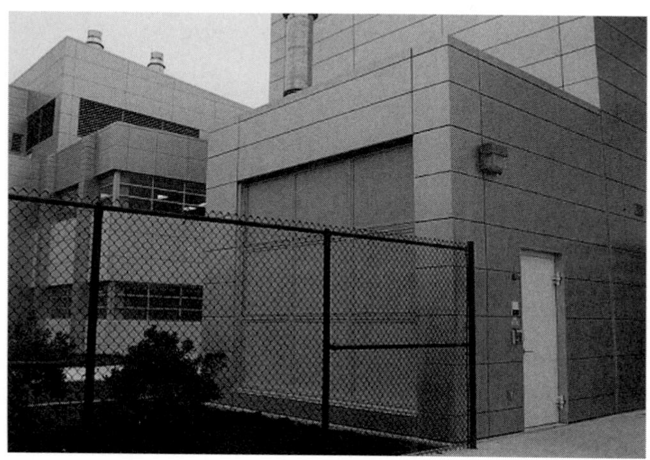

FIGURE 8.14 *The pyrophoric bunker at the Birck Nanotechnology Center. In addition to the blow-out wall shown, the ceiling will blow out in an explosion, dissipating the energy of the blast.*

hazard. The gas rooms have explosion-proof electrical components, and flammable gases are in a separate room from toxic gases.

All hazardous gases—gases rated 3 or higher on the NFPA scale in any category—are to be located in gas cabinets within the gas rooms. These rooms are maintained under a negative pressure relative to the hallway and outside world, and the gas cabinets are at negative pressure relative to the room.

These cabinets are automated-purge cabinets with redundant safety features such as excess-flow sensors, reduced-flow orifices, and system-failure shutdown protocols. They utilize high-turbulence construction with high exhaust flow—200 cubic feet per minute at 0.02 inches of water pressure differential. These are monitored by automated sensors and manometers with a visual readout at the cabinet location. All cabinets contain fire sprinklers (Figures 8.15 and 8.16).

The next area of vulnerability is the distribution piping carrying the hazardous gases to their points of use. The piping used is coaxial stainless steel tubing with an inert gas—argon—filling the interstitial region between the tubing. The tubing runs are located in protected areas—in pipe racks and ceiling chases—with control bars (like those in a parking garage) to prevent access by equipment that is tall enough to contact the piping runs.

To back up the engineering controls described above, a dual monitoring system has been implemented. The overall system consists of two sub-systems that are joined together for alarm purposes. One subsystem is a gas-sensing

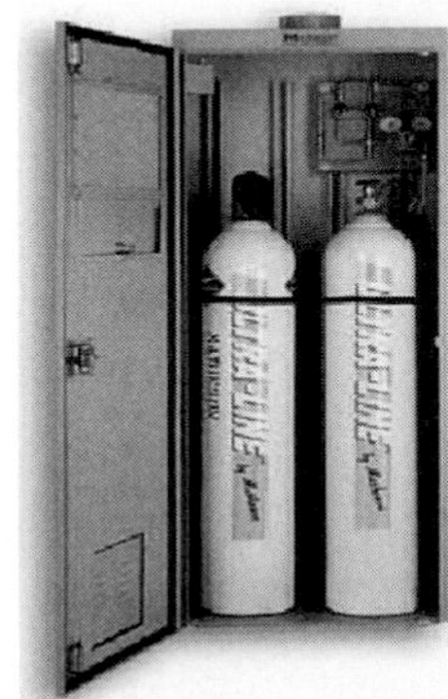

FIGURE 8.15 *The interior of a BNC gas cabinet. Only gases that are compatible and of like hazard may share a multiple–cylinder cabinet. Generally, these are different dilutions of the same material.*

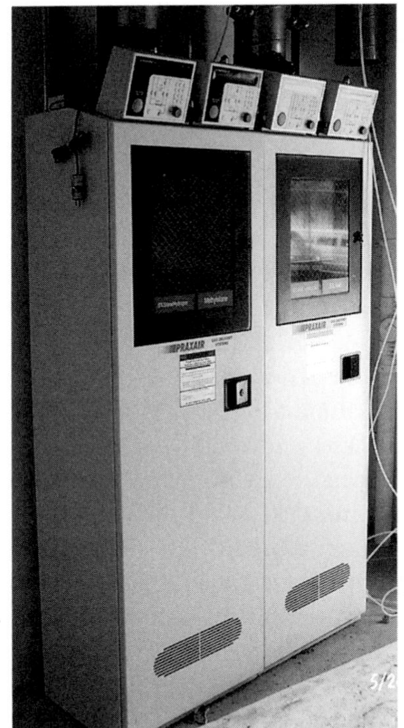

FIGURE 8.16 *Automated-purge gas cabinets used in BNC. These cabinets are required for all gases rated 3 or above in any NFPA hazard category. The cabinets are located in secure, isolated rooms at the perimeter of the facility. In addition, each cabinet is locked to provide additional security.*

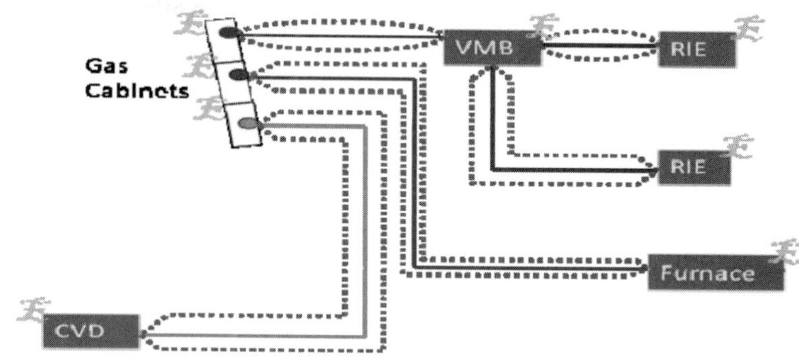

FIGURE 8.17 *A combination of gas monitoring (sniffing) sensors and pressure sensors are used to ensure the detection of any leak. Automated monitoring provides notification automatically should a leak occur.*

system that draws air from various points, passes that air over a chemically coated tape and looks for a color change on the tape. Tapes are sensitive to specific families of gases, such as hydrides or oxidizers. For gases where the tape technology is inappropriate, such as flammables, pellistor (catalytic) sensors are used (Figure 8.17).

The sensing system is activated by the presence of the hazardous gas and is able to provide quantitative information. This allows alarm levels to be set by concentration points. In BNC, 50% of the threshold limit value (TLV) for toxic gases and/or 25% of the lower explosive limit (LEL) is used for the warning level and 100% of the TLV and/or 50% of the LEL is used for the danger level. A warning level triggers a page to appropriate staff members who will respond to correct the situation. A danger level triggers a building evacuation and alerts emergency responders.

The sensing system is used anywhere outside of the coaxial piping system, such as gas cabinets, valve manifold boxes (VMBs), and equipment enclosures. The sensors are placed in the exhaust ductwork immediately downstream of the potential leak point. This ensures that the highest concentration of the gas will be sensed by the system, providing maximum sensitivity in the event of a leak. This design allows the monitoring of the efficacy of the engineering control, preventing the possibility of personnel exposure.

The second subsystem is the interstitial pressure monitoring system. This system monitors the inert-gas pressure in the interstitial region between the delivery tubing and the containment tubing. The interstitial pressure is set at 50% of the delivery-gas pressure and the system is sealed.

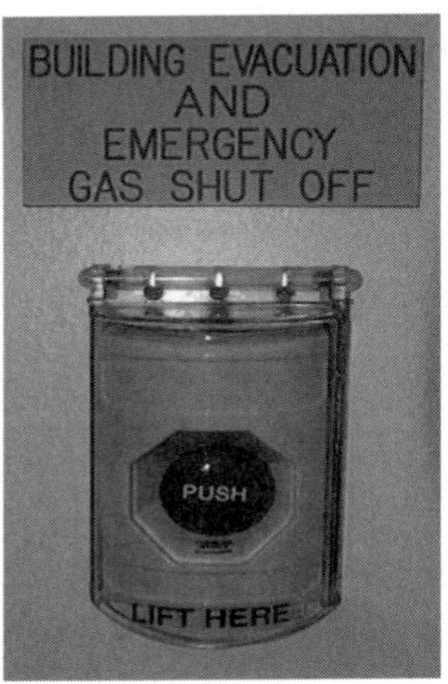

FIGURE 8.18 *An emergency gas shutoff box. All people in the facility are empowered to use these push stations in the event of an emergency.*

A drop in pressure indicates a leak in the outer-containment tubing. An increase in pressure indicates a leak in the delivery tubing. Either of these incidents triggers a page to the appropriate engineering staff member. A sudden pressure drop to atmosphere indicates a catastrophic failure of a piping run and triggers a building evacuation and activates emergency responders.

In the event of a failure of all other systems, certainly a highly unlikely scenario, a hazardous situation may be recognized by an occupant of the facility. Emergency annunciation boxes are located at strategic points around the facility. These boxes contain a covered mushroom switch—lifting the cover and pushing the mushroom switch shuts down all hazardous gases in the facility and announces a building evacuation. This also triggers emergency responders to come to the facility (Figure 8.18).

The last level of protection for hazardous gases is PPE. For short-term maintenance operations and cylinder changes, self-contained breathing apparatus (SCBA) is used. For long-term maintenance activities, an air-line cart attached to an SCBA is used. At least two people must be present—buddy system—with both wearing SCBA.

8.5 SUMMARY

The Birck Nanotechnology Center accommodates a relatively large population across diverse cultures and technical backgrounds. This provides particular challenges to occupant safety, in that an individual's depth of knowledge may be shallow in certain areas while world-leading in other areas. Cultural differences in dealing with mistakes and accidents also present challenges to safe facility operation. Additionally, the facility is open to the general public during normal business hours, expanding the number of people in the building at any given time.

The concept of mitigating potentially hazardous situations in the facility design process was an effective way of dealing with these facility-operational challenges. By designing systems and barriers into the initial building design, many of these challenges can be reduced to an insignificant level. The development of redundant elements can eliminate the risks in many cases.

While designed and constructed before the "Prevention through Design initiative," the Birck Nanotechnology Center in Discovery Park at Purdue University provides numerous examples of the principles of PtD. One scenario that exemplifies the implementation of those principles is the development of designs that mitigate the risks involved in dealing with hazardous gases. An in-depth look at the design elements used in this mitigation provides an effective case study in the implementation of Prevention through Design.

As was stated previously, the most prevalent risks in a nanotechnology facility come from chemical and biological exposures. For this reason, the emphasis on safety designs and operational programs is placed there. The lack of agreement in the level of hazards in nanoscale materials drives the need for prudence here as well. The simplest and most logical approach is to prevent the exposure of personnel to nanoparticles altogether, but this is not practical. Instead, a hierarchy of controls beginning with isolation of nanomaterials, progressing through the control of their aerosol properties, and ending with personal protective equipment is utilized.

It is highly recommended that the designers of nanotechnology facilities implement the principles outlined in this chapter. While specific applications of those principles will vary among facilities, the overall concepts apply to a wide variety of facilities. The specific example of hazardous gas management will apply in many facilities, but beyond that, direct applications are the methods of hazard analysis and facility-level controls that were implemented in the BNC.

The overall message of this chapter is that safety needs to be prevalent from the early planning stages of a facility through design, construction and startup. This will allow the operational safety program to function more efficiently and more effectively. This commitment in the early stages of facility design will have significant long-term payoffs throughout the life of the facility.

It is very important that the flexibility to add further engineering controls be comprehended in the facility design. A prime example is the ventilation system design. Designing enough capacity to add additional glove boxes and fume hoods as engineering controls greatly reduces the cost of adding these controls in the future and allows the flexibility to add controls as new information regarding nanomaterials emerges.

NIOSH defines Prevention through Design (PtD) as,

> *Addressing occupational safety and health needs in the design process to prevent or minimize the work-related hazards and risks associated with the construction, manufacture, use, maintenance, and disposal of facilities, materials, and equipment.*[4]

The principles involved in this initiative are very important to nanotechnology facility design and have been embodied in the Birck Nanotechnology Center.

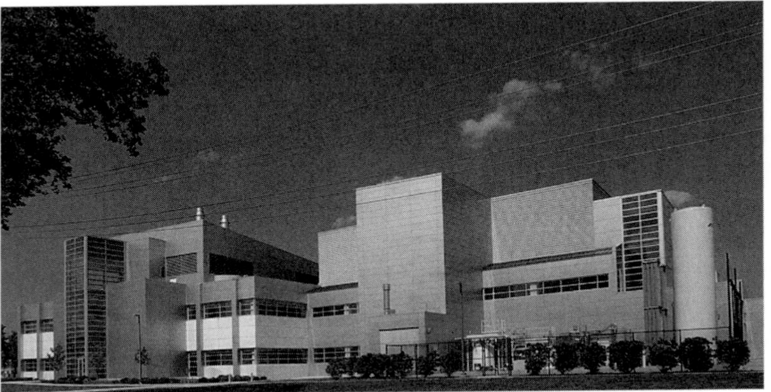

The west side of the Birck Nanotechnology Center. The cleanroom portion of the facility is in the foreground, with the laboratory areas to the left.

[4] Please see www.cdc.gov/niosh/topics/ptd/ for further information regarding Prevention through Design. This quotation is taken from this web site.

Index

Q

R

S

T

U

V

W